European School of Oncology

Monographs

Series Editor: U. Veronesi

The European School of Oncology gratefully acknowledges financial support for the production of this monograph received from Farmacia (Hellas) SA, Schering-Plough SA, Sandoz (Hellas) AEBE, Lederle (Hellas) AE, Roche (Hellas) AE, and Schering AG.

Springer
Berlin
Heidelberg
New York
Barcelona
Budapest
Hong Kong
London
Milan
Paris
Tokyo

G. A. Pangalis (Ed.)

Malignant Lymphomas: Biology and Treatment

An Update

With 29 Figures and 47 Tables

Springer

Gerassimos Alexander Pangalis

Associate Professor in Haematology and Medicine
National and Kapodistrian
University of Greece School of Medicine
Laikon General Hospital
Athens 115 27, Greece

Visiting Clinical Associate Professor
University of Southern California
School of Medicine
Los Angeles, CA 90033, USA

Library of Congress Cataloging-in-Publication Data
Malignant lymphomas: biology and treatment; an update / G.A. Pangalis (ed.)
(Monographs / European school of oncology)
Includes bibliographical references.
ISBN-13: 978-3-642-79915-0 e-ISBN-13: 978-3-642-79913-6
DOI: 10.1007/ 978-3-642-79913-6
1. Lymphomas. I. Pangalis, Gerassimos A. II. Series: Monographs
(European School of Oncology)
[DNLM: 1. Lymphoma--therapy. 2. Lymphoma--physiopathology. WH 525 M2483 1995]
RC280.L9M336 1995
616.99'442--dc20
DNLM/DLC
for Library of Congress

Softcover reprint of the hardcover 1st edition 1995

Typesetting: Camera ready by editor

SPIN: 10128698 19/3133 - 5 4 3 2 1 0 — Printed on acid-free paper

Dedicated to all those,
who strive with love and care,
as expressed by the Greek word
έρως [eros]
against malignant lymphomas

Foreword

The European School of Oncology came into existence to respond to a need for information, education and training in the field of the diagnosis and treatment of cancer. There are two main reasons why such an initiative was considered necessary. Firstly, the teaching of oncology requires a rigorously multidisciplinary approach which is difficult for the Universities to put into practice since their system is mainly disciplinary orientated. Secondly, the rate of technological development that impinges on the diagnosis and treatment of cancer has been so rapid that it is not an easy task for medical faculties to adapt their curricula flexibly.

With its residential courses for organ pathologies and the seminars on new techniques (laser, monoclonal antibodies, imaging techniques etc.) or on the principal therapeutic controversies (conservative or mutilating surgery, primary or adjuvant chemotherapy, radiotherapy alone or integrated), it is the ambition of the European School of Oncology to fill a cultural and scientific gap and, thereby, create a bridge between the University and Industry and between these two and daily medical practice.

One of the more recent initiatives of ESO has been the institution of permanent study groups, also called task forces, where a limited number of leading experts are invited to meet once a year with the aim of defining the state of the art and possibly reaching a consensus on future developments in specific fields of oncology.

The ESO Monograph series was designed with the specific purpose of disseminating the results of these study group meetings, and providing concise and updated reviews of the topic discussed.

It was decided to keep the layout relatively simple, in order to restrict the costs and make the monographs available in the shortest possible time, thus overcoming a common problem in medical literature: that of the material being outdated even before publication.

Umberto Veronesi
Chairman Scientific Committee
European School of Oncology

Contents

Contents

Introduction

The continuous and rather voluminous influx of new information regarding the biology and treatment of malignant lymphomas requires a frequent updating of this topic. It is especially the progress made in the biology of these diseases which gives us a better understanding of their development, enables us to improve their classification and introduces us to a new era of therapeutic manipulation (biological response modifiers and monoclonal antibodies). Furthermore, due to advances made in supportive bone marrow and peripheral stem cell transplantation - after mobilization with growth factors - more intensive treatment may be delivered in an attempt to improve the current moderate results in certain lymphoma subtypes.

In this monograph an international panel of experts on lymphoma and related disorders contribute their experience to an update of the biology and treatment of malignant lymphomas. This book is the product of an advanced seminar on malignant lymphomas organized by the Athens Office of the European School of Oncology, held in October 1993 at Vouliagmeni, Attiki, Greece, in collaboration with the Lymphoma Clinic, First Department of Internal Medicine of the National and Kapodistrian University School of Medicine of Greece.

Gerassimos Alexander Pangalis, M.D.

Associate Professor,
Lymphoma Clinic,
Laikon General Hospital, Athens, Greece
Visiting Clinical Associate Professor,
University of Southern California

Histopathology of Non-Hodgkin's Malignant Lymphomas

Constantine S. Papadimitriou [1] and Christos N. Kittas [2]

1 Department of Pathology, Aristotelian University of Thessaloniki, School of Medicine, Thessaloniki 54006, Greece
2 Department of Histology, University of Athens School of Medicine, Goudi, Athens 11526, Greece

Histopathology forms the basis for the diagnosis, classification, treatment and prognosis of non-Hodgkin malignant lymphomas. Nowadays several reliable methods are being used in the pathology laboratories for the identification of the various cell types of the normal lymphoid tissues and their neoplastic counterparts; such methods are aimed at a better understanding of the nature of the malignant lymphomas and their reasonable classification. They include classic morphology, histochemistry, immunohistochemistry, image analysis/ flow cytometry and molecular pathology techniques such as gene rearrangement methodology, polymerase chain reaction (PCR), *in situ* hybridisation and DNA clonality [1].
Morphology is the mainstay of the malignant lymphoma examination process. It includes the cell morphology itself as well as the patterns of homing of either T or B zones of the lymphoid tissues by the neoplastic cells. Although cell morphology can be used to identify accurately only some cell types (e.g. plasma cells), in most instances it can provide substantial information on the B or T-cell nature of the lymphomatous cells. It is undoubtedly sufficient to distinguish substantial morphological categories of malignant lymphoma (e.g. centroblastic/centrocytic, lymphoplasmacytoid/cytic, and some types of peripheral T-cell lymphomas). It seems unreasonable to use more sophisticated methods of investigating lymphomas when they are not preceded and supported by the data of the traditional morphological methods which are more simple, inexpensive and offer significant directory possibilities. Cytochemical and histochemical (on frozen or paraffin sections) enzyme stains are useful to reach a differential diagnosis. Acid phosphatase [2], acid non-specific esterase [3], chloroacetate esterase [4] and terminal deoxynucleotidyl transferase (TdT) [5] are the most valuable ones. Not only mere enzyme positivity but also the pattern of their intracellular distribution is of importance. For example acid phosphatase and acid non-specific esterase are negative or finegranularily positive in B cells and strongly and diffusely positive in histiocytes. T lymphocytes show a focal spotty positivity for both enzymes. In particular, acid phosphatase is present in the lymphoid cells of the central lymphoid organs (e.g. thymocytes) and in peripheral T-cell lymphocytes as well, while acid non-specific esterase characterizes only the peripheral T lymphocytes and mainly CD4 helper T cells. Chloroacetate esterase positivity is expressed by cells of granulocytic series and mast cells. TdT characterizes the lymphoid cells of thymic and prethymic stage as well as those of Pre-B type. These enzyme stainings are being applied less and less and are substituted by the immunohistochemical use of monoclonal antibodies either against enzymes or, more importantly, against epitopes characterizing various cell categories of lymphocytic, monocytic or even myelocytic origin.
Of great help in the differential diagnosis of malignant lymphomas is the immunohistochemical demonstration of various surface or cytoplasmic markers: immunoglobulins, enzymes such as TdT, lysozyme and elastase of leukocytes as well as antigens characterizing various categories of cells (e.g. antigens of lymphocyte differentiation, antigens specific for T or B cells, antigens of monocytes/histiocytes, CALLA, HLA-antigens, antigens of IL-2R, TCR etc). It must be emphasized that new monoclonal antibodies are being produced that recognize special cell subcategories such as the follicular centre lymphoid cells, the helper (CD4) and

Table 1. Kiel classification (updated)

B-cell ML	T-cell ML
Low-grade ML	**Low-grade ML**
Lymphocytic	Lymphocytic
chronic lymphocytic leukaemia	chronic lymphocytic leukaemia
prolymphocytic leukaemia	prolymphocytic leukaemia
hairy-cell leukaemia	Small cell, cerebriform
Lymphoplasmacytic/cytoid (immunocytoma)	mycosis fungoides, Sezary's syndrome
Plasmacytic	Lymphoepithelioid (Lennert's)
Centroblastic/centrocytic	Angioimmunoblastic (AILD)
follicular ± diffuse	T-zone lymphoma
diffuse	Pleomorphic, small cell (HTLV-1±)
Centrocytic (mantle cell)	
Monocytoid (including marginal zone cell)	
High-grade ML	**High-grade ML**
Centroblastic	Pleomorphic, medium-sized and large cell (HTLV-1±)
Immunoblastic	
Burkitt's lymphoma	Immunoblastic (HTLV-1±)
Large cell anaplastic (Ki-1+)	Large cell anaplastic (Ki-1+)
Lymphoblastic	Lymphoblastic
Rare types	Rare types

Table 2. International Working Formulation

Low grade	Intermediate grade	High grade
A. *Malignant lymphoma* *Small lymphocytic* consistent with CLL plasmacytoid	**D.** *Malignant lymphoma, follicular* *Predominantly large cleaved cell* diffuse areas sclerosis	**H.** *Malignant lymphoma* *Large cell, immunoblastic* plasmacytoid clear cell polymorphous epithelioid cell component
B. *Malignant lymphoma, follicular* *Predominantly small cleaved cell* diffuse areas sclerosis	**E.** *Malignant lymphoma, diffuse* *Small cleaved cell* sclerosis	**I.** *Malignant lymphoma* *Lymphoblastic* convoluted cell non-convoluted cell
C. *Malignant lymphoma, follicular* *Mixed, small cleaved and large cell* diffuse areas sclerosis	**F.** *Malignant lymphoma, diffuse* *Mixed, small and large cell* sclerosis epithelioid cell component	**J.** *Malignant lymphoma* *Small non-cleaved cell* Burkitt's follicular areas
	G. *Malignant lymphoma, diffuse* *Large cell* cleaved cell non-cleaved cell	

suppressor (CD8) T cells, the follicular dendritic cells (FDRC), the interdigitating reticulum cells (CD6), the NK cells (CD57), etc. In addition, monoclonal antibodies which can recognize on paraffin sections epitopes characterizing B or T cells, dendritic cells and monocytes/histiocytes (e.g. CD20, LN1, LN3, UCHL1, beta F1, CD21, CD68, MAC etc.) [6-11] become more and more numerous.

Even with the use of various specific monoclonal antibodies a certain percentage of malignant lymphomas remain negative for both B and T-cell markers, thus deserving the designation of "null cell" lymphomas. The use of molecular pathology techniques [12-15] offers a substantial aid in such instances as well as in problems concerning cell origin, aetiopathogenicity and prognosis. In fact, gene rearrangement analysis has shown that many of the "null" lymphoblastic malignant lymphomas have rearrangements of the immunoglobulin genes while a considerable number of "null" large cell lymphomas have T-cell receptor rearrangements [12-16]. *In-situ* hybridization is useful for the demonstration of specific RNA or DNA corresponding to cellular or viral components (Igs-RNA, EBER and EBNA for EBV etc.). It must be emphasized that the polymerase chain reaction (PCR) and *in-situ* hybridization can in many instances be applied to paraffin-embedded material [17,18]. Moreover, the PCR technique can be used to raise the sensitivity of *in-situ* hybridization in paraffin sections.

An applicable classificaton should combine scientific correctness with a high prognostic value, a high rate of reproducibility and significant clinical and epidemiological correlation. During the past few decades several more or less successful attempts to classify lymphomas have been made. Two classifications prevail: the Kiel classification (Table 1) [19-20] and the international working formulation, IWF (Table 2) [21]. The use of one or both of these classifications is necessary since pathologists and clinicians require a common reference. However, it must be stressed that in many cases the two classifications are not automatically interchangeable and therefore the degree of the pathologist's experience is decisive [22]. Both classifications apply better to lymph node malignant lymphomas, since the extranodal lymphomas frequently display significant peculiarities in their morphology, phenotype, genotype and clinical behaviour. Such cases are lymphomas of the gastrointestinal tract and the so-called MALTomas in general [23,24], lymphomas of the skin [25,26], large cell lymphomas of the mediastinum [27,28], and lymphomas of the nasal cavities [29].

Both classifications, Kiel and IWF, have their advantages and disadvantages. The Kiel classification has the advantages of a) incorporating morphology and immunology and distinguishing categories of B and T-cell lymphomas; b) separating lymphomas into low and high grade of malignancy; c) subdividing T-cell malignant lymphomas into several groups; d) including peculiar categories of lymphomas such as marginal zone/B-monocytoid cell and large cell (Ki-1+) anaplastic lymphomas. The only disadvantage of the Kiel classification is that it designates as low-grade malignant lymphomas some entities like centrocytic (mantle cell), AILD-like, T-zone and peripheral pleomorphic small T-cell lymphomas, although their course is either relatively aggressive or unpredictable. The IWF classification, on the other hand, is purely descriptive and does not distinguish between B and T-cell entities. The T-cell distinction is completely absent. In addition to high and low grade of malignancy, the IWF distinguishes a third, intermediate grade. This distinction seems unnecessary as most of the lymphomas belonging to this latter group behave and are treated like those of high-grade malignancy [30,31], while some of them should be placed in the low-grade category.

In the present work the Kiel classification is used primarily, and an attempt is made to correlate it with the IWF. Some peculiar lymphoma entities of histopathogenic, prognostic or differential diagnostic importance which are difficult to incorporate into either of the above classifications are described separately.

Low Grade Malignant Lymphomas

Low-grade malignant lymphomas are histologically characterized by the presence of small or medium-sized lymphoid cells. Sometimes they are mixed with limited numbers of larger blastic cells, for example in the so-called centroblastic-centrocytic malignant lymphomas.

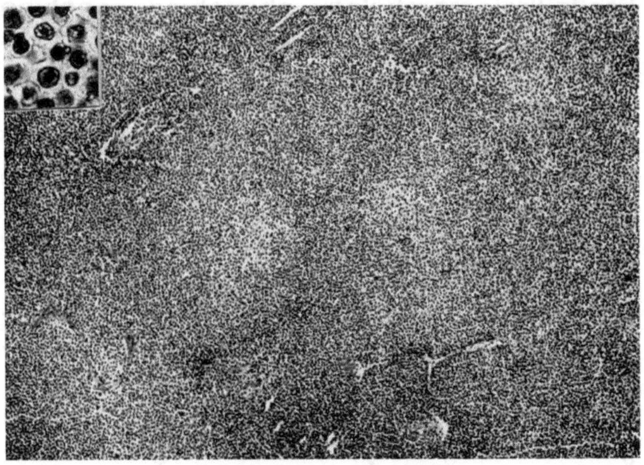

Fig. 1. B-CLL with apparent proliferation centres. H+E, X80
Inset: prolymphocytes/para-immunoblasts. H+E, X400

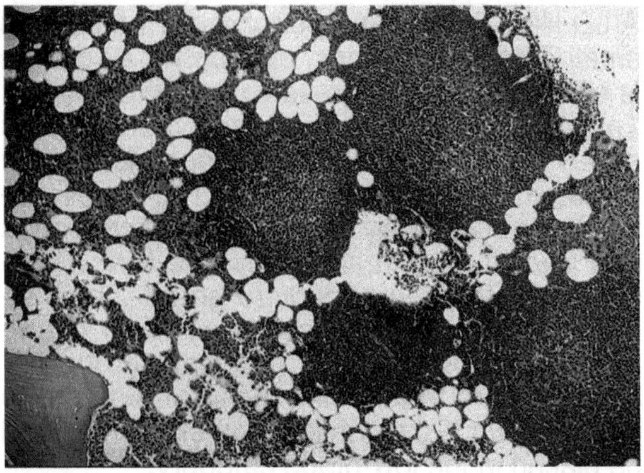

Fig. 2. B-CLL. Nodular infiltration of bone marrow. H+E, X80

Lymphocytic Lymphoma

The malignant lymphomas included in this group consist mainly of lymphocytes or their forms of prolymphocytes and hairy cells. They belong more frequently to the B than to the T-cell lineage.

Chronic lymphocytic leukaemia of B-cell type (B-CLL)

This is characterized by infiltrations with B lymphocytes that do not show any transformation to Ig-secretory cells such as lymphoplasmacytoid and plasmacytic cells. This interruption of maturation could be attributed partly to defective CD4+ helper T cells and partly to an increased activity of CD8+ suppressor T cells [32]. Immunohistochemically [33] the neoplastic lymphocytes express the B-cell antigens CD20, CD22 and CD23, are either kappa or lambda monoclonal and show SIg of the IgM class, frequently together with IgD. However, not rarely B-CLL lymphocytes especially after micro-wave retrieval may show some intracytoplasmic Ig-positivity. This fact, in conjuction with the positivity for CD5 antigen, raises the possibility of B-CLL and lymphoplasmacytoid immunocytoma being variants of the same entity [34]. They seem to be histogenetically related to CD5-positive lymphocytes of the primary follicle or the follicular mantle zone [35]. B-CLL does not occur in subjects under 20 years of age. It shows generalized lymphadenopathy and usually a leukaemic picture with bone marrow infiltration. According to Rappaport's group cases of lymphocytic lymphoma [32,36] may exist without any synchronous or metachronous leukaemic picture. Effacement of the normal lymph node structure is observed histologically due to diffuse infiltration with maturing lymphocytes [34,36-38]. Among these larger lymphocytes, the prolymphocytes [39], are found with less dense chromatin and prominent nucleoli as well as large cells, the paraimmunoblasts with basophilic cytoplasm, oval nuclei and central, prominent nucleoli. They are sometimes dispersively distributed but more frequently form clusters (pseudofollicular foci or proliferation centres, Fig. 1). Mitoses and positivity for the proliferation antigen Ki-67 are present only in prolymphocytes and paraimmunoblasts where also most of the *p53* oncoprotein positivity is expressed [40]. The greater the proliferation centres, the more tumorous is the appearance of the lymph nodes. About 4% of the cases eventually develop into true, high-grade malignant lymphoma, usually immunoblastic (Richter's syndrome) [41]. In some cases a development of giant cells similar to Hodgkin and Sternberg-Reed cells superimposes the B-CLL morphology. Such cells are positive for Epstein-Barr virus elements (LMP, EBER) and Ki-1 (CD30) antigen, a fact which renders possible a relationship of such cases with Hodgkin's disease [42].
Patients usually survive for many years without any substantial therapy. The extent of bone marrow infiltrates and their way of distri-

bution are of particular importance [43]. More favourable prognosis have the cases with nodular patterns (Fig. 2) while cases with diffuse distribution survive less. The prognosis also seems to depend on the size and number of proliferation centres in the lymph nodes [44].

Chronic lymphocytic leukaemia of T-cell type (T-CLL)

In T-CLL the lymph nodes are less pronounced and the spleen enlargement is more prominent than in B-CLL. The bone marrow is not always infiltrated while skin involvement is frequent. The diffusely infiltrated lymph nodes show proliferation of postcapillary venules. Proliferation centres are absent. The neoplastic lymphocytes have morphological and immunohistochemical characteristics of either CD4+ helper or CD8+ suppressor T cells [45,46]. Rare cases show a mixed immunophenotype with simultaneous CD4 and CD8 positivity in the same cells.

Hairy cell leukaemia

Hairy cells often show hair-like projections of their cytoplasm [47] on haematological smears and imprints. These projections are better recognized by electron microscopy. In the majority of cases the cells represent a peculiar, not fully defined B-cell variety [48,49]. Some authors relate hairy cells to B-monocytoid marginal zone cells of the lymph node cortex and to centrocyte-like cells of mucosa-associated lymphoid tissue [50,51]. In very rare instances the hairy cells reveal characteristics of a T-cell [52] or even a monocytic [53,54] phenotype. Hairy cells are identified by their positivity to tartrate-resistant acid phosphatase and to acidify non-specific esterase [55]. In addition, monoclonal antibodies exist which recognize antigenic epitopes on hairy cells [56]. The usual immunophenotype of hairy cells corresponds to CD22, CD20 and CD29 positivity and CD5 and CD23 negativity. Hairy cells are also stained for HML-1 antibody, which was initially found to recognize intraepithelial T lymphocytes [57]. They also show positivity for CD11c (KiM1 and KiM1P in frozen and paraffin sections, respectively).
Hairy cells are larger than typical lymphocytes with irregular ellipsoid or reniform nuclei. They stay apart from each other because of their

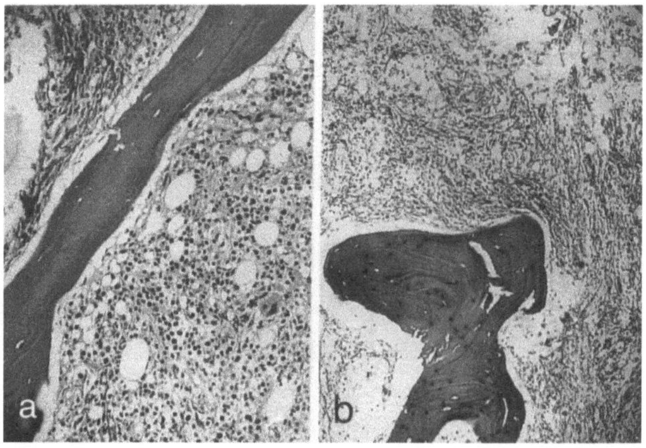

Fig. 3. Hairy cell leukaemia: a) Bone marrow infiltration. H+E, X120; b) Gomori's reticulin fiber stain X80

relatively abudant cytoplasm which is hardly recognizable in H+E stained paraffin sections [47]. Lymph nodes are involved in advanced stages of the disease. Organs which are infiltrated early and whose biopsy contributes to the establishment of the diagnosis are bone marrow, spleen and liver. In bone marrow (Fig. 3) reticulin fibers and even fibrosis are abundant [47] and responsible for the dry-tap reported by haematologists. In the spleen the infiltrates mainly occupy the cords of the expanded red pulp. The picture of the peripheral blood is not always clearly leukaemic.
Hairy cell leukaemia in which the HTLV-2 virus has in some way been implicated [58] displays a rather indolent and long lasting course especially after appropriate therapy. The percentage of Ki-67-positive hairy cells is very low. However, second malignancies do occur in hairy cell leukaemia patients [59].

Lymphoplasmacytic/Lymphoplasmacytoid Lymphoma (LP-Immunocytoma)

Histologically, LP-immunocytoma resembles B-CLL. In addition it shows various numbers of Ig-secreting cells of plasmacytic or lymphoplasmacytoid appearance [34]. The latter have moderate to abundant cytoplasm with rough endoplasmic reticulum-like plasma cells and a nucleus reminiscent of lymphocytes. PAS-positive intranuclear inclusions, representing Igs, are often found. Immunohistochemically (Fig. 4)

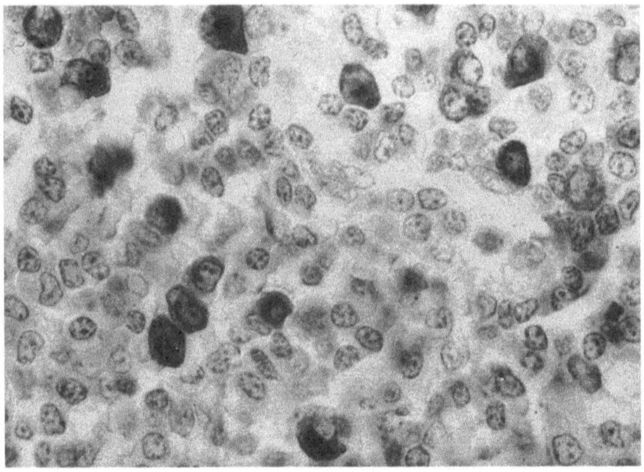

Fig. 4. Lymphoplasmacytoid immunocytoma. Cytoplasmic monoclonality for K-light chains. PAP method X500

plasmacytic and plasmacytoid cells reveal cytoplasmic monoclonal immunoglobulin [34,60, 61], which in descending frequency belongs to IgM, IgG or IgA. In 35% of the cases a paraproteinaemia is present. LP-immunocytoma is the tissue ground of the so-called macroglobulinaemia of Waldenström. In rare cases neoplastic cells produce only heavy or light chains of Igs, resulting in heavy (IgM, IgG) or light-chain disease, respectively. Two histological subtypes of LP-immunocytoma are described. The lymphoplasmacytoid subtype is morphologically and immunophenotypically more like B-CLL. It shows lymphoplasmacytoid cells and a phenotype of $CD19^+$, $CD20^+$, $CD22^+$, $CD5^+$ and $CD23^+$ [62]. It not infrequently shows a leukaemic picture and borderline cases to B-CLL exist [34].

The lymphoplasmacytic subtype includes among the other neoplastic lymphocytes classic monoclonal plasma cells. The phenotype of neoplastic cells corresponds to $CD19^+$, $CD20^+$, $CD22^+$, $CD5^-$ and $CD23^{+/-}$. The presence of follicular dendritic cells, a feature reminiscent of MALTomas, characterizes more than half of the cases of the lymphoplasmacytic subtype [63,64]. The prognosis of LP-immunocytoma is slightly more unfavourable than that of B-CLL. Accordingly, the percentages of Ki-67-positive lymphoid cells are slightly higher in LP-immunocytoma than in B-CLL. Paradoxically it seems that leukaemic cases have a better prognosis than aleukaemic cases [65]. The high-grade malignant lymphomas which may develop from LP-immunocytomas are usually immunoblastic.

Plasmacytic Lymphoma (Plasmacytoma)

Plasmacytes represent the end stage of differentiation of B cells after antigenic stimulation. From this point of view plasmacytoma must be considered as a kind of lymphoma. Here we mainly discuss the extramedullary plasmacytomas [66], which more frequently involve the upper respiratory tract. However, plasmacytomas of the gastrointestinal tract, the testes and the lungs, among other organs, are no curiosities. Primary lymph node plasmacytoma represents about 0.8% of non-Hodgkin lymphomas. The neoplastic plasma cells display immunohistochemically monoclonal CIg, usually of the IgA, less frequently of the IgG and rarely of the IgM class [66]. Their immunophenotype corresponds to $CD19^-$, $CD20^-$, $CD22^-$ and PCA1/$CD38^+$ [67,68]. Not infrequently, however, they express one or more haematopoietic and non-haematopoietic antigens, thus complicating the differential diagnosis [69]. Basically there is no histogenetic difference between extramedullary plasmacytomas and multiple myelomas. Moreover, solitary plasmacytomas of the bone occur [70,71] and extramedullary plasmacytomas may develop typical multiple myeloma. Extramedullary plasmacytomas do not often display paraproteinaemia. Their prognosis is much better than that of multiple myelomas.

Mantle Cell Lymphoma

This type, formely called centrocytic lymphoma [72], corresponds to intermediate lymphocytic lymphoma of the Rappaport group [73,74]. It has been proved that it derives from mantle cells of the follicles and has nothing to do with the centrocytes of the follicular (germinal) centres [75,76]. Histologically, the neoplasm consists of small to medium-sized centrocyte-like cells (Fig. 5a) with irregular, cleaved nuclei [72,74]. By definition no neoplastic cells with blastic appearance are found among the cleaved cells. Instead, a small number of T cells can be found. Very often the vessel wall, mostly of the capillaries, is thickened and hyalinized. The growth pattern is rather diffuse,

Table 3. The three categories of centrocyte cells

Cell markers	Mantle cells	Marginal zone cells	B-monocytoid cells
IgM	+	+	+
IgD	+	-	-
CD45R (KiB3)	-	-	+
CD5	+	-	-
AP-ase	-	+	-
KiM1P	-	+	+

but not infrequently a nodularity is seen. In early stages of growth a mantle-like neoplastic infiltration around reactive germinal centres is observed. Immunophenotypically they are strongly and simultaneously positive for surface IgM and IgD [75-77]. Their phenotype corresponds to a subtype of cells of the follicular mantle zone being CD19+, CD20+, CD22+ and especially CD5+ and CD23-. The phenotypes of the various categories of centrocyte-like cells are given in Table 3.

The mean number of mitoses and Ki67-positive neoplastic cells is much higher than that found in B-CLL, LP-immunocytoma and centroblastic/centrocytic malignant lymphoma. Mantle cell lymphoma can also be distinguished from the latter on the basis of molecular genetic differences. It shows the translocation t(11;14) (q13;q32) causing *bcl*-1 gene rearrangement, while very often centroblastic/centrocytic lymphoma (especially the nodular type) shows the translocation t(14;18) causing *bcl*-2 gene rearrangement [75,78]. Mantle cell lymphoma has a much worse prognosis than B-CLL, LP-immunocytoma and centroblastic/centrocytic lymphomas [79]. It has been shown that t(11;14) chromosomal translocation occurring in mantle cell lymphoma results in overexpression of a cyclin gene, PRAD1 [80]. The median survival time is less than 4 years. Mantle cell lymphomas represent 10% of non-Hodgkin lymphomas and the great majority occur at ages over 20.

According to the IWF classification most of the cases of mantle cell lymphoma can be categorized as either "diffuse small cleaved cell" or "diffuse large cleaved cell" lymphoma, although the reverse does not apply.

Centroblastic/Centrocytic Lymphoma

This neoplasm derives from follicular (germinal) centres. The neoplastic population consists of variable numbers of centroblasts and centrocytes. Among these histiocytes and especially

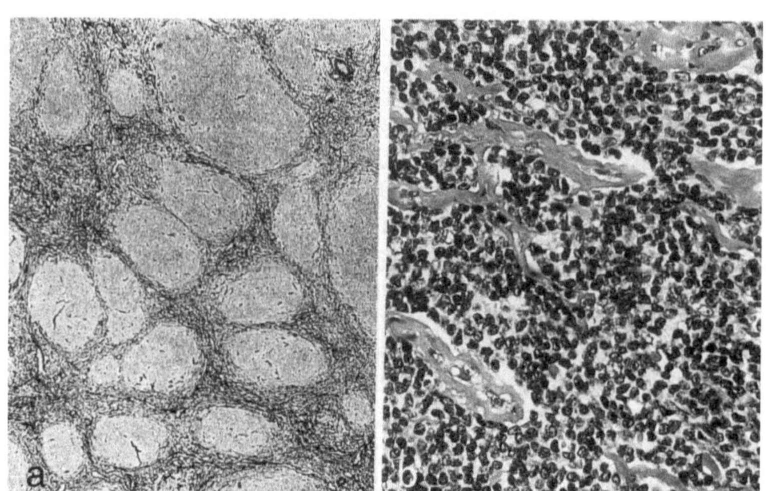

Fig. 5. a) Mantle cell lymphoma with hyalinization of the vascular walls. H+E, X250;
b) Follicular centroblastic/centrocytic lymphoma. Comoris reticulin stain, X80

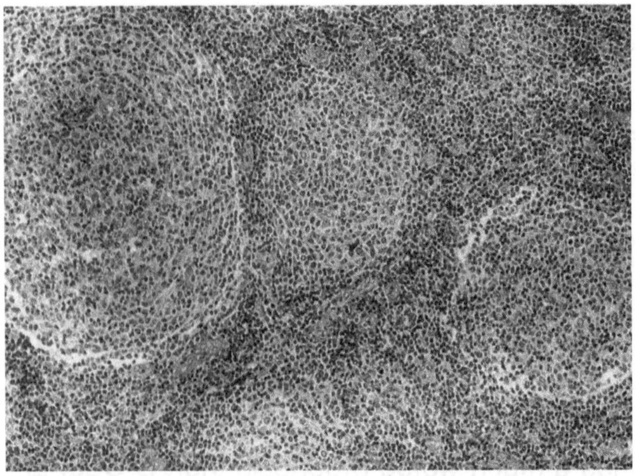

Fig. 6. Follicular centroblastic/centrocytic lymphoma. H+E, X120

follicular dendritic cells are found. The latter are more easily recognized after appropriate immunohistochemical staining (anti-DRC antibodies, CD21) [81]. Three histological subtypes are distinguished: a) a type with small centrocytes and low numbers of centroblasts; b) a type with small centrocytes and numerous centroblasts; c) a type with large centrocytes and numerous centroblasts.

In over 60% of the cases a complete or partial nodular (follicular) pattern (Figs. 5b and 6) of the neoplastic tissue is observed [82-85]. Among and within the neoplastic nodular structures substantial numbers of T cells are found. CD4-positive helper cells predominate [3,86]. Sclerosis may also be present [87] and is considered an indicator of good prognosis.

Neoplastic cells show SIgs and not infrequently CIgs which mostly belong to the IgM and IgD classes [86,88]. Those with follicular distribution are consistently positive for CD19, CD20, CD22 and CD10 (CALLA). Neoplastic cells within diffuse patterns of growth show negativity for CD10 and positivity for CD23. Centrocytes are CD5 negative. Immunohistochemically the *bcl*-2 oncoprotein is expressed in follicular centroblastic-centrocytic lymphoma because of *bcl*-2 gene rearrangement due to the translocation t(14;18) which frequently occurs in this type of lymphoma [89-91]. The *bcl*-2 oncoprotein inhibits cell apoptosis and is normally present in the small lymphocytes of the follicle mantle while it is absent from reactive germinal centres. Although *bcl*-2 oncoprotein expression is not exclusively related to t(14;18) and may occur in non-lymphoid tissues as well, its presence is considered to be helpful in distinguishing reactive follicles from neoplastic follicular structures [89,90,92,93].

Centroblastic-centrocytic lymphoma is rare in young persons and very rare in childhood [94]. Paraproteinaemia is rare while a leukaemic picture is observed in over 30% of cases. In peripheral blood smears the characteristic cleaved cells can be recognized.

Centroblastic/centrocytic lymphoma has the most favourable prognosis after B-CLL. Prognosis is much better in nodular (follicular) subtypes and especially in those with very many centrocytes and very few centroblasts [95,96]. Survival drops significantly when transformation to high-grade centroblastic lymphoma occurs, irrespectively of the nodular or diffuse pattern of growth.

According to the IWF the diffuse subtypes are of intermediate grade of malignancy. The subtype in the Kiel classification with "numerous small centrocytes and a few centroblasts" is categorized in the IWF as "diffuse small cleaved cell lymphoma". According to the IWF nodular subtypes are of low-grade malignancy except for those with "predominantly large cells" [97].

Monocytoid B-Cell Lymphoma

This is a rare lymphoma. The neoplastic cells correspond to the cells of so-called "immature sinus histiocytes", which are of B-cell origin and are referred to as monocytoid B cells (parafollicular) [98-100]. In most cases the neoplastic cells present a pattern of intrasinusoidal distribution. The monocytoid B cells are usually of medium size (Fig. 7) although a large cell variety has been described [101]. Their cytoplasm is moderately abundant and the nuclei are round to oval and somewhat cleaved. Small numbers of monoclonal Ig-positive immunoblasts can also be found. Variable numbers of rather neoplastic plasma cells and a few neutrophils are dispersed among the monocytoid cells: a picture simulating that of reactive immature sinus histiocytosis. The tumour cells are mostly IgM positive. Their immunophenotype corresponds to CD19+, CD20+, CD22+, KiB3+ and CD5-. On paraffin sections the B-monocytoid cells show a characteristic granular cytoplasmic positivity for KiM1P [102].

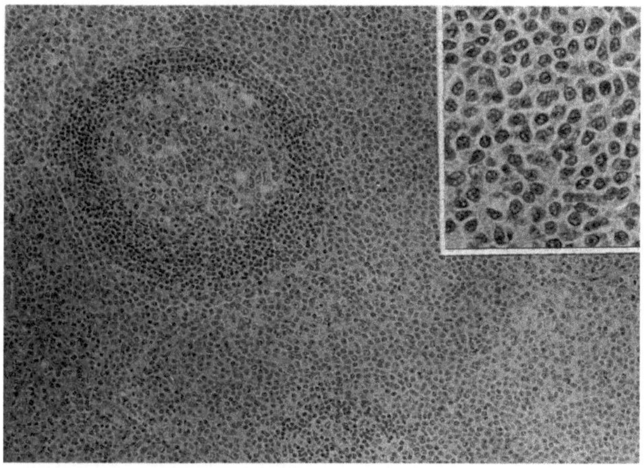

Fig. 7. Monocytoid B-cell lymphoma, with dense extensive infiltrates and a remaining reactive germinal centre. H+E, X120. Inset: X320

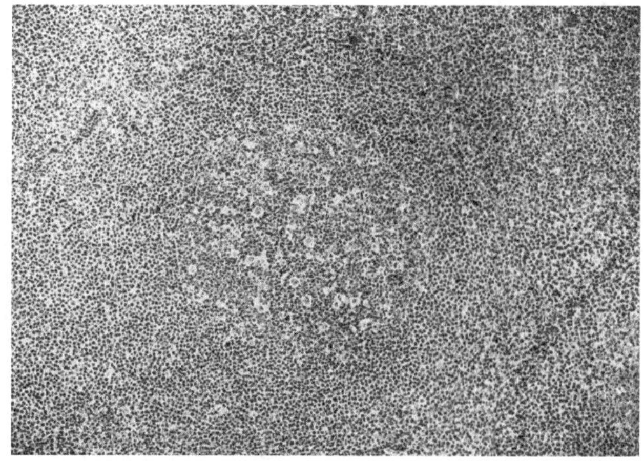

Fig. 8. Marginal zone cell lymphoma with a reactive germinal centre surrounded by neoplastic marginal zone cells. H+E, X80.

Lymphomas with monocytoid B-cell appearance at extranodal sites including the gastrointestinal tract, salivary glands and thyroid gland have also been described [103-105]. This can be explained by the close histogenetic relationship of the above categories with each other and with the marginal zone cells [38,104, 106-109]. It seems that circulating B lymphocytes enter the primary follicles and become a normal component of the follicular mantle zone. After antigenic stimulation these cells transform into centroblasts, which then differentiate to centrocytes. Centrocytes coming into contact with the antigen trapped on the surface of follicular dendritic cells differentiate to plasma cell precursors and memory B cells. The former, when leaving the germinal centres, become plasma cells in medullary cords of the lymph nodes or even in the lamina propria of gut mucosa, the spleen red pulp and the bone marrow. Memory B cells migrate to the marginal zone and become marginal B cells. The latter usually intermingle with the mantle zone cells, but not in the spleen and mesenterial lymph nodes where they form a rather separate outer zone in the follicular lymphocyte corona [38,108]. After stimulation they may become larger and develop into monocytoid B cells. This development can occur in lymph nodes (parafollicular cells, immature sinus histiocytosis) or at extranodal sites such as mucosa-associated lymphoid tissue (MALT) of the gut, bronchi, salivary glands, thyroid gland and other epithelial organs. Marginal zone cells directly or through the monocytoid B-cell stage are able to differentiate into plasma cells [100, 110-113]. The sites that prefer to home the above precursors of plasma cell genesis depend on special surface receptors on their own surface or in venules and other stromal tissue components [114-116]. Because of the close histogenetic and functional relationship between marginal zone cells and monocytoid B cells, many authors include marginal zone cell lymphomas (Fig. 8) and monocytoid B-cell lymphomas in the same category [117].

Monocytoid B-cell lymphoma is not listed in the IWF. Although these lymphomas often show moderate to high numbers of mitoses and, according to the IWF, could morphologically be categorized as intermediate grade of malignancy diffuse lymphomas (either small or large cell, non-cleaved/cleaved), their prognosis seems to be better in many instances. However, relapses and development of high-grade lymphomas do occur [99,100,113,117-119].

Mycosis Fungoides and Sezary's Syndrome

These two types represent, together with T-CLL, the classic example of low-grade T-cell lymphomas, which all belong to the peripheral T-cell lymphomas. They derive from peripheral T lymphocytes [120], in contrast to T-lymphoblastic lymphomas which derive from central T cells of the thymic or prethymic stage.

Mycosis fungoides primarily involves the skin. Lymph nodes and other organs are infiltrated in advanced stages. The T lymphocytes of MF show a cerebriform, gyroid nucleus (Lutzner cells). In most cases they belong to helper CD4-positive cells and only exceptionally they are CD8-positive. Some cases with expression of both phenotypes have been described [121]. Sometimes the functional stimulation of the neoplastic CD4-cell clone on reactive B lymphocytes induces B-cell clonal expansion with monoclonal plasma cells on the tissue level and a paraprotein in blood serum [122].
Skin lesions exhibit 3 stages of development [123,124]. Firstly the premycotic stage, which histologically is easily confused with inflammatory lichenoid infiltrates. In such cases immunohistochemistry is of significant help since in reactive inflammatory cases intraepidermal and dermal cell infiltrates are of the same phenotype. In cases of neoplastic MF lesions a discrepancy in the phenotype expression between the two cell groups may be found because of neoplastic loss of some surface markers [123,125,126] which seems to occur exclusively in intraepidermal T cells [127].
The second, infiltrative stage is histologically diagnostic as it shows dense cell infiltration of the dermis and clear epidermotropism with the characteristic Pautrier's microabscesses. Among the dermal infiltrates there are numerous inderdigitating reticulum cells with a simultaneous hyperplasia of Langerhans cells in the overlying epidermis. Both are characterized immunohistochemically by their positivity for S100-protein and CD1-antigen .
In the third, tumour stage the neoplastic infiltrates consist of larger transformed Lutzner cells and/or large immunoblastic cells in various numbers. The histological picture is compatible with any one of the various types of high-grade malignant peripheral T-cell lymphomas. T-immunoblastic cells and anaplastic large T-cell forms are usually positive for Ki-1 antigen.
Sezary's syndrome can be regarded as the leukaemic variety of mycosis fungoides. In both conditions bone marrow involvement is seldom seen and only in advanced stages.
The lymph nodes initially show lesions typical of dermatopathic lymphadenopathy with prominent interdigitating reticulum cells in expanded T-cell areas. Neoplastic infiltration of lymph nodes, which occurs in later stages, is considered a bad prognostic sign [128]. It is marked by the infiltration of the T-zone areas by varying numbers of atypical cerebriform cells. The infiltrates are denser and more monomorphic in cases of Sezary's syndrome while interdigitating cells are more prominent in cases of mycosis fungoides. The relatively high numbers of Ki-67-positive cells, as well as DNA flow cytometry findings and TCR rearrangement [129-130] facillitate the documentation of neoplastic lymph node infiltration.

T-zone Lymphoma

This is a rare lymphoma. It is the counterpart of the follicular centroblastic/centrocytic lymphoma [131], in the sense that in the early stages of growth the non-neoplastic germinal centres of the lymph node remain intact while the extrafollicular T-areas with the proliferating post-capillary venules represent the neoplastic sites. The nuclei of the neoplastic T lymphocytes are usually monomorphic and occasionally slightly pleomorphic. Their cytoplasm is scanty. However, some larger cells with clear cytoplasm or immunoblastic characteristics (T-immunoblast) can also be found. Islands of plasmacytoid monocytes and occasional eosinophils and/or epithelioid cells may be observed. Immunohistochemically the neoplastic cells show a mature T-cell phenotype: CD22+, CD23+, CD5+ and mostly CD4+.
T-zone lymphomas sooner or later transform into high-grade malignant lymphomas mostly of the T-immunoblastic type. However, patients with T-zone lymphomas have a higher survival rate than patients with high-grade malignant T-cell lymphomas [132].
T-zone lymphoma is not listed in the IWF. Some of the cases could be categorized as malignant lymphoma - diffuse, mixed small and large cell.

Lymphoepithelioid Lymphoma (Lennert's Lymphoma)

This is a rare lymphoma with an incidence peak in middle age. It is usually characterized by a generalized lymphadenopathy. Skin, liver and spleen involvement is common [133]. Histologically, the lymph nodes are diffusely infiltrated. There are numerous epithelioid cells distributed singly or in small foci. Among them various numbers of small to medium-sized neoplastic T cells are found (Fig. 9). They are relatively atypical and show mitoses. Immunohistochemically these cells display a phenotype of mature T cells: CD2+, CD3+, CD5+ and CD4+ [133,134]. Ki-67 positivity is almost exclusively seen in the CD4-positive neoplastic cells and not in the coexistent CD8-positive reactive cells. TCR gene rearrangement studies have confirmed the T-cell origin of Lennert's lymphoma [135,136]. Some neoplastic cells have a pale to clear cytoplasm and may even become larger and immunoblastic. In very rare cases may the cells resemble Sternberg-Reed cells. Small numbers of eosinophils and plasma cells may be found. Formely this kind of lymphoma was confused with Hodgkin's disease and angioimmunoblastic lymphadenopathy [137,138] or even with LP-immunocytoma [134, 138] containing numerous epithelioid cells. Development into a high-grade malignant lymphoma of the T-immunoblastic, Ki-1+ large cell anaplastic and large T-cell pleomorphic type is not infrequent [133,139]. The prognosis of Lennert's lymphoma is rather unfavourable. Survival depends on the clinical stage of the disease and its median value does not exceed 12 months. It is said that sufficiently aggressive therapy may improve the survival rates [140, 141].

According to the IWF Lennert's lymphoma in its typical form could be categorized as "diffuse, mixed small and large cell malignant lymphoma".

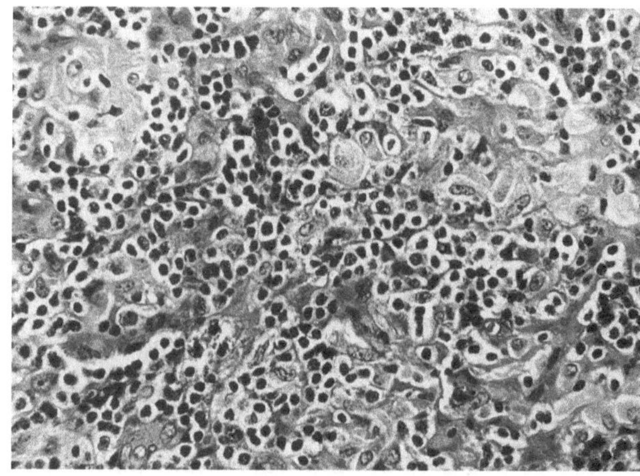

Fig. 9. Lennert's lymphoma. Abundant epithelioid cells intermingled with T-cell infiltrates. H+E, X320

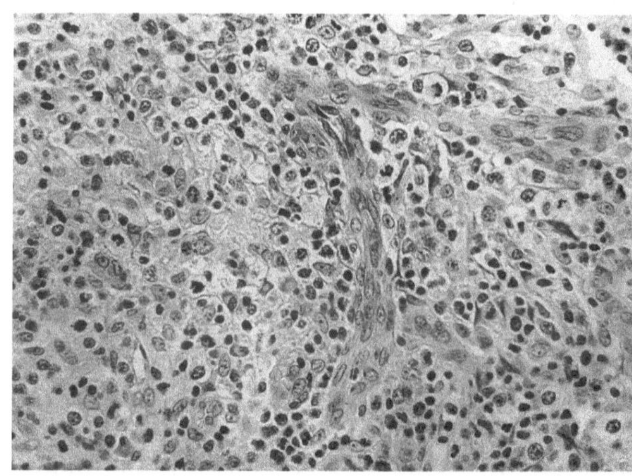

Fig. 10. AILD-like T-cell lymphoma with proliferating post-capillary venules and atypical clear T cells. H+E, X320

T-cell Lymphoma of AILD Type (AILD-like ML)

Immunoblastic [142] or angioimmunoblastic [143] lymphadenopathy appears clinically as a systemic disease with generalized lymphadenopathy, spleen and liver enlargement, Coombs-positive haemolytic anaemia, polyclonal hyperglobulinaemia, drug hypersensitivity and skin eruptions. Histologically the effacement of the lymph node architecture is complete or almost complete. Some "burnt-out" [143] pale stained germinal centres may be found. Arborizing vessels of the post-capillary venule type show strong proliferation even outside the lymph-nodal capsule. PAS-positive amorphous material in thickened vascular walls and among cells characterizes most of the cases. The infiltrating cell population is polymorphic, consisting of lymphocytes, plasma cells, dispersed immunoblasts, histiocytes and eosinophils [142-144]. In some cases the presence of epithelioid cells is prominent [142, 145]. AILD, occurring more frequently in elderly patients, was initially considered as a hyperimmune reaction [142-143] due to drugs or other immunogens. After the first description in Japan of peripheral T-cell lymphoma resembling immunoblastic lymphadenopathy [146], it became gradually obvious that the majority of so-called AILD represent a real T-cell lymphoma. The elements which favour such a view are: a) in most cases and in the vicinity of the proliferating vessels accumulations of atypical T cells with clear cytoplasm are found (Fig. 10); b) in many cases chromosomal abnormalities (trisomy 3 or 5) are documented [147,148]; c) TCR gene rearrangement methods have demonstrated clonality of T cells regarding TCR-ß and TCR-γ chain genes [149-151]. However, in part of the cases there is an additional IgH-chain gene rearrangement [149].

Immunohistochemically the proliferating T cells (Ki-67+) are most frequently CD4 positive whereas in a minority of cases the proliferating cells show CD8 positivity [149]. The latter is related to the presence of IgH chain gene rearrangement. Another histological and immunohistochemical characteristic of AILD-type lymphoma is the abundance of hyperplastic follicular dendritic cells [152] inside as well as outside the "burnt-out" germinal cells, even among the arborizing vessels.

Although non-neoplastic, immunoreactive cases of AILD occur [144], the prognosis is generally poor, especially for cases of AILD-type T-cell lymphoma. The mean survival time was about 24 months after combined prednisone and chemotherapy [153]. It seems that the group with CD8 positivity and IgH chain gene rearrangement has a relatively better prognosis [149]. In over 10% of AILD-type T-cell lymphomas transformation into high-grade malignant lymphoma of the large T-cell pleomorphic, T-immunoblastic or large cell anaplastic (Ki-1+) type occurs. The finding of light chain (κ or λ) monoclonal plasma cells and immunoblasts [154,155] could be explained either as a true B-cell lymphoma or as reactive B-cell clonal expansion induced by the helper activity of the CD4-positive neoplastic cell clone.

Aetiopathogenetically AILD-type T-cell lymphoma has been related to viruses such as rubella [156], herpes-like [157] and Mazon-Pfizer monkey virus [158].

Pleomorphic Small T-cell Lymphoma

Although occurring also in childhood, pleomorphic small T-cell lymphoma shows its incidence peak after 60 years of age. The tumour cells may be HTLV-1 positive, especially in Japan and the Caribbean area. Histologically the lymph nodes are diffusely involved by small-sized (Fig. 11a) pleomorphic cells. Their nuclei are gyroid, indented or irregular with small nucleoli. The cytoplasm is rather scarce and pale to clear [20,120,159]. Skin involvement is common. Usually, all types of peripheral T-cell lymphomas show more mitoses than their morphological analogues among B-cell lymphomas. In addition, they frequently show epidermotropism/epitheliotropism and angiotropism. Immunohistochemically they have the phenotype of helper CD4-positive T cells (Fig. 11b). With molecular methods they reveal clonal gene rearrangement for TCR-γ or TCR-ß. Despite the "cytic" appearance of the neoplastic cells and the initial absence of "blastic" cells, the prognosis of pleomorphic small T-cell lymphomas is poor. Neoplastic cells undergo an early activation and transformation to large cells, resulting in

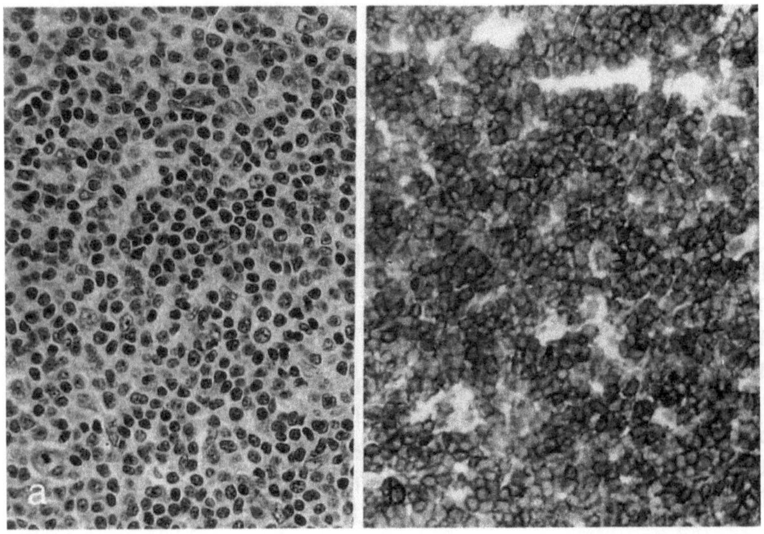

Fig. 11. Pleomorphic small T-cell lymphoma. a) H+E, X320; b) Immunostaining for CD4, X320

development of high-grade malignant T-cell lymphoma.
Pleomorphic small T-cell lymphoma is rather difficult to be categorized in the IWF.

High Grade Malignant Lymphomas

Most of the high-grade malignant lymphomas consist of neoplastic lymphoid cells with "blastic" appearance. They are either primary or secondary, and in the latter case preceded by a low-grade malignant lymphoma.

Centroblastic Lymphoma

This is the most frequent high-grade malignant lymphoma [160]. It occurs at all ages with a peak after 60 years. Histologically it is exclusively or partially composed of centroblasts. Lymph nodes are usually diffusely infiltrated although a complete or partial follicular growth pattern is not infrequent [97]. Macrophages with tingible bodies may be dispersed among centroblasts, giving a "starry sky" picture. Dendritic cells [81], even after appropriate immunohistochemical staining, are seen only in small numbers in the cases with a diffuse growth pattern. Cells with centrocytic or immunoblastic appearance may be found in varying numbers.
On the basis of the cell components of the lymphomatous infiltrates 4 subtypes of centroblastic lymphoma have been distinguished [160]: a) the monomorphic subtype (Fig. 12a), consisting mostly (>60%) of medium-sized or large, typical centroblasts. They have round pale nuclei with the nucleoli frequently attached to the nuclear membrane. Immunoblasts, when present, must not exceed 10% of the neoplastic cell population; b) the polymorphic subtype (Fig. 13a), showing a mixed neoplastic popula-

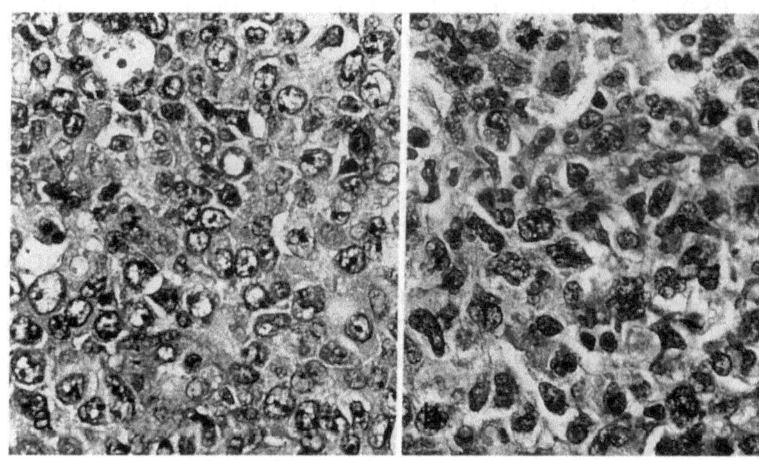

Fig. 12. Centroblastic lymphoma. a) Monomorphic, b) multilobated. H+E, X500

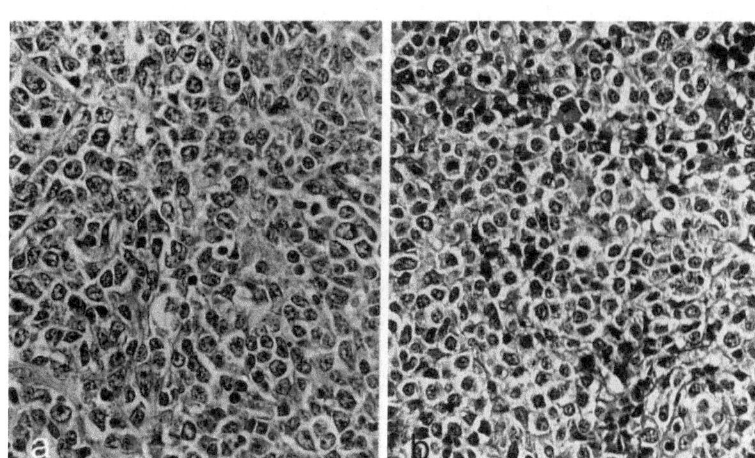

Fig. 13. Centroblastic lymphoma. a) Polymorphic, b) centrocytoid. H+E, X320

tion composed of centroblasts, immunoblasts and cells of centrocytic character. It is the most common type of centroblastic lymphoma. Centroblasts must represent at least 10% of the cell population; c) the multilobated subtype (Fig. 12b), where multilobated centroblasts predominate or at least represent more than 20% of the neoplastic population. The nucleoli are frequently indiscernible. Although multilobated cells were first regarded as a characteristic of T-cell lymphomas, it is now acknowledged that the majority of such lymphomas belong to the B-cell lineage [161-165]; d) the centrocytoid subtype (Fig.13b), in which the predominant neoplastic cells show intermediate morphological features between centrocytes and centroblasts. They are medium to large-sized with angular to oval nuclei and centrally located nucleoli.

Immunohistochemically the majority of the neoplastic cells are positive for surface IgMk. About 10% of the cases, however, are negative for SIg. Cytoplasmic immunoglobulin can also be observed. The immunophenotype corresponds to CD19, CD20 and CD22 positivity. Most of the cases are CD5 negative. CD10 (CALLA) positivity is observed in part of the cases.

Although Ki67-positive neoplastic cells may be very numerous, centroblastic lymphomas as a rule have the best prognosis among all types of high-grade malignant lymphomas [166,167].

In the IWF most centroblastic lymphomas are included in the group of intermediate-grade malignancy under the terms "follicular, predominantly large cell" [97] and "diffuse large cell, cleaved and non-cleaved" [168]. Some cases of polymorphic centroblastic lymphoma with numerous immunoblasts could be classified as "large cell immunoblastic, polymorphous or with epithelioid cell component" [169].

Immunoblastic Lymphoma

This type is composed of B or T-immunoblasts. These are usually large cells with a relatively abundant basophilic cytoplasm [160, 170]. Their large nuclei contain one or more large, centrally located nucleoli (Fig. 14a). On purely morphological grounds it is difficult to distinguish B from T-cell immunoblastic lymphomas. Only cases with plasmablastic/plasmacytic differentiation (Fig. 14b) can be readily classified as B-cell immunoblastic lymphomas. In other cases at least immunohistochemistry is needed for such a distinction. Morphological features such as irregular nuclei, clear cytoplasm and epithelioid cell content are no exclusive characteristic of lymphomas of either B or T-cell origin. Moreover, follicular dendritic reticulum cells or interdigitating reticulum cells are either absent or very scarcely present in immunoblastic lymphomas.

Immunohistochemically B-immunoblastic lymphomas are positive for CD19, CD20 and CD22. CD5 positivity is usually found in cases developed secondary to B-CLL/LP-immunocytomas. Most cases show SIg, mainly of the IgM class. Over 50% of the cases display cytoplasmic immunoglobulin positivity even in paraffin sections. T-immunoblastic

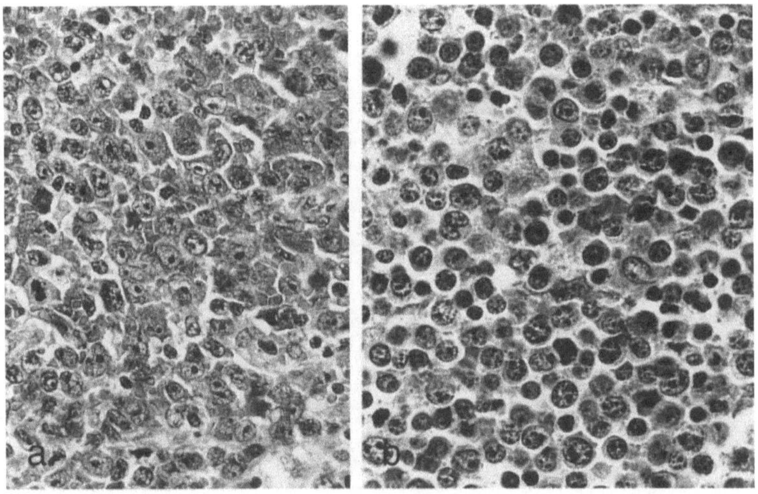

Fig. 14. Immunoblastic lymphoma. a) Without and b) with plasmablastic/ plasmacytic differentiation. H+E, X400

lymphomas are positive for UCHL1, CD2, CD3, CD5 and in their great majority express CD4 and only rarely CD8. Secondary cases originating from pleomorphic T-cell lymphomas may show positivity for HTLV-1. B and more frequently T-immunoblastic lymphomas may show CD30 positivity, a feature which makes it difficult to distinguish these types from anaplastic large cell lymphomas [160,171]. In some cases B as well as T-cell immunoblastic lymphomas may lose their appropriate phenotypic markers. In such instances molecular methods for Ig and TCR gene rearrangements are needed to distinguish B from T-cell types [13].

B-immunoblastic lymphomas are more frequent than T-immunoblastic lymphomas. The former can be divided into 3 histological subtypes with histogenetic relevance [160]: a) B-cell immunoblastic lymphoma without plasmacytic differentiation, of intra- or extrafollicular origin; b) B-cell immunoblastic lymphoma with plasmablastic/plasmacytic differentiation, mainly of extrafollicular origin; c) B-cell immunoblastic lymphoma with a high lymphocyte content (Fig. 8b) developed secondarily to a B-CLL/LP immunocytoma.

The bone marrow is infrequently infiltrated and a leukaemic picture is very rare, occurring in about 15% of B-cell immunoblastic lymphoma cases.

The prognosis of immunoblastic lymphomas in adults is worse than that of other high-grade malignant lymphomas. It is even more unfavourable in cases of T-cell origin [141].

Regarding the classification of immunoblastic lymphomas there is general agreement between the Kiel classification and the IWF. Some cases with cell polymorphism might be classified according to the Kiel classification as polymorphic centroblastic and according to the IWF as polymorphous immunoblastic lymphoma. However, this discrepancy has no influence on therapy.

Lymphoblastic Lymphoma

Malignant lymphomas of this category consist of medium-sized blastic cells with scanty to moderate, variably basophilic cytoplasm. The nuclei show finely dispersed chromatin. Cells corresponding to their normal counterparts are hardly seen in adult lymphoid tissue. The term "lymphoblast" is applied here in the way it is used for the blast cells of acute lymphoblastic leukaemia in haematology. They correspond to immunophenotypes and genotypes of early stages of B and T-cell lymphogenesis [172-175]. Accordingly, the lymphoblastic lymphomas are either of B or T-cell lineage. In both groups the lymph node architecture is diffusely effaced. Mitoses and Ki-67-positive cells are numerous. The nuclei of the neoplastic cells may be irregular, indented or convoluted. Although convolutions were formely considered as characterizing T-cell lymphoblastic lymphomas [176] (Fig. 15), they are encountered in B-cell types as well [160]. Lymphoblastic neoplasms begin either as aleukaemic tumour masses or are indistinguishable from acute lym-

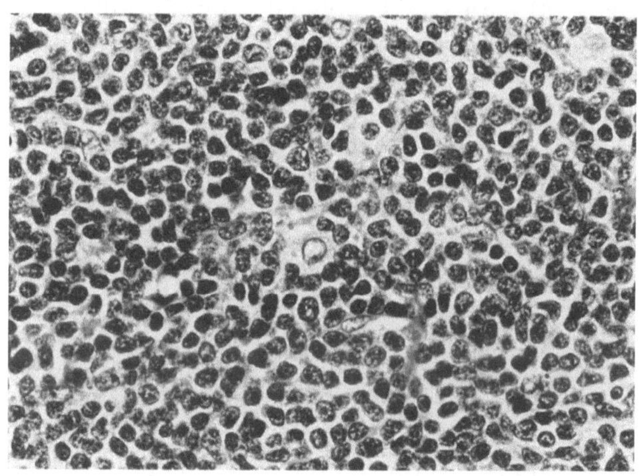

Fig. 15. T-cell lymphoblastic lymphoma convoluted type. H+E, X400

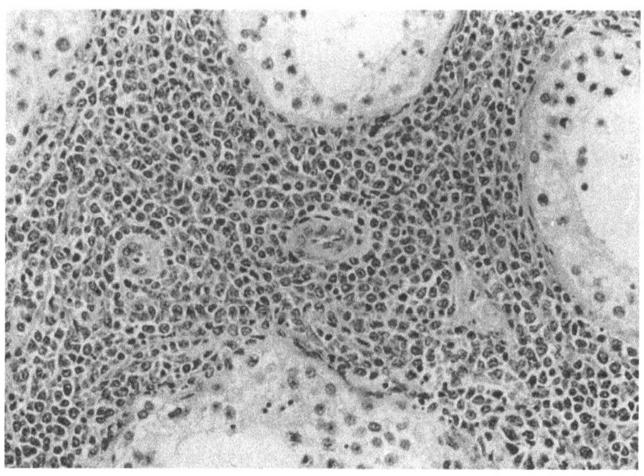

Fig. 16. Lymphoblastic lymphoma with testicular infiltration. H+E, X320

phoblastic leukaemia especially in children (Fig. 16). Additionally some cases of acute myelogenous leukaemia or blastic crises of chronic myelogenous leukaemia may show a predominant lymphoblastic cell component in some stages. Non-leukaemic lymphoblastic lymphomas are much less frequent than their leukaemic counterparts [160]. Histologically it is impossible on purely morphological grounds to distinguish the above two groups from each other as well as B-cell from T-cell types.

Lymphoblastic lymphomas of B-cell type express a pre-B or mature B-cell phenotype. The pre-B-cell phenotype is characterized by expression of cytoplasmic IgM (light chains not detectable), Pan-B antigens CD19 and CD20 and TdT [177,178]. There is also a less mature phenotype, the so-called Pre-pre-B, with positivity only for CD19 and TdT and negativity for IgM. The so-called "null" cell lymphoblastic lymphomas, which are negative for IgS and Pan-B antigens and positive for CALLA (CD10) and TdT, have been proved by Ig-gene rearrangement methods to be primarily of B-cell lineage [179]. The mature B-cell lymphoblastic lymphomas express surface immunoglobulins and Pan-B antigens while they are negative for TdT. Lymphoblastic lymphomas of T-cell type show phenotypes corresponding to prothymocyte ($CD2^+$,$CD7^+$), cortex thymocyte ($CD1^+$,$CD5^+$, cytoplasmic $CD3^+$, and simultaneously $CD4^+$ and $CD8^+$) and thymocyte (surface $CD3^+$, $CD4^+$ or $CD8^+$) stage of normal lymphogenesis [179-181]. CD7 is the earliest T-cell antigen [182].

TCR gene rearrangement methods have demonstrated in T-cell lymphoblastic lymphomas some patterns corresponding to the stages of normal lymphogenesis. It seems that TCR-δ chain gene rearrangement occurs first followed by TCR-γ, then TCR-β and lastly TCR-α chain gene rearrangements [175]. In the medullary thymocyte stage all TCR genes are rearranged. By means of molecular biology techniques most cases can be classified as either B or T-cell lymphoblastic lymphomas. However, we must keep in mind that in some cases of B-cell lymphoblastic lymphoma no gene rearrangement can be found [175,183,184].

Chromosomal abnormalities are not rare in lymphoblastic lymphomas [185-187]. Mostly they are translocations involving the antigen receptor genes and closely related to oncogenes tcl-1,2,3,5. Translocation t(9:22) seems to be related to a bad prognosis [186].

Burkitt's Lymphoma

This type of lymphoma is best referred to by the name of the man who first described it [188] because the exact origin of the neoplastic cells is unknown. Burkitt's lymphoma has been categorized by Lukes and Collins [189] as "small non-cleaved follicular centre cell lymphoma". Although there are some immunophenotypic and morphologic findings favouring a germinal centre cell origin [190,191], this view cannot be considered definitive. The rare, partially follicular pattern could be regarded as secondary neoplastic involvement of preexisting germinal centres [192]. Preceding infiltration of the mantle zone has been observed in some cases [192]. The IWF distinguishes two types of so-called "small non-cleaved cell lymphoma": Burkitt's and non-Burkitt's type. The second type is clinically closer related to other adult high-grade non-Hodgkin lymphomas of B-cell origin. However, in many cases its histological distinction from Burkitt's type is very difficult. Particularly in children these two types of SNC lymphoma are clinically and biologically indistinguishable [193-195]. The Kiel classification subdivides Burkitt's lymphoma into the typical form and "Burkitt's lymphoma with cytoplasmic immunoglobulin". The latter may include cases which could be designated as SNC non-Burkitt lymphoma in the American literature. The distinction of these two types of Burkitt's lymphoma is in many cases difficult if not impossible. It rather seems to be a continuum as the neoplastic cells of typical Burkitt's lymphoma transform into immunoblasts [196,197] and SNC lymphoma of Burkitt's type can assume an immunoblastic appearance in AIDS patients [198].

Histologically, Burkitt's lymphoma in its typical form shows a diffuse pattern of infiltration with homogeneously uniform cells (Fig. 17a). They are medium-sized, round to oval in shape, have a moderate amount of basophilic cytoplasm and form a cohesive pattern. The nuclei are not larger than those of the adjacent tingible body macrophages. Their chromatin is coarsely dispersed with 2-5 prominent, centrally located, basophilic nucleoli. Another histological feature is the "starry sky" picture due to the presence

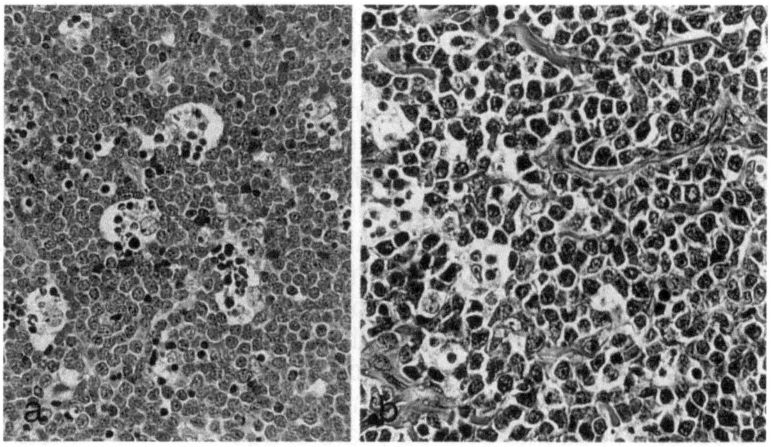

Fig. 17. Burkitt's lymphoma. a) Classic type, b) with plasmablastic differentiation. H+E, X400

of macrophages among the tumour cells. Their cytoplasm contains many phagocytosed neoplastic cells and nuclear remnants as the rate of cell apoptosis is very high. Similarly the number of mitoses is high and the Ki-67-positive, proliferating tumour cells exceed 80% [199-200]. In imprints the tumour cells show many cytoplasmic vacuoles. Immunophenotypically the neoplastic lymphoid cells express SIgs (usually IgM), Pan-B cell antigens such as CD19 and CD22, the CD10 (CALLA) antigen and the CD77 antigen. The latter has been seen only in germinal centre cells [190]. Follicular dendritic reticulum cells are very seldom seen [200].

Two distinct clinicopathological subtypes of Burkitt's lymphoma are recognized. The endemic or African subtype occurs more often in children and shows large extranodal masses involving the jaw bones and abdominal viscera [201]. The sporadic or non-endemic, non-African subtype includes significant numbers of adult cases [202] and more frequently presents with an abdominal mass involving the abdominal lymph nodes, ileocaecal region, retroperitoneum and ovaries [202]. The jaws are less commonly involved. A leukaemic picture is not frequent (5-10%), occurring mostly as a terminal phenomenon [203].

Epstein-Barr virus infection has been implicated in the aetiology of Burkitt's lymphoma, especially of the endemic subtype. Over 90% of the cases of this subtype show lymphomatous cells containing copies of the EBV-DNA genome [204], which is in contrast with the low percentages (about 15%) in the non-endemic subtype. Immunohistochemically, the pattern of EBV protein expression is LMP negative and EBNA-2 negative, distinct from the pattern (LMP positive and EBNA-2 negative) found in undifferentiated nasopharyngeal carcinoma [205,206]. Cytogenetically, Burkitt's lymphoma, either endemic or sporadic, shows characteristic chromosomal translocations involving chromosome 8 and chromosomes 2, 14 or 22. Translocation t(8;14) occurs most frequently, while translocation t(2;8) and t(8;22) are less common [207]. Characteristically, the locus 8q24 of the *c-myc* oncogene is involved in chromosome 8, while in the other chromosomes the loci 14q32 for the IgH gene, 2p11 for the Igκ gene or 22q11 for the Igλ gene are involved. These translocations bring the *c-myc* sequence in juxtaposition to one of the immunoglobulin genes resulting in subsequent transcription of *c-myc*. *C-myc* oncoprotein stimulates the neoplastic cells to proliferate. Some differences in chromosomal breakpoints in t(8;14) have been observed between the endemic and non-endemic subtypes [208,209]. In both subtypes the chromosome 14 breakpoint occurs within the region of the IgH chain gene while the chromosome 8 breakpoint occurs either far 5' to *c-myc* (endemic Burkitt's lymphoma) or within the *c-myc* gene (sporadic Burkitt's lymphoma). There is an exception regarding sporadic Burkitt's lymphoma of the ileocaecal region. Here the breakpoint on chromosome 14 is similar to that occurring in endemic Burkitt's lymphoma [210].

Burkitt's lymphoma with cytoplasmic immunoglobulin is histologically characterized by diffuse growth of medium-sized, basophilic lymphoid cells intermingled with small and large forms. Giant cell forms are occasionally found. Thus the nuclear variation and cellular pleomorphism are greater than in typical Burkitt's lymphoma (Fig. 17b). Additionally, a variable number of cells show features of plasmablastic differentiation. Immunohistochemically, cytoplasmic immunoglobulin can be detected even in paraffin sections. CD10 (CALLA) is not consistently expressed [211]. This type of lymphoma is closely related to non-endemic Burkitt's lymphoma. However, the CIg-positive form is less frequently extranodal than the CIg-negative form of Burkitt's lymphoma and affects most often patients over 60 years of age.

Small non-cleaved cell lymphoma, non-Burkitt type according to the IWF, is histologically characterized by a greater cell variation than Burkitt's lymphoma. Giant cell forms may occasionally be found. Immunohistochemically there is a strong resemblance to Burkitt's lymphoma [200].

Without therapy the prognosis is very poor. After appropriate therapy long-lasting remissions have been achieved. Non-endemic and EBV-negative forms show the greatest resistance to therapy.

Pleomorphic Medium-Sized and Large T-Cell Lymphoma

This is the most common type of peripheral T-cell lymphomas caused by the retrovirus HTLV-1 [212,213]. HTLV-1 is also aetiologically implicated in some cases of peripheral T-cell immunoblastic or pleomorphic small T-cell lymphomas. HTLV-1 selectively infects T cells. Viral DNA is found in the neoplastic T cells but not in the reactive B cells [214]. Pleomorphic medium-sized and large T-cell lymphoma caused by HTLV-1 is identical to adult T-cell leukaemia/lymphoma (ATLL). It has been described in Japan first [215-216] and later in Eastern China and in the Caribbean. It has also been observed in Europe and the United States [217-220]. A proportion of the population in endemic areas, ranging from 15% to 40%, show seropositivity for the ATLL antigen and are HTLV-1 carriers [221,222]. ATLL occurs in individuals older than 40 years with a mean age of 57 years. It represents over 80% of all cases of non-Hodgkin lymphomas in Japan [215,223].

There exists an HTLV-1-negative form of pleomorphic medium-sized and large T-cell lymphoma [120,159,173,224] which occurs sporadically in all geographic areas but mainly in the western countries. The elderly are affected most frequently. Histologically it is very difficult to distinguish HTLV-1-negative from HTLV-1-positive cases [224]. In the HTLV-1-negative, sporadic form, involvement of lymph nodes, skin, tonsils and other tissues may be seen. The growth of the neoplastic cells is diffuse. They are medium-sized or large pleomorphic (Fig. 18) with moderately abundant, lightly stained basophilic cytoplasm [120,159,213, 218]. The nuclei are gyroid, irregularly indented and bizarre (Fig. 16a). The chromatin is fine to coarse and the nucleoli in many cells are prominent. The number of mitoses and Ki67-positive cells is high. Gene rearrangement methods reveal clonal rearrangement of TCR-α, TCR-β and TCR-γ [225-227]. Immunohistochemically

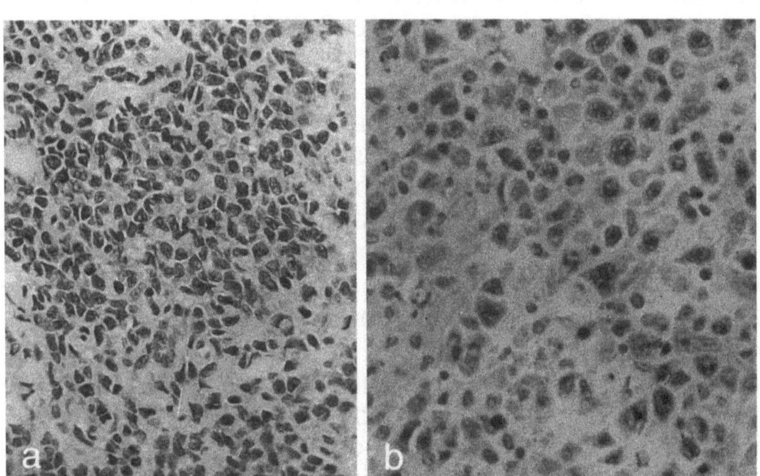

Fig. 18. Pleomorphic T-cell lymphoma. a) Medium-sized, b) large cell

the neoplastic cells show a phenotype of mature peripheral T cells: CD2+, CD3+, CD5+ and CD4+ or CD8+. In part of the cases the cells express CD25 (IL-2R) and CD7 [218]. In HTLV-1-positive, endemic (ATLL) cases the histology is much more pleomorphic. The neoplastic cells differ from one case to another not only in shape but also in size [224]. Mitoses are numerous. By molecular methods gene rearrangements of TCR-α, β and γ are demonstrated [215,220]. Lymphadenopathy, spleen and liver enlargement and skin involvement are frequent. The prognosis is more unfavourable in ATLL than in HTLV-1-negative cases [228].
Peripheral pleomorphic large T-cell lymphoma is not listed in the IWF. It could be classified either as "large cell immunoblastic, polymorphic" or as "diffuse large cell, cleaved and noncleaved".

Large Cell Anaplastic Ki-1+ Lymphoma

This lymphoma type occurs at all ages. Histologically it is characterized (Fig. 19a) by large to giant cells with varying degrees of nuclear irregularity and abundant cytoplasm [229-233]. The chromatin is finely distributed and the nucleoli are prominent, solitary or multiple. Cells indistinguishable from typical Sternberg-Reed cells may be found. The tumour cell growth pattern is similar either to Rappaport's malignant histiocytosis [234] or to carcinomas. They are designated as anaplastic cells because of their atypia and the lack of a normal lymphoid cell counterpart. Erythrophagocytosis may be observed in reactive histiocytes and rarely in neoplastic cells. Eosinophils and plasma cells are present in varying numbers. Some authors [231,233] identify 2 histological subtypes with some prognostic relevance: subtype I has more irregular neoplastic cells. Among them giant forms are not infrequent. Subtype II shows tumour cells that are less irregular in shape.
Immunohistochemically almost all neoplastic cells are CD30 (Ki-1) positive [229,235]. However, CD30 positivity is not a prerequisite for the diagnosis of anaplastic large cell lymphomas as some cases are practically CD30 negative. In addition, other high-grade NHLs of either T or B-cell origin may show significant CD30 positivity [235]. Immunophenotypically 3 subtypes are recognized: a) the T-cell subtype, which is the most frequent. Tumour cells express CD2, CD3 and CD4 as well as activation antigens CD25 and HLA-DR. Molecular biology methods reveal rearrangements of TCR-γ and TCR-β [236]; b) the B-cell subtype. Neoplastic cells express the antigens CD19 and CD22. IgS expression is very rare although DNA analysis demonstrates IgH gene rearrangement. Expression of the activation antigens CD25 and HLA-DR is frequent; c) the null cell subtype. Neoplastic cells do not express any phenotypic B or T-cell markers. DNA analysis frequently shows TCR gene rearrangements. However, in a significant number of cases no rearrangements of either TCR or Ig genes are observed. Such cases present difficulties in differential diagnosis from carcinomas inasmuch as LCALs positive for keratin [237] and non-lymphomatous neoplasms posi-

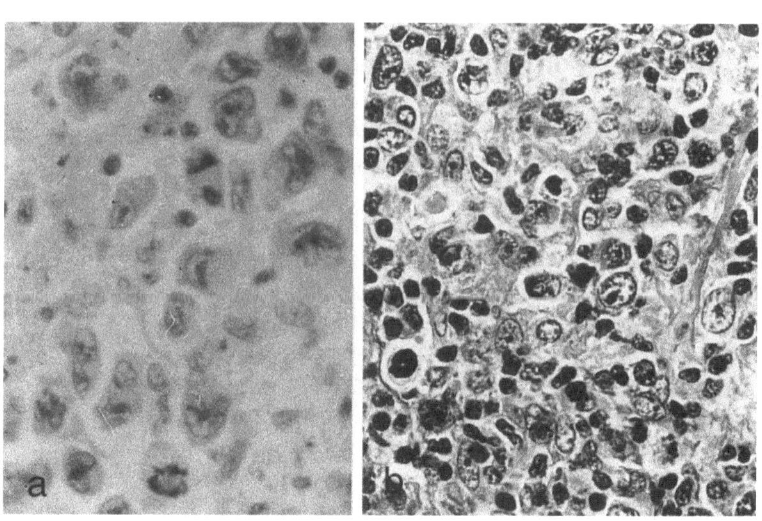

Fig. 19. a) Large cell, anaplastic (Ki-1+) lymphoma, H+E, X 400; b) enteropathy T-cell lymphoma, H+E, X 500

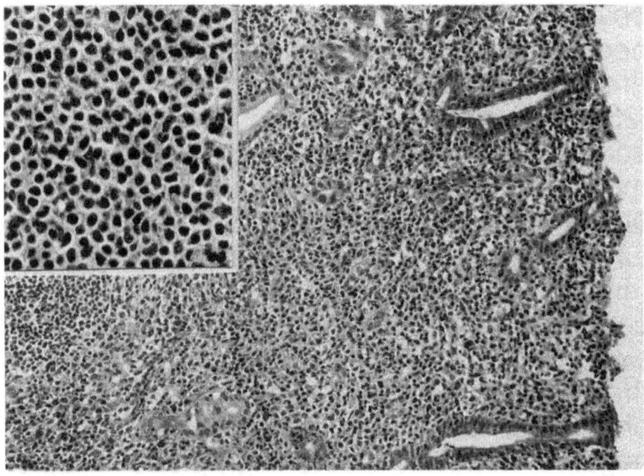

Fig. 20. MALToma of the stomach. H+E, X80. Inset: centrocyte-like morphology X320

tive for CD30 [238] have been observed. Cytogenetically, LCALs frequently show chromosomal abnormalities such as translocations t(2:5) (p23:q35) and t(2:13) (p23;q34) [230, 239,240].

LCAL can be divided into primary and secondary forms. The latter develop most frequently from low and high-grade T-cell NHL and Hodgkin's disease [235,241].

The prognosis of LCAL is variable and in most cases the disease is aggressive. Prognosis is much better in primary cases, in children, in histological subtype II, in skin cases and in secondary cases developed from Hodgkin's disease [231-233,242]. It seems that expression of interleukin-9 is associated with the anaplastic appearance and tumour proliferation in LCAL [243].

Other Types of Malignant Lymphomas

Malignant Lymphomas of Mucosa-Associated Lymphoid Tissue (MALTomas)

In their typical form these belong to the low-grade lymphomas most frequently involving the gastrointestinal tract [244]. It is believed that the normal counterparts of neoplastic MALToma cells are the post-germinal centre cells, which are morphologically similar, irrespective of their nodal or extranodal location [107,245-247]. Their specific homing capacity depends on surface receptors primarily of lymphoid cells but also of stromal and vascular tissue elements [114,115,248]. It seems that post-germinal centre cells of MALT home to lymphoid tissue not only of the usual mucosal sites (e.g. stomach, intestine) but also of other extranodal epithelium-bearing sites such as the skin, breasts, salivary glands, thyroid gland, bladder, kidney, female genitals, prostate, thymus, conjuctiva [24,249-258]. The cells usually have a centrocyte-like configuration, are closely related to marginal zone cells and B-monocytoid cells [26,100,105,107,109,245] and represent the cell source for local memory cell reaction and local immunity.

MALTomas have various components in their cell population. Depending on the predominant cell type, MALTomas (Fig. 20) may histologically resemble B-CLL, lymphoplasmacytoid/lymphoplasmacytic immunocytoma, marginal zone cell or B-monocytoid cell lymphoma [35, 245,255]. Additional histological features of low-grade MALTomas are multifocal distribution in gastric or intestinal mucosa, disorganized or fully neoplastically occupied germinal centres and lymphoepithelial lesions [259-261].

Immunohistochemically MALTomas express monoclonal SIg and not infrequently CIg [35, 260]. They show positivity for Pan-B antigens CD19 and CD20. They are negative for CD5 and CD10 (CALLA) antigens, in contrast to B-CLL and centroblastic/centrocytic lymphomas, respectively. In paraffin sections they exhibit granular positivity for KiM1P. For a high-grade malignant lymphoma [23] to be classified as MALToma it must show areas with a residual component of typical low-grade MALToma. However, typical lymphoepithelial lesions have also been observed in high-grade malignant lymphomas [262]. This finding facilitates the appropriate classification. High-grade malignant lymphomas developing from a MALToma usually have the histological features of either centroblastic or immunoblastic lymphomas. It must be emphasized that, even in cases of low-grade appearance, MALTomas show numbers of blasts interspersed between the other neoplastic cells.

MALTomas have a striking tendency to remain localized for long periods of time and to be cured with local therapy. Even when they relapse, usually after prolonged disease-free intervals, they either continue to remain localized or relapse at other extranodal sites bearing epithelial tissues [263-265]. *Helicobacter pylori* has recently been implicated in the aetiopathogenesis of MALTomas [266]. Isaackson underlines the similarities between α-heavy chain disease of the small intestine and gastric lymphomas of MALT type.

Signet Ring Cell Lymphoma

This type is nodular (follicular) or diffuse, mainly of B and rarely of T-cell origin [267,268]. The vacuoles are usually filled with PAS-positive material which in cases of B-cell (centroblastic/centrocytic) lymphoma corresponds to immunoglobulins. Its resemblance to signet ring cell mucin producing carcinomas is obvious.

Malignant Angioendotheliomatosis

This is also called angioendotheliotropic or angiotropic lymphoma and intravascular lymphomatosis [269-272]. It is a systemic intravascular lymphoproliferative disease with occlusion of the small vessels of the skin and various other organs. The cells are large with irregular nuclei and an immunoblastic appearance in most cases. Immunohistochemical and gene rearrangement studies have confirmed that the neoplastic cells usually are of B-cell origin [271] and only rarely of T-cell origin [272].

Lymphomatoid Granulomatosis and Angiocentric Lymphoma

This is an angiodestructive form of lymphoid cell proliferation. Lymphomatoid granulomatosis was initially described by Liebow as involving the lungs [273]. Later it was found to occur also in the skin, brain and other organs. Jaffe's group included it under the name of "angiocentric immunoproliferative lesion" diseases formerly called lymphomatoid granulomatosis, midline reticulosis, midline granuloma or polymorphic reticulosis [274,275]. Histologically the lesions are characterized by a polymorphic cell population containing atypical lymphoid cells of small and medium size. Evolution to large cell lymphoma of high-grade malignancy is not infrequent. Immunohistochemically most cases show a T-cell phenotype. B-cell phenotype is rare [275-277]. Gene rearrangement studies were unable to demonstrate a consistent T or B-cell genotype in the majority of cases [16, 276,277]. In many cases EBV-DNA was found, especially with the PCR technique [276, 277].

Mediastinal Large Cell Lymphoma

This lymphoma type is located in the mediastinum and seems to develop mainly extranodally. Histologically it consists of large cells (Fig. 21a) mostly similar to centroblasts [278-280]. There is significant sclerosis and a frequent carcinoma-like pattern. This lymphoma seems to derive from the B cells of the thymus. Immunohistochemically the neoplastic cells show a B-cell phenotype: $CD20^{+}$, $CD22^{+}$, $CD19^{+/-}$, $CD5^{-}$, CIg^{-}, $SIg^{+/-}$ [27,28,278,281]. Differential diagnosis must distinguish this type from Hodgkin's disease, anaplastic large cell lymphomas and carcinomas.

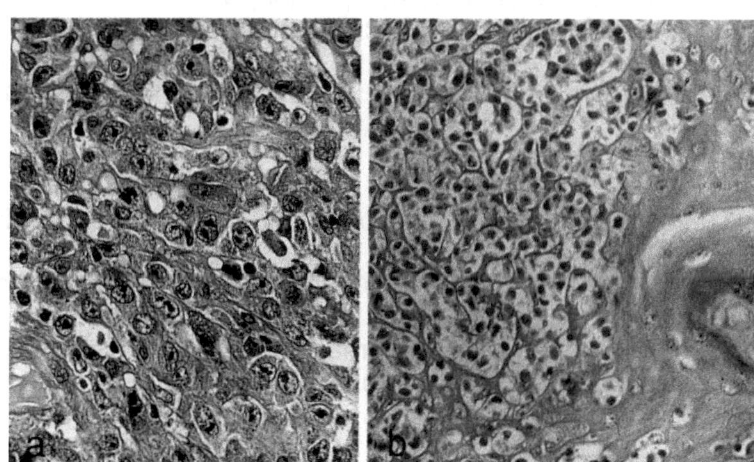

Fig. 21. a) Mediastinal large cell lymphoma. H+E, X400; b) Lymphomatoid papulosis with carcinoma-like appearance

The prognosis is rather poor. Complete remissions, however, have been achieved with chemotherapy [28,280].

Filiform or Microvillous Large Cell Lymphoma

Histologically these lymphomas resemble large cell anaplastic lymphomas but they are not CD30 (Ki-1) positive [282,283]. Immunophenotypically they belong to the B-cell lymphomas. Electron microscopy shows numerous cytoplasmic processes. Typical large cell anaplastic, Ki-1+ lymphomas, however, may also show such numerous cytoplasmic processes.

Splenic Lymphoma with Villous Lymphocytes

This is characterized by spenomegaly without substantial lymphadenopathy. In peripheral blood smears and spleen tissue imprints medium-sized lymphocytes with short cytoplasmic villi are found [284,285]. Splenic lymphoma with villous lymphocytes does not represent a distinct entity and is closely related to lymphoplasmacytic immunocytoma. It frequently expresses monoclonal serum Igs. Histologically the spleen shows mainly involvement of the white pulp [286]; when the bone marrow is involved it displays a nodular or interstitial/mixed pattern. Neoplastic cells show significant lymphoplasmacytoid/cytic differentiation. Their immunophenotype corresponds to: SIg^+, CIg^+, $CD20^+$, $CD22^+$ and $CD5^-$, $CD23^-$. Cytogenetically they frequently show the translocation t(11;14) (q13;q32) analogous to that found in mantle cell lymphomas [287,288].

Composite Lymphoma

This name is given to combinations in the same lymph node of either Hodgkin's disease with a non-Hodgkin lymphoma or two different non-Hodgkin lymphomas [289-292]. In most cases, however, the second lymphoma is a high-grade malignant blastic transformation of the same cell clone occurring in the low-grade malignant component.

T-cell Lymphoma in Enteropathy (Celiac Disease)

These are the most frequent T-cell lymphomas of the gastrointestinal tract (Fig. 19b). They were initially characterized as "malignant histiocytosis" of the intestine [293] and were reported in certain countries, particularly England, while they were practically absent from other countries, including Greece [294]. Today immunohistochemical and genotypic studies have proved the T-cell origin [295,296]. They show the immunophenotype of the intraepithelial T lymphocytes of gastrointestinal mucosa: $CD4^-$, $CD8^-$, HML-1+ [293,297,298].

Lymphomatoid Papulosis

In the early stages this lymphoma shows a clinical resemblance to mycosis fungoides. Differential diagnosis between the two entities is difficult. In later stages lymphomatoid papulosis is characterized by episodic eruptions of papules and nodules which may become necrotic [106]. Despite its prolonged benign clinical course, final development of high-grade malignant lymphoma is not uncommon. Histologically the infiltrates are densely distributed in the dermis and are composed of lymphocytes, histiocytes and large atypical lymphoid cells (Fig. 21b) which are positive for CD30 (Ki-1) and T-cell markers [299,300]. Their T-cell origin is confirmed by the demonstration of TCR gene rearrangements [301,302]. There seems to be a continuum from lymphomatoid papulosis to large cell anaplastic (Ki-1+) lymphomas of the skin [303].

True Histiocytic Lymphoma and Malignant Histiocytosis

This lymphoma type is rare and has the tendency to involve not only lymph nodes but also skin and bone marrow [304]. The majority of neoplasms which were formerly, on morphological grounds, classified as malignant histiocytosis have immunohistochemically and genotypically been proved to represent T-cell, large cell lymphomas (mostly Ki-1+) and in rare cases B-cell lymphomas [160,171,304,305].

B-cell Lymphoma with High T-cell Content

It may be difficult histologically to distinguish this type from Hodgkin's disease as it consists of large monoclonal B cells lying among numerous T lymphocytes [9,306,307]. Reactive T cells may even be pleomorphic or atypic, while the large neoplastic B cells display either a centroblastic or immunoblastic morphology. However, similar histological appearance may show true peripheral small T-cell lymphomas with induction (helper activity) of monotypic reactive B-cell proliferation. In other instances analogous histology may be the result of a composite T and B-cell lymphoma or the development of a high-grade B-cell lymphoma from a nodular lymphocyte-predominant Hodgkin's disease [308,309].
An accurate diagnosis requires a combined morphological, immunohistochemical and even genotypic analysis.

Lymphomas of the Nasal Cavities

These lymphomas deserve separate mention because of their immunophenotypic, genotypic and morphological peculiarities. They may be classified into two categories: T-cell lymphomas of the midline reticulosis group and other lymphomas of the nasal and paranasal cavities. The latter mostly display a T-cell phenotype, are usually of high-grade malignancy, may show CD30 (Ki-1) positivity and present difficulties in differential diagnosis from carcinomas [310-312].
Genotypic analysis in most cases shows a germ-line configuration of either TCR or Ig genes. Additionally the presence of an EBV genome in neoplastic cells is frequent [313].

Lymphohistiocytic Lymphoma

This has been defined by Lennert's group as a lymphoma consisting of a polymorphous cell population including lysozyme-positive histiocytes, plasma cells, CD4-positive lymphocytes and varying numbers of large CD30+ cells [314]. Their prognosis is unpredictable, ranging from good to the evolution of large cell, anaplastic lymphoma.

Differential Diagnosis and Prognostic Evaluation of Malignant Lymphomas

Of great significance in everyday practice are: 1) the differential diagnosis of a non-Hodgkin lymphoma from Hodgkin's disease, other non-lymphomatous neoplasms, reactive lymphoproliferative conditions and other types of pseudolymphomas; 2) the prognostic evaluation of each form and each case of non-Hodgkin lymphomas.

Distinction of NHL from HD

Putting aside the instances of composite lymphomas, where a B-cell lymphoma develops from lymphocyte-predominant Hodgkin's disease, the histological forms of NHL with a high risk to be diagnostically confused with Hodgkin's disease are: follicular centre cell malignant lymphoma with Sternberg-Reed (S-R)-like giant cell forms, T-cell-rich B-cell lymphoma, histiocyte-rich B-cell lymphoma, mediastinal large B-cell lymphoma with sclerosis, peripheral pleomorphic large T-cell lymphoma, AILD-like T-cell lymphoma, anaplastic large cell (Ki-1+) lymphoma and B-cell/lymphocytic lymphoma with S-R cells [9,28,42,142,143,224,229,235, 241,280]. Features helping in distinguishing NHL from Hodgkin's disease are either morphological or phenotypic/genotypic (Table 4). As regards morphology, cellular monotony favours an NHL while abundance of H/S-R cells and extensive necrosis and/or sclerosis render HD more likely. Immunophenotypically, the presence of either B or T-cell surface markers in the majority of neoplastic cells favours the diagnosis of an NHL, while the reverse is more compatible with Hodgkin's disease [6,10,11,13, 315]. By definition CD30 expression by the majority of neoplastic cells occurs almost exclusively in large cell anaplastic lymphoma, Hodgkin's disease (all subtypes except nodular lymphocyte predominant subtype) and lymphomatoid papulosis [235,300,316]. Genotypically most B and T-cell lymphomas show consistent Ig and TCR gene rearrangement, respectively. By contrast, DNA analysis in most cases of HD is inconsistent or debatable regarding Ig and TCR gene rearrangements [317-319].

Table 4. Features distinguishing NHL from HD

MORPHOLOGY

	S-R and H cells	Focal sclerosis	Necrosis	Cellular monotony
NHL	Sparse	-/+	-/+	+/+++
HD	Rather numerous	±/+++	+/+++	-/+

PHENOTYPE/GENOTYPE

		CD45 (LCA)	CD20	Other B-markers	UCHL-1 (CD45 RO)	CD3	CD15 (LeuM1)	CD30 (Ki-1)	IgH gene rearrange-ment	TCR gene rearrange-ment
NHL	B	+++	+++	+++	-/±	-	-/±	-/+	+++	-/±
	T	+++	-/(±)	-	+++	±/+++	-/+	-/+	-/±	+++
HD		-/±	-/+	-/+	-/±	-/±	+/+++	++/+++	inconsistent	inconsistent
Nodular LPHD		+/+++	+++	±/++	-	-	-	-/±	debatable	-

Distinction of NHL from Other Neoplasms

Care must be taken to distinguish NHL from various types of carcinomas and melanomas and in rare cases sarcomas (Table 5). As regards the morphology only some features characterizing certain types of neoplasms (melanin and tubule formation with mucin secretion) may be decisive for the diagnosis. Other carcinoma-like features, such as cell cohesiveness and intrasinusoidal pattern, may be observed in large cell lymphomas as well [235,280,320]. Immunohistochemically lymphomatous cells typically express surface lymphoid cell (B or T-cell) markers while carcinomas and other non-lymphomatous neoplasms bear epithelial and other characteristic markers. However, it must be kept in mind that in rare cases epithelial cells may express CD20 (L26) antigen [321] while some lymphomas may display not only EMA but also keratin positivity [237,323]. CD30 antigen, being a proliferation antigen, may be present not only in neoplastic cells of HD and NHL but also in embryonic and undifferentiated carcinomas [238]. In such equivocal cases gene rearrangement studies may solve, although not always [324], the differential diagnostic problem.

NHL and Reactive Lymphoproliferations

The first important group of reactive lymphoproliferations causing diagnostic problems are those simulating low-grade malignant B-cell lymphomas. Such lesions occur usually in the lungs, ileum, stomach, ocular adnexa and glands [325-331]. Despite the presence of some morphological and immunohistochemical features which favour a diagnosis of either pseudolymphomatous hyperplasia or malignant lymphoma, such features do not represent absolute diagnostic criteria. Germinal centres, if present, are considered to favour a diagnosis of reactive lymphoproliferation. However, MALTomas, particularly of the gastrointestinal tract, are histologically characterized by a multifocal distribution and the presence of numerous intact or neoplastically occupied germinal centres [259,260]. Lymphoepithelial lesions immunohistochemically consisting of B cells can be used as a strong diagnostic element for the diagnosis of gastrointestinal MALTomas but not of those of the thyroid gland. It is said that deep mural infiltration distinguishes gastric MALTomas from reactive lymphoid hyperplasia. There are, however, pseudolymphomas of the ileum with very significant deep infiltration of the intestinal wall [327]. Immunohistochemical

Table 5. Distinction of NHL from other neoplasms (carcinomas, melanomas, rarely sarcomas)

MORPHOLOGY

	Sheets, tubes, mucin, melanin	Fibrosis	Cohesion	Intra-sinusoidal pattern	Necrosis
NHL	-	+	+	+	±
Neoplasms	+	+	+	+	+

PHENOTYPE/GENOTYPE

	LCA (CD45)	B- or T-cell markers	EMA	Keratin	S-100	CD3 (Ki-1)	CD15 (LeuM1)	Endocrine and other markers	Vimentin
NHL	+	+	-/+	-/+	-	-/+	-/+	-	-/+
Neoplasms	-	- (L26+)	+/-	+/-	-/+	-/+	-/+	+	-/+

Ig polyclonality even in paraffin sections is a strong criterion for a diagnosis of reactive lymphohyperplasia. In ocular lymphoproliferations Ig polyclonality does not predict the final course and the remote prognosis of the lesions [325].

The second important group of pseudolymphomas are those which may be diagnostically confused with true T-cell NHL. Such pathological lesions may involve either the lymph nodes or extranodal sites. The former are represented by angioimmunoblastic lymphadenopathy [332,333] and the latter by skin pseudolymphomas, which like true skin T-cell lymphomas are divided into lichenoid (MF-like) and nodular (patchy) histological forms [25]. Some morphological and immunohistochemical features favour a diagnosis of true T-cell lymphomas. These are: significant epidermotropism (epitheliotropism), loss of T-cell markers particularly from intraepithelial cell infiltrates [127], and cell pleomorphism. The last feature, however, may be present to some extent in patchy pseudolymphomas of the skin [25]. On the other hand, although the presence of a polymorphic cell population usually characterizes the histology of pseudolymphomas, it may also be found in patchy true T-cell lymphomas of the skin [25].

Polyclonal B-immunoblastic hyperplasia [333] involving lymph nodes and extranodal sites, particularly bone marrow, must be distinguished from fully developed high-grade malignant lymphomas. The criteria for diagnosing polyclonal B-immunoblastic hyperplasia are the lack of morphological features characteristic of malignancy and the presence of numerous immunohistochemically polyclonal (polytypic) B-immunoblasts. They are the result of viral infections and abnormal immunoreactions. Their course is rather unpredictable. Genotypic analysis may reveal the true (reactive or neoplastic) nature of the lesions.

Prognostic Parameters of NHL

Classic morphological features and histopathological subcategories in conjuction with immunohistochemical data on frozen and paraffin sections remain the most important prognostic parameters in everyday practice of lymphoma management. It must be emphasized, however, that pathologists and clinicians should not limit themselves to using the lymphoma classification of their preference. They must know the pathological entities and individualize each case of lymphoma. For this purpose complementary parameters should be used. The most important seem to be the mitotic indices which include the pyknotic (apoptotic) index and expression of Ki-67, Brdu, PCNA, MIB1, and KiS antigens [167,334-336], which are closely related to cell proliferation activity. A high index

(>50%) is related to high-grade malignancy and aggressive course. Most of these proliferation antigens can be demonstrated even on paraffin sections by using the appropriate antibodies and microwave retrieval techniques [337]. Some oncogenes, particularly *c-myc* and *p53*, have been found mainly in high-grade malignant lymphomas, in B or T-immunoblastic lymphomas, in paraimmunoblasts of B-CLL and in S-R cells. However, no adequate survival data have been reported to date. The *bcl*-2 oncoprotein has been related to the regulation of chemoresistance in NHL [40,338-340]. DNA cytometry in sections and cell imprints are very promising methods but, like morphometric analysis, are not usable because relevant studies are still limited and their results are certainly not standardized for practical use [334,341-344]. Additionally, it seems that demonstration of cytokine expression may help to evaluate morphologic heterogeneity, tumour progression and therapeutic control [345,346].

With respect to the contribution of genotyping in non-Hodgkin lymphomas it must be emphasized that this is not always decisive because lineage infidelity may be observed. So, simultaneous TCR and IgH gene rearrangements may be seen in part of the AILD cases [149] as well as in other forms of low-grade malignant lymphomas. Monotypic B-cell proliferation may be induced by reactive or neoplastic CD4-positive lymphocytes with helper activity. Moreover, oligoclonal T-cell proliferation even with TCR gene rearrangement has been observed as a result of host reaction against lung carcinomas [347,348]. Translocations such as t(14;18) and *bcl*-2 and JH gene rearrangements, considered as being typical of follicular centre-cell lymphomas, may also be seen in other diffuse non-Hodgkin lymphomas and in S-R cells of Hodgkin's disease [75,78,349, 350]. Their presence in follicular lymphadenopathy could be partly attributed to false technique [351]. In conclusion, it must be underlined that classification and evaluation of prognosis have to be based on many parameters especially in difficult cases because 1) monoclonality as well as absence of monoclonality, even after usage of the finest methods, do not establish or exclude neoplasia, respectively, and 2) almost none of the biological markers exclusively characterize a certain group of normal or neoplastic cells. It must always be kept in mind that histopathology remains the strong basis for diagnosis and treatment of malignant lymphomas.

After the completion of this manuscript a new consensus classification appeared in the literature under the acronym R.E.A.L. (Revised European American Lymphoma) [352]. This classification is based on the evaluation of the morphological, immunophenotypic and genetic features of the involved cells as well as the clinical presentation of the disease (nodal - extranodal).

According to the group of investigators who presented the REAL classification it contains nothing new except consensus, it can be used together with the Working Formulation and it aims to improve international communication. The REAL Classification is given in Table 6.

Table 6. Comparison of the REAL Classification with the Kiel Classification and the Working Formulation

Revised European American Lymphoma Classification
Precursor B-lymphoblastic lymphoma/leukaemia
B-cell chronic lymphocytic leukaemia/prolymphocytic leukaemia/small lymphocytic lymphoma
Lymphoplasmacytoid lymphoma
Mantle cell lymphoma
Follicular centre lymphoma, follicular
• Grade I
• Grade II
• Grade III
Follicular centre lymphoma, diffuse, small cell (provisional)
Extranodal marginal zone B-cell lymphoma (low-grade B-cell lymphoma of MALT type)
Nodal marginal zone B-cell lymphoma (provisional)
Splenic marginal zone B-cell lymphoma (provisional)
Hairy cell leukaemia
Plasmacytoma/myeloma
Diffuse large B-cell lymphoma
Primary mediastinal large B-cell lymphoma
Burkitt's lymphoma
High grade B-cell lymphoma, Burkitt-like (provisional)
Precursor T-lymphoblastic lymphoma/leukaemia
T-cell chronic lymphocytic leukaemia/prolymphocytic leukaemia
Large granular lymphocytic leukaemia
• T-cell type
• NK-cell type
Mycosis fungoides/Sezary syndrome
Peripheral T-cell lymphomas, unspecified (including provisional subtype: subcutaneous panniculitic T-cell lymphoma)
Hepatosplenic γ–δ T-cell lymphoma (provisional)
Angioimmunoblastic T-cell lymphoma

REFERENCES

1 Goldfarb AN and Litz CE: A novel approach to clonality analysis. Alterations in genomic methylation of Epstein-Barr virus transformed lymphocytes. Pathol Res Pract 1993 (189):312-315

2 Jackila AJ, Lic Y, Lam KW, Yam LT: The cytochemistry of tartrate-resistant acid phosphatase. Technical considerations. Am J Clin Pathol 1978 (70): 45-55

3 Papadimitriou CS and Papacharalampous NX: Distribution of T-lymphocytes in follicular lymphomas as revealed by acid a-naphtol acetate esterase. J Clin Pathol 1979 (32):808-813

4 Leder LD: Ueber die selectieve Ferment cytochemische Darstellung von neutrophile myeloischen Zellen und Gewabsmastzellen im Paraffinschnitt. Klin Wschr 1964 (42):553

5 Bollum FJ: Terminal desoxynucleotidyl transferase as a hematopoetic cell marker. Blood 1979 (54): 1203-1215

6 Andrade RE, Wick MR, Frizzera G, Gazl-Peczalska KJ: Immunophenotyping of hematopoietic malignancies in paraffin sections. Hum Pathol 1988 (89): 488-492

7 Kasai K, Kameya T, Ono M et al: Relationships among expression, transcription and rearrangement of T-cell receptor ß gene in T-cell lymphomas. Virch Arch (A) 1990 (419):57-65

8 Tabrizchi H, Hansmann ML, Parwaresch MR, Lennert K: Distribution pattern of follicular dendritic cells in low grade B-cell lymphomas of the gastrointestinal tract immunostained by Ki-FDC1p: A new paraffin-resistant monoclonal antibody. Modern Pathology 1990 (3):470-478

9 Kamel OW, Gelb AB et al: Leu 7 (CD57) reactivity distinguishes nodular lymphocyte predominance Hodgkin's disease from nodular sclerosing Hodgkin's disease, T-cell lymphoma and follicular lymphoma. Am J Pathol 1993 (142):541-546

10 Krajewsi AS, Myskow MW et al: Diagnosis of T-cell lymphoma using beta F1 and anti-T-cell receptor beta chain antibody. Histopathology 1989 (15):239-247

11 Norton AJ and Isaacson PG: Lymphoma phenotyping in formalin-fixed and paraffin wax-embedded tissues. I. Range of antibodies and staining patterns. Histopathology 1989 (13):437-446

12 Cleary ML, Tela MJ, Weiss LM, Warnke RA, Sklar J: Most null large cell lymphomas are B cell neoplasms. Lab Invest 1985 (53):521-525

13 Chen Y-T, Godwin TA et al: Immunohistochemistry and gene rearrangement studies in the diagnosis of malignant lymphomas: a comparison of 152 cases. Hum Pathol 1991 (22):1249-1257

14 Lardelli Pilar, Swaby RF et al: Determination of lineage and clonality in diffuse lymphomas using the polymerase chain reaction technique. Hum Pathol 1991 (22):685-689

15 Wu AM, Winberg CD et al: Genotype and phenotype: a practical approach to the immunogenetic analysis of lymphoproliferative disorders. Hum Pathol 1990 (21):1132-1141

16 Weiss LM, Picker LJ, Copenhaver CM, Warnke, RA, Sklar J: Large-cell hematolymphoid neoplasms of uncertain lineage. Hum Pathol 1988 (19):967-973

17 Weiss LM, Movahed LA et al: Detection of immunoglobulin light-chain mRNA in lymphoid tissues using a practical in situ hybridization method. Am J Pathol 1990 (137):979-988

18 Anagnostopoulos I, Herbst H, Niedobitek G, Stein H: Demonstration of monoclonal EBV genomes in Hodgkin's disease and Ki-1 positive anaplastic large cell lymphoma by combined Southern blot and in situ hybridization. Blood 1989 (74):810-819

19 Stansfeld AG, Diebold J et al: Updated Kiel classification for lymphomas. Lancet 1988 (1):292-293

20 Hastrup N, Hamilton-Dutoit S et al: Peripheral T-cell lymphomas: an evaluation of reproducibility of the updated Kiel classification. Histopathology 1991 (18):99-105

21 Ersboll J, Schultz HB et al: Comparison of the working formulation of non-Hodgkin's lymphomas with the Rappaport, Kiel and Lukes and Collins classifications. Cancer 1985 (55):2442-2458

22 Stel HV, Vroom Th M et al: Therapy-relevant discrepancies between diagnosis of institutional pathologists and experienced hematopathologists in the diagnosis of malignant lymphoma. Path Res Pract 1989 (184):242-247

23 Chan JKC, Ng CS, Peter G: Relationship between high-grade lymphoma and low-grade B-cell mucosa-associated lymphoid tissue lymphoma (MALToma) of the stomach. Am J Pathol 1990 (136):1153-1164

24 Mielke B and Moller P: Histomorphologic and immunophenotypic spectrum of primary gastro-intestinal B-cell lymphomas. Int J Cancer 1991 (47):334-343

25 Rijlaarsdam JU, Scheffer E et al: Cutaneous pseudo-T-cell lymphomas. A clinicopathologic study of 20 patients. Cancer 1992 (69):717-724

26 Santucci M, Pimpinelli N et al: Primary cutaneous B-cell lymphoma: a unique type of low-grade lymphoma. Clinicopathologic and immunologic study of 83 cases. Cancer 1991 (67):2311-2326

27 Davis RE, Dorfman RF et al: Primary large-cell lymphoma of the thymus: a diffuse B-cell neoplasm presenting as primary mediastinal lymphoma. Hum Pathol 1990 (21):1262-1268

28 Jacobson JO, Aisenberg BC et al: Mediastinal large cell lymphoma, an uncommon subset of adult lymphoma curable with combined modality therapy. Cancer 1988 (62):1898-1899

29 Gorp JV, Weiping L, Jacobse K et al: Epstein-Barr virus in nasal T-cell lymphomas (polymorphic reticulosis/midline malignant reticulosis) in western China. J Pathol 1994 (173):81-87

30 Longo DL, Glatstein E, Duffey PL et al: Treatment of localized aggressive lymphomas with combination chemotherapy followed by involved-field radiation therapy. J Clin Oncol 1989 (7):1295-1302

31 Warnke RA, Strauchen JA, Burke JS, Hoppe RT, Campbell BA, Dorfman RF: Morphologic types of diffuse large-cell lymphoma. Cancer 1982 (50):690-695

32 Perri RT and Kay NE: Large granular lymphocytes from B-chronic lymphocytic leukemia patients inhibit normal B-cell proliferation. Am J Hematol 1989 (31):166-172

33 Batata A and Shen B: Immunophenotyping of subtypes of B-chronic (mature) lymphoid leukemia. A study of 242 cases. Cancer 1992 (70):2436-2443

34 Papadimitriou CS, Muller-Hermelink V, Lennert K: Histologic and immuno-histochemical findings in the differential diagnosis of chronic lymphocytic leukemia of B-cell type and lymphoplasmacytic/lymphoplasmacytoid lymphoma. Virch Arch (A) 1979 (384):149-158

35 Zukerberg L, Medeiros L, Ferry J, Harris NL: Diffuse low grade B-cell lymphomas: identification of four major immunophenotypic subtypes. Lab Invest 1991 (62): 87A (abstract)

36 Pangalis GA, Nathwani BN, Rappaport H: Malignant lymphoma, well differentiated lymphocytic. Its relationship with chronic lymphocytic leukemia and macroglobulinemia of Waldenström. Cancer 1977 (39):999-1010

37 Ellison DJ, Nathwani BN, Cho SY, Martin SE: Interfollicular small lymphocytic lymphoma: the diagnostic significance of pseudofollicles. Hum Pathol 1989 (20):1108-1118

38 Orfao A, Gonzalez M. San Miguel JF et al: B-cell chronic lymphocytic leukemia: Prognostic value of the immunophenotype and the clinico-haematological features. Am J Hematol 1989 (31):26-31

39 Melo JV, Catovsky D, Galton DAG: The relationship between chronic lymphocytic leukemia and prolymphocytic leukemia II. Patterns of evaluation of "prolymphocytoid" transformation. Br J Haematol 1986 (64):77-86

40 Said JW, Barrera R, Shintaku IP, Nakamura H, Koeffler HP: Immuno-histochemical analysis of P53 expression in malignant lymphomas. Am J Pathol 1992 (141):1343-1348

41 Foucar K and Rydell RE: Richter's syndrome in chronic lymphocytic leukemia. Cancer 1980 (46): 118-134

42 Momose H, Jaffe ES, Shin S-S, Chen Y-Y, Weiss LM: Chronic lymphocytic leukemia/small lymphocytic lymphoma with Reed-Sternberg like cells and possible transformation to Hodgkin's disease. Mediation by Epstein-Barr virus. Am J Surg Pathol 1992 (16):859-867

43 Pangalis GA, Roussou PA, Kittas C et al: B chronic lymphocytic leukemia. Prognostic implication of bone marrow histology in 120 patients; experience from a single hematology unit. Cancer 1987 (59): 761-771

44 Brittinger G, Bartels H, Fulle HH et al: Clinical and prognostic relevance of the Kiel classification of non-Hodgkin lymphomas: results of a prospective multicenter study by the Kiel lymphoma study group. Hematol Oncol 1984 (2):269-306

45 Brouet JC, Flandrin G, Sasportes M, Preud'Homme JL, Seligmann M: Chronic lymphocytic leukemia of T-cell origin. Lancet 1975 (2):890-893

46 Raziuddin S, Sheikha A et al: T-cell chronic lymphocytic leukemia. T-cell function and lymphokine secretion. Cancer 1992 (69):1146-1152

47 Naeim F: Hairy cell leukemia. Characteristic of the neoplastic cells. Hum Pathol 1988 (19):375-388

48 Hsu SM, Yang K, Jaffe ES: Hairy cell leukemia: a B-cell neoplasm with a unique antigenic phenotype. Am J Clin Pathol 1983 (80):421-425

49 Anderson KC, Boyd AW, Fisher DC et al: Hairy cell leukemia: a tumor of preplasma cells. Blood 1985 (65):620-623

50 van Krieken JHJM, Vonschilling C, Kluin M, Lennert K: Splenic marginal lymphocytes and related cells in the lymph node: A morphologic and immunohistochemical study. Hum Pathol 1989 (20):320-325

51 Stroup R and Sheibani K: Antigenic phenotypes of hairy cell leukemia and monocytoid B-cell lymphoma: an immunohistochemical evaluation of 66 cases. Hum Pathol 1992 (23):172-177

52 Semenzato G, Basso G, Cartei G et al: Hairy cell leukemia with T-cell features. Br J Haematol 1980 (46):491-493

53 Van der Planken M, Peetermans M: Acid alpha naphtyl acetate esterase and beta-glucuronidase in hairy cell leukemia. Blut 1980 (41):137-140

54 Coasguen S, Le Prise PY, Lablay R et al: Adherence properties of hairy cells. Nouv Rev Fr Hematol 1983 (25):97-101

55 Tolksdorf G and Stein H: Acid alpha-naphtyl acetate esterase in hairy cell leukemia cells and other cells of the hematopoietic system. Blut 1979 (39):165-179

56 Saati T, Caspar S, Brousset P, Chittal S, Caveriviere P: Production of anti-B monoclonal antibodies VDBB.42, DBA.44, DNA.7 and DND.53 reactive on paraffin embedded tissues with a new B-lymphoma cell line grafted into athymic nude mice. Blood 1989 (74):2746-2785

57 Micklem KJ, Dong Y et al: HML-1 antigen on mucosa associated T cells, activated cells, and hairy leukemic cells is a new integrin containing the ß7 subunit. Am J Pathol 1991 (139):1297-1301

58 Rosenblatt JD, Golde DW, Wachsman W et al: A second isolate of HTLV-II associated with atypical hairy-cell leukemia. N Engl J Med 1986 (315):372-377

59 Jacobs RH, Vokes EE, Colomb HM: Second malignancies in hairy cell leukemia. Cancer 1985 (56): 1462-1467

60 Martinsson V, Sundstrom C, Grimelius B: Immunophenotype analysis of B-CLL lymphoma and immunocytoma. AFMIS 1989 (97):1025-1032

61 Pangalis GA, Natwani BN, Rappaport H: Detection of cytoplasmic immunoglobulin in well-differentiated lymphoproliferative diseases by the immunoperoxidase method. Cancer 1980 (45):1334-1339

62 Lennert K, Tamm I, Wacker H-H: Histopathlogy and immunocytochemistry of lymph node biopsies in chronic lymphocytic leukemia and immunocytoma. Leukemia and Lymphoma 1991 (5):157-160

63 Hall PA, D'Ardenne AJ, Richards MA, Stansfeld AG: Lymphoplasmacytoid lymphoma: an immunohistological study. J Pathol 1987 (153):213-223

64 Harris NL and Bhan AK: B-cell neoplasms of the lymphocytic, lympho-plasmacytoid and plasma cell types: immunologic analysis and clinical correlation. Hum Pathol 1985 (16):829-837

65 Kimby E and Mellstedt H: Chlorambucil/prednison versus CHOP in symptomatic chronic lymphocytic leukemia of B-cell type. A randomized trial. Leukemia and Lymphoma 1991 (5):93-96

66 Papadimitriou CS and Schwarze EW: Extramedullary non-gastrointestinal plasmacytoma. An im-

munohistochemical study of 16 cases. Path Res Pract 1983 (176):306-312
67 Shimizu S, Takiguchi T, Fukutoku M et al: Establishment of a CD4-positive plasmacytoma cell line (AMO1). Leukemia 1993 (7):274-280
68 Tamamori T, Nakayama F, Sugimoto H, Fenxiang J, Iwatsuki K, Takigawa M: Extramedullary plasmacytoma: cytological and genotypic studies. Br J Dermatol 1993 (129):468-472
69 Petruch VR, Horny H-P, Kaiserling E: Frequent expression of haemopoietic and non-haemopoietic antigens by neoplastic plasma cells: an immunohistochemical study using formalin-fixed, paraffin-embedded tissue. Histopathology 1992 (20):35-40
70 Holland J, Trenkner DA, Wasserman Th, Fineberg B: Plasmacytoma. Treatment results and conversion to myeloma. Cancer 1992 (69):1513-1517
71 Wiltshaw E: Extramedullary plasmacytoma. Br Med J 1971 (II):319-328
72 Swerdlow SH, Habeshaw JA, Murray LJ, Dhaliwal HS, Lister TA, Stansfeld AG: Centrocytic lymphoma: a distinct clinicopathologic and immunologic entity. A multiparameter study of 18 cases at diagnosis and relapse. Am J Pathol 1983 (113):181-197
73 Weisenburger DD, Nathwani BN, Diamond LW, Winberg CD, Rappaport H: Malignant lymphoma intermediate lymphocytic type: a clinicopathologic study of 42 cases. Cancer 1981 (48):1415-1425
74 Strickler JG, Medeiros LJ, Copenhaver CM et al: Intermediate lymphocytic lymphoma. An immunophenotypic study with comparison to small lymphocytic lymphoma and diffuse small cleaved cell lymphoma. Hum Pathol 1988 (19):550-554
75 Banks PM, Chan J, Cleary ML et al: Mantle cell lymphoma. A proposal for unification of morphologic, immunologic and molecular data. Am J Surg Pathol 1992 (16):637-640
76 Abe M, Ono N, Tominaga K et al: Histogenesis of diffuse small cleaved cell lymphoma. An immunohistochemical and molecular genetic (bcl-2 gene) study with comparison to follicular small cleaved cell lymphoma and mantle zone lymphoma. Cancer 1992 (70):821-829
77 Weisenburger DD, Duggan MJ, Perry DA, Sanger WG, Armitage JO: Non-Hodgkin's lymphomas of mantle zone origin. Pathol Ann 1991 (26):139-158
78 Vandenberghe E, De Wolf-Peeters C, Van den Dord J et al: Translocation (11:14): a cytogenetic anomaly associated with B-cell lymphomas of non-follicle centre cell lineage. J Pathol 1991 (163):13-18
79 Meusers P, Engelhard M, Bartels H et al: Multicentre randomized therapeutic trial for advanced centrocytic lymphoma: Anthracycline does not improve the prognosis. Hematol Oncol 1989 (7): 365-380
80 Rosenberg C, Lwong E, Petty E et al: Overexpression of PRAD1, a candidate BCL1 breakpoint region oncogene, in centrocytic lymphomas. Proc Natl Acad Sci USA 1991 (88):9638-9642
81 Mori N, Oka K, Kojima M: DRC antigen expression in B-cell lymphomas. Am J Clin Pathol 1988 (89): 488-492
82 West KP, Potter LJ, Henderson SD et al: A retrospective study of follicular lymphomas. Histopathology 1989 (14):629-636
83 Chittal SM, Caveriviere P, Voigt JJ et al: Follicular lymphoma with abundant PAS-positive extracellular material. Immunohistochemical and ultra-structural observations. Am J Surg Pathol 1987 (11):618-624
84 Kerrigan DP, Foucar K, Dressler L: High grade non-Hodgkin lymphoma relapsing as a low grade follicular lymphoma: so-called downgraded lymphoma. Am J Hematol 1989 (30):36-41
85 Foucar K, Armitage JO, Dick FR: Malignant lymphoma, diffuse mixed small and large cell. A clinicopathologic study of 47 cases. Cancer 1983 (51): 2090-2099
86 Swerdlow SH, Murray LJ, Habeshaw JA, Stansfeld AG: B- and T-cell subsets in follicular centroblastic centrocytic (cleaved follicular center cell) lymphoma: an immunohistologic analysis of 26 lymph nodes and three spleens. Hum Pathol 1985 (16): 339-352
87 McCurley TL, Gay RE, Gay S et al: The extracellular matrix in "sclerosing" follicular center cell lymphomas. An immunohistochemical and ultrastructural study. Hum Pathol 1986 (17):930-938
88 Harris NL, Nadler LM, Bhan AK: Immunohistologic characterization of two malignant lymphomas of germinal center type (centroblastic/centrocytic and centrocytic) with monoclonal antibodies. Follicular and diffuse lymphomas of small-cleaved cell type are related but distinct entities. Am J Pathol 1984 (117):262-272
89 Pezzella F, Tse AGD, Cordell JL, Pulford KAF, Gatter KC, Mason DY: Expression of the bcl2 oncogene protein is not specific for the 14;18 chromosomal translocation. Am J Pathol 1990 (137):225-232
90 Wotherspoon AC, Pan L, Diss TC, Isaackson PG: A genotypic study of low grade B-cell lymphomas, including lymphomas of mucosa associated lymphoid tissue (MALT). J Pathol 1990 (162):135-140
91 Clark HM, Jones DB et al: Cytogenetic and molecular studies of t(14;18) and t(14;19) in nodal and extranodal B-cell lymphoma. J Pathol 1992 (166): 129-137
92 Pezzella F, Gatter KC, Mason DY, Bastard C, Duval C et al: Bcl 2 protein expression in follicular lymphomas in absence of 14:18 translocation. Lancet 1990 (I):1510-1511
93 Lu Q-L, Poulsom R, Wong L, Hanby AM: Bcl-2 expression in adult and embryonic non-haematopoietic tissues. J Pathol 1993 (169):431-437
94 Frizzera G and Murphy SB: Follicular (nodular) lymphoma in childhood: A rare clinical-pathological entity. Report of eight cases from four cancer centers. Cancer 1979 (44):2218-2235
95 Meuge C, Hoerni B, de Mascarel A et al: Non-Hodgkin malignant lymphomas. Clinicopathologic correlations with the Kiel classification. Retrospective analysis of a series of 274 cases. Eur J Cancer 1978 (14):587-592
96 Molenaar WM, Bartels H, Koudstaal J: Histological, epidemiological and clinical aspects of centroblastic/centrocytic lymphomas subdivided accord-

ing to the "working formulation". Br J Cancer 1984 (49):263-268
97 Garcia CF, Warnke RA, Weiss LM: Follicular large cell lymphoma. An immunophenotype study. Am J Pathol 1986 (123):425-431
98 Cousar JB, McCinn DL, Glick AD, List AF, Collins RD: Report of an unusual lymphoma arising from parafollicular B-lymphocytes or so-called "monocytoid" lymphoyctes. Am J Clin Pathol 1987 (87): 121-128
99 Sheibani K, Burke J, Swartz W, Nademanee A, Winberg C: Monocytoid B-cell lymphoma. Clinicopathologic study of 21 cases of a unique type of low grade lymphoma. Lab Invest 1988 (58):84-88
100 Nathwani BN, Mohrmann RL et al: Monocytoid B-cell lymphomas: an assessment of diagnostic criteria and a perspective on histogenesis. Hum Pathol 1992 (23):1061-1071
101 Plank L, Hansmann M-L, Fischer R: The cytological spectrum of the monocytoid B-cell reaction: recognition of its large cell type. Histopathology 1993 (23):425-431
102 Radzun HJ, Hansmann ML, Heidebrecht HJ et al: Detection of a monocyte/macrophage differentiation antigen in routinely processed paraffin-embedded tissues by monoclonal antibody Ki-M1P. Lab Invest 1991 (65):306-315
103 Cogliatti S, Lennert K, Hansmann M, Zwingers T: Monocytoid B cell lymphoma: clinical and prognostic features of 21 patients. J Clin Pathol 1990 (43):619-625
104 Nizze H, Cogliatti S, von Schilling C, Feller A, Lennert K: Monocytoid B-cell lymphoma: morphological variants and relationship to low-grade B-cell lymphoma of the mucosa-associated lymphoid tissue. Histopathology 1991 (18):403-414
105 Aozasa K, Matsumoto M et al: Monocytoid B-cell lymphoma arising in extranodal organs. Cancer 1991 (67):2305-2310
106 Isaacson P, Spencer J: Monocytoid B-cell lymphomas. Am J Surg Pathol 1990 (14):888-891
107 Spencer J, Finn T, Pulford K, Mason D, Isaacson P: The human gut contains a novel population of B lymphocytes which resemble marginal zone cells. Clin Exp Immunol 1985 (62):607-612
108 Van den Oord JJ, De Wolf-Peeters C, Desmet VJ: The marginal zone of the human reactive lymph node. Am J Clin Pathol 1986 (86):475-479
109 Shin S, Sheibani K, Fishleder A et al: Monocytoid B-cell lymphoma in patients with Sjogren's syndrome: a clinicopathologic study of 13 patients. Hum Pathol 1991 (22):422-430
110 MacLennan I, Liu Y, Oldfield S, Ahang J, Lane P: The evolution of B-cell clones. Curr Top Microbiol Immunol 1990 (159):37-63
111 Liu Y-J, Oldfield S, MacLennan I: Memory B cells in T-cell dependent antibody responses colonise the splenic marginal zones. Eur J Immunol 1988 (18): 355-362
112 Liu Y-J, Johnson G, Gordon J, MacLennan I: Germinal centers in T-cell dependent antibody responses. Immunol Today 1992 (13):1-39
113 Spencer J, Finn T, Pulford KAF, Mason DY, Isaacson PG: The human gut contains a novel population of B-lymphocytes which resembles marginal zone cells. Clin Exp Immunol 1985 (62): 607-612
114 Gallatin W, Weissman I, Butcher E: A cell-surface molecule involved in organ-specific homing of lymphocytes. Nature 1983 (304):30-34
115 Butcher E: Cellular and molecular mechanisms that direct leukocyte traffic. Am J Pathol 1990 (136):3-12
116 Stevens SK, Weissman IL, Butcher EC: Differences in the migration of B and T lymphocytes: Organ selective localization in vivo and the role of lymphocyte-endothelial recognition. J Immunol 1982 (128):844-851
117 Harris NL: Low grade B-cell lymphoma of mucosa-associated lymphoid tissue and monocytoid B-cell lymphoma. Related entities that are distinct from other low-grade B-cell lymphomas. Arch Pathol Lab Med 1993 (117):771-775
118 Fransila KO, Jaser N, Sivula A: Gastrointestinal non-Hodgkin's lymphoma. A population-based clinicopathological study of 111 adult cases with a follow-up of 10-15 years. APMIS 1993 (101):631-641
119 Ngan B-Y, Warnke RA, Wilson M, Takagi K, Cleary M, Dorfman R: Monocytoid B-cell lymphoma: a study of 36 cases. Hum Pathol 1991 (22):409-421
120 Pinkus GS, O'Hara CJ, Said JW: Peripheral post-thymic T-cell lymphoma: A spectrum of disease. Cancer 1990 (65):971-998
121 Kansu E and Hauptman SP: Suppressor cell population in Sezary syndrome. Clin Immunol Immunopathol 1979 (12):341-350
122 Kovary PM, Niedorf H, Sommer G et al: Paraproteinaemia in Sezary syndrome. Dermatologica 1977 (154):138-146
123 Ralfkiaer E, Wantzin GL, Mason DY et al: Phenotypic characterization of lymphocyte subsets in mycosis fungoides. Comparison with large plaque parapsoriasis and benign chronic dermatoses. Am J Clin Pathol 1985 (84):610-619
124 Sterry W: Mycosis fungoides. Curr Top Pathol 1985 (74):167-223
125 Kernohan NM and Smart LM: Anomalous phenotype of cutaneous T-cell infiltrates. J Pathol 1990 (160): 81-82
126 Picker LJ, Weiss LM, Medeiros LJ, Wood GS, Warnke RA: Immunophenotypic criteria for the diagnosis of non-Hodgkin's lymphoma. Am J Pathol 1987 (187):181-191
127 Michie SA, Abel EA, Hoppe RT, Warnke RA, Wood GS: Discordant expression of antigens between intraepidermal and intradermal T-cells in mycosis fungoides. Am J Pathol 1990 (137):1447-1451
128 Matthew MJ: Surgical pathology of mycosis fungoides and Sezary syndrome. In: Jaffe ES (ed) Surgical Pathology of the Lymph Nodes and Related Organs. Major Problems in Pathology, Vol. 16. Saunders, Philadelphia, 1985 pp 329-356
129 Schefter E, Mejer CJLM, Van Vloten WA: Dermatopathic lymphadenopathy and lymph node involvement in mycosis fungoides. Cancer 1980 (45):137-148
130 Weiss LM, Hu E, Wood GS et al: Clonal rearrangements of T-cell receptor genes in mycosis fungoides and dermatopathic lymphadenopathy. N Engl J Med 1985 (313):539-544

131 Helbron D, Brittinger G, Nennert K: T-zonen Lymphom. Klinishes Bild, Therapie und Prognose. Blut 1979 (39):117-131

132 Nakamura S and Suchi T: A clinicopathologic study of node-base, low-grade, peripheral T-cell lymphoma. Angioimmunoblastic lymphoma, T-zone lymphoma and lymphoepithelioid lymphoma. Cancer 1991 (67):2565-2578

133 Patsouris E, Noel H et al: Histological and immunohistological findings in lymphoepithelioid cell lymphoma (Lennert's Lymphoma). Am J Surg Pathol 1988 (12):341-350

134 Spier CM, Lippman SM, Miller TP, Crogan TM: Lennert's lymphoma. A clinicopathologic study with emphasis on phenotype and its relationship to survival. Cancer 1988 (61):517-524

135 Feller AC, Griesser GH, Mak TW, Lennert K: Lymphoepithelioid lymphoma (Lennert's lymphoma) is a monoclonal proliferation of helper/inducer T-cells. Blood 1986 (68):663-667

136 O'Connor NTJ, Feller AC, Wainscoat JS et al: T-cell origin of Lennert's lymphoma. Br J Haematol 1986 (64):521-528

137 Noel H, Helbron D, Lennert K: Epithelioid cellular lymphogranulomatosis (lymphoepithelioid cell lymphoma). Histologic and clinical observations. In: Van den Tweel JG (ed) Malignant Lymphoproliferative Diseases. Leiden University Press, The Hague 1980 pp 433-445

138 Patsouris E, Noel H, Lennert K: Lymphoplasmacytic/lymphoplasmacytoid immunocytoma with a high content of epithelial cells. Histologic and immunohistochemical findings. Am J Surg Pathol 1990 (14):660-670

139 Palutke M, Tabaczka P, Weise RW et al: T-cell lymphomas of large cell type. A variety of malignant lymphomas "histiocytic" and mixed lymphocytic "histiocytic". Cancer 1980 (46):87-101

140 Spier CM, Lippman et al: Lennert's lymphoma. A clinicopathologic study with emphasis on phenotype and its relationship to survival. Cancer 1988 (61):517-524

141 Succhi T, Lennert K, Tu LY et al: Histopathology and immunohistochemistry of peripheral T-cell lymphomas: a proposal for their classification. J Clin Pathol 1987 (40):995-1015

142 Lukes RJ and Tindle BH: Immunoblastic lymphadenopathy. A hyperimmune entity resembling Hodgkin's disease. N Engl J Med 1975 (292):1-8

143 Frizzera G, Moran EM, Rappaport H: Angioimmunoblastic lymphadenopathy. Diagnosis and clinical course. Am J Med 1975 (59):803-818

144 Knecht H: Angioimmunoblastic lymphadenopathy: ten years experience and state of current knowledge. Semin Haematol 1989 (26):208-215

145 Patsouris E, Noel H, Lennert K: Angioimmunoblastic lymphadenopathy-type of T-cell lymphoma with a high content of epithelioid cells. Histopathology and comparison with lymphoepithelioid cell lymphoma. Am J Surg Pathol 1989 (13): 262-275

146 Shimoyama M, Tobinai K, Minato K, Watanabe S: Immunoblastic lymphadenopathy (IBL)-like T-cell lymphoma. Recent Results Cancer Res 1987 (23): 161-170

147 Schlegelberger B, Feller AC, Godde-Salz E, Grote W, Lennert K: Stepwise development of chromosomal abnormalities in angioimmunoblastic lymphadenopathy. Cancer Genet Cytogenet 1990 (50):15-29

148 Godde-Salz E, Feller AC, Lennert K: Chromosomal abnormalities in lymphogranulomatosis X (LgrX)/ angioimmunoblastic lymphadenopathy (AILD). Leuk Res 1987 (11):181-190

149 Feller AC, Griesser H, Von Schilling C, Walker HH, Dallenbach F et al. Clonal gene rearrangement patterns correlate with immunophenotype and clinical parameters in patients with angioimmunoblastic lymphadenopathy. Am J Pathol 1988 (133): 549-557

150 Weiss LM, Strickler JG, Dorfman RF et al: Clonal T-cell populations in angioimmunoblastic lymphadenopathy and angioimmunoblastic-like lymphoma. Am J Pathol 1986 (122):392-398

151 Takagi N, Nakamura S et al: A phenotypic and genotypic study of three node-based, low-grade peripheral T-cell lymphomas: angioimmunoblastic lymphoma, T-zone lymphoma and lymphoepithelioid lymphoma. Cancer 1992 (69):2571-2582

152 Leung CY, Ho FCS, Strivastava G, Loke SL, Liu YT, Chan ACL: Usefulness of follicular dendritic cell pattern in classification of peripheral T-cell lymphomas. Histopathology 1993 (23):433-437

153 Siegert W, Nerl C, Meuthen I et al: Recombinant human interferon-alpha in the treatment of angioimmunoblastic lymphadenopathy. Results in 12 patients. Leukemia 1991 (5):892-895

154 Pangalis GA, Moran EM, Nathwani BN, Zelman RJ, Kim H, Rappaport H: Angioimmunoblastic lymphadenopathy. Long-term follow-up study. Cancer 1983 (52):318-321

155 Lennert K, Knecht H, Burkert M: Vorstadien maligner Lymphome. Verh Dtsch Ges Pathol 1979 (63): 170-196

156 Krueger GRF, Bergholz M, Bartsch HH, Fischer R, Schauer A: Rubella virus antigen in lymphocytes of patients with angioimmunoblastic lymphadenopathy. J Cancer Res Clin Oncol 1979 (95):87-91

157 Dumont J, Thiery JP, Mazabraud A: Adenopathies angio-immuno-blastiques: étude ultrastructurale des ganglions. Discussion sur le role eventuel du virus d'Epstein-Barr (EBV). Nouv Rev Fr Hematol 1979 (21):257-282

158 Shamoto M and Suchi T: Intracytoplasmic type A virus-like particles in angioimmunoblastic lymphadenopathy. Cancer 1979 (44):1641-1643

159 Winberg CD, Krance R, Scheibani K, Rappaport H: Peripheral T-cell lymphoma. Cancer 1986 (57): 2329-2342

160 Hui PK, Feller AC, Lennert K: High-grade non-Hodgkin's lymphoma of B-cell type. Histopathology 1988 (12):127-143

161 Pinkus GS, Said JW, Hargreaves HK: Malignant lymphoma, T-cell type: A distinct morphologic variant with large multilobated nuclei: Report of four cases. Am J Clin Pathol 1979 (72):540-550

162 Weinberg DA and Pinkus GS: Non-Hodgkin's lymphomas of large multilobated cell type. A clinicopathologic study of ten cases. Am J Clin Pathol 1981 (76):190-196

163 Baroni CD, Pascarmona E, Calogero A et al: B- and T-cell non-Hodgkin's lymphomas with large multilobated cells: morphological, phenotypic and clinical heterogeneity. Histopathology 1987 (11): 1121-1132
164 Chan JKC, Ng CS, Tung S: Multilobated B-cell lymphoma, a variant of centroblastic lymphoma. Report of four cases. Histopathology 1986 (10): 601-612
165 Weiss RL, Ashwood ER, Kjeldsberg CR: Multilobated B-cell lymphoma. Arch Pathol Lab Med 1990 (114):28-33
166 Strauchen JA, Young RC, DeVita VT Jr, Anderson T, Fantone JC, Berard CW: Clinical relevance of the histopathological subclassification of diffuse "histiocytic" lymphoma. N Engl J Med 1978 (299): 1382-1387
167 Del Vecchio MT, Leoncini L et al: Diffuse centrocytic and/or centroblastic malignant non-Hodgkin's lymphomas: a comparison of mitotic and pyknotic (apoptotic) indices. Int J Cancer 1991 (47):38-43
168 Azar HA, Jaffe ES, Berard CW et al: Diffuse large cell lymphoma. Correlation of morphologic features with functional markers. Cancer 1980 (46):1428-1441
169 Ng CS, Chan JKC, Hui PK et al: Large B-cell lymphomas with a high content of reactive T-cells. Hum Pathol 1989 (20):1145-1154
170 Schneider DR, Taylor CR, Parker JW et al: Immunoblastic sarcoma of T- and B-cell types. Morphologic description and comparison. Hum Pathol 1985 (16):885-900
171 Penny RJ, Blaustein JC et al: Ki-1 positive large cell lymphomas, a heterogenous group of neoplasms. Morphologic, immunophenotypic, genotypic and clinical features of 24 cases. Cancer 1991 (68):326-373
172 Pangalis GA, Nathwani BN, Rappaport H, Rosen RB: Acute lymphoblastic leukemia. The significance of nuclear convolutions. Cancer 1979 (43): 551-557
173 Cossman J, Chused TM, Fisher RI et al: Diversity of immunological phenotypes of lymphoblastic lymphoma. Cancer 1983 (43):4486-4490
174 Brownell MD, Sheibani K, Battifora H et al: Distinction between undifferentiated (small non-cleaved) and lymphoblastic lymphoma. An immunohistologic study on paraffin-embedded, fixed tissue sections. Am J Surg Pathol 1987 (11):779-787
175 de Villartay J-P, Pullman A, Andrade R et al: γ/δ lineage relationship within a consecutive series of human precursor T-cell neoplasms. Blood 1989 (74): 2508-2518
176 Lukes RJ and Collins RD: A functional approach to the classification of malignant lymphoma. Recent Results Cancer Res 1974 (46):18-30
177 Mc Caffrey R, Harrison TA, Parkman R, Baltimore D: Terminal deoxynucleotidyl transferase activity in human leukemic cells and in normal human thymocytes. N Engl J Med 1975 (292):775-780
178 Braziel R, Keneklis T, Donlon JA et al: Terminal deoxynucleotidyl transferase in non-Hodgkin's lymphoma. Am J Clin Pathol 1983 (80):655-659
179 Korsmeyer SJ, Hieter PA, Ravetch JV, Poplack DG, Waldmann TA, Leder P: Developmental hierarchy of immunoglobulin gene rearrangements in human leukemic pre-B-cells. Proc Natl Acad Sci USA 1981 (78):7096-7100
180 Knowles DM: Phenotypic markers and gene rearrangement analysis in T-T-cell neoplasia. Am J Surg Pathol 1988 (12):160-163
181 Feller AC, Parwaresch MR, Stein H, Ziegler A, Herbst H, Lennert K: Immunophenotyping of T-lymphoblastic lymphoma/leukemia: correlation with normal T-cell maturation. Leuk Res 1986 (10):1025-1031
182 Pittaluga S, Raffeld M, Lipford EH, Cossman J: 3A1 (CD7) precedes Tß gene rearrangements in precursor T (lymphoblastic) neoplasma. Blood 1986 (68): 134-139
183 Kitchingman GR, Rovigatti U, Mauer AM, Melvin S, Murphy SB, Stass S: Rearrangement of immunoglobulin heavy chain genes in T-cell acute lymphoblastic leukemia. Blood 1985 (65):725-729
184 Weiss LM, Bindl JM, Picozzi VJ, Link MP, Warnke RA: Lymphoblastic lymphoma: an immunophenotype study of 26 cases with comparison to T-cell acute lymphoblastic leukemia. Blood 1986 (67): 474-478
185 Haluska FG, Finger LR, Kagan J, Croce CM: Molecular genetics of chromosomal translocations in B- and T-lymphoid malignancies. In: Cossman J (ed) Molecular Genetics in Cancer Diagnosis. Elsevier, New York 1990 pp 154-158
186 Fletcher JA, Lynch EA, Kimball VM, Donnelly M, Tantravahi R, Sallan SE: Translocation (9;22) is associated with extremely poor prognosis in intensively treated children with acute lymphoblastic leukemia. Blood 1991 (77):435-439
187 Thirman MJ, Gill HJ, Burnett RC et al: Rearrangement of the MLL gene in acute lymphoblastic and acute myeloid leukemias with 11q23 chromosomal translocations. N Engl J Med 1993 (329): 909-914
188 Burkitt D. A sarcoma involving the jaws in African children. Br J Surg 1958 (46):218-223
189 Lukes RJ and Collins RD: New approaches to the classification of the lymphomata. Br J Cancer 1975 (31):1-28
190 Fellous M, Cartron J-P, Wiels J, Tursz T: A monoclonal antibody against a Burkitt lymphoma associated antigen has an anti-PK red blood cell specificity. Br J Haematol 1985 (60):559-565
191 Mann RB, Jaffe ES, Braylan RC et al: Non-endemic Burkitt's lymphoma. A B-cell tumor related to germinal centers. N Engl J Med 1976 (295):685-691
192 Pallesen G: Burkitt's lymphoma: diagnostic and taxonomic aspects. In: Molander D (ed) Diseases of the Lymphatic System. Springer Verlag, Berlin 1983 pp 89-102
193 Wilson JF, Kjeldsberg CR, Sposto R et al: The pathology of non-Hodgkin's lymphoma of childhood. II. Reproducibility and relevance of the histologic classification of "undifferentiated" lymphomas (Burkitt's versus non-Burkitt's). Hum Pathol 1987 (18): 1008-1014
194 Miliauskas JR, Berard CW, Young RC, Garvin AJ, Edwards BK, De Vita VT: Undifferentiated non-Hodgkin's lymphomas (Burkitt's and non Burkitt's

types). The relevance of making this distinction. Cancer 1982 (50):2115-2121
195 Grogan TM, Warnke RA, Kaplan HS: A comparative study of Burkitt's and non-Burkitts's "undifferentiated" malignant lymphoma: immunologic, cytochemical, ultrastructural, cytologic, histopathologic, clinical and cell culture features. Cancer 1982 (49):1817-1828
196 Rowe M, Rooney CM, Rickinson AB et al: Distinctions between endemic and sporadic forms of Epstein-Barr virus-positive Burkitt's lymphoma. Int J Cancer 1985 (35):435-441
197 Kelly DR, Nathwani BN, Griffith RC et al: A morphologic study of childhood lymphoma of the undifferentiated type. The Pediatric Oncology Group experience. Cancer 1987 (59):1132-1137
198 Egerter DA and Beckstead JH: Malignant lymphomas in the acquired immunodeficiency syndrome. Additional evidence for a B-cell origin. Arch Pathol Lab Med 1988 (112):602-606
199 Weiss LM, Strickler JG, Medeiros LJ, Gerdes J, Stein H, Warnke RA: Non-Hodgkin's lymphomas: proliferative rate as assessed by Ki-67 antibody. Hum Pathol 1987 (18):1155-1159
200 Garcia CF, Weiss LM, Warnke RA: Small noncleaved cell lymphoma: an immunophenotypic study of 18 cases and comparison with large cell lymphoma. Hum Pathol 1986 (17):454-461
201 Wright DH: Gross distribution and haematology. In: Burkitt DP and Wright DH (eds) Burkitt's Lymphoma. Livingstone, Edinburgh 1970 pp 64-81
202 Banks PM, Arseneau JC, Gralnick HR, Canellos GP, DeVita VT Jr, Berard CW: American Burkitt's lymphoma: a clinicopathologic study of 30 cases. II. Pathologic correlations. Am J Med 1975 (58): 322-329
203 Ziegler JL: Burkitt's Lymphoma. N Engl J Med 1981 (305):735-745
204 Ziegler JL, Andersson M, Klein G, Henle W: Detection of Epstein-Barr virus DNA in American Burkitt's lymphomas. Int J Cancer 1976 (17):701-706
205 Klein G: Viral latency and transformation. The strategy of Epstein-Barr virus. Cell 1989 (58):5-8
206 Pallesen G, Hamilton-Dutoit SJ, Rowe M, Young LS: Expression of Epstein-Barr virus latent gene products in tumour cells of Hodgkin's disease. Lancet 1991 (337):320-322
207 Leder P, Battey J, Lenoir G et al: Translocations among antibody genes in human cancer. Science 1983 (222):765-771
208 Pelicci P-G, Knowles DM, Magrath IT, Dalla-Favera R: Chromosomal breakpoints and structural alterations of the c-myc locus differ in endemic and sporadic forms of Burkitt lymphoma. Proc Natl Acad Sci USA 1986 (83):2984-2988
209 Neri A, Barriga F, Knowles DM, Magrath IT, Dalla-Favera R: Different regions of the immunoglobulin heavy-chain locus are involved in chromosomal translocations in distinct pathogenetic forms of Burkitt lymphoma. Proc Natl Acad Sci USA 1988 (85):2748-2752
210 Van Krieken JHJM, Raffeld M, Raghoebier S, Jaffe ES, Van Ommen GJB, Kluin PhM: Molecular genetics of gastrointestinal non-Hodgkin's lymphomas: unusual prevalence and pattern of c-myc rearrangements in aggressive lymphomas. Blood 1990 (76):797-800
211 Payne CM, Grogan TM, Cromey DW, Bjore JR CG, Kerrigan DP: An ultrastructural morphometric and immunophenotypic evaluation of Burkitt's and Burkitt's like lymphomas. Lab Invest 1987 (57): 200-218
212 Stansfeld AG, Diebold J, Kapanci Y, Kelenyi G, Lennert K et al: Updated Kiel classification for lymphomas. Lancet 1988 (I):292-293
213 Su JJ, Wang CH, Cheng AL et al: Characterization of the spectrum of postthymic T-cell malignancies in Taiwan. A clinicopathologic study of HTLV-1 positive and HTLV-1 negative cases. Cancer 1986 (61):2060-2070
214 Gallo RC and Wong-Staal F: Retroviruses as etiologic agents of some animal and human leukemias and lymphomas and as tools for elucidating the molecular mechanism of leukemogenesis. Blood 1982 (60):545-557
215 Uchiyama T, Yodoi J, Sagqawa K, Takatsuki K, Uchino H: Adult T-cell leukemia: clinical and hematologic features of 16 cases. Blood 1977 (50): 481-492
216 Takatsuki K, Ychiyama T, Sagqawa K, Yodoi J: Adult T-cell leukemia in Japan. Excerpta Medica International Congress Service 1976 (415):73-74
217 Swerdlow SH, Habeshaw JA, Rohatiner AZS, Lister TA, Stansfeld AG: Caribbean T-cell lymphoma/ leukemia. Cancer 1984 (54):687-696
218 Jaffe ES, Blattner WA, Blayney DW et al: The pathologic spectrum of adult T-cell leukemia/ lymphoma in the United States. Am J Surg Pathol 1984 (8):263-275
219 Blayney DW, Jaffe ES, Blattner WA et al: The human T cell leukemia/lymphoma virus associated with American adult T cell leukemia/lymphoma. Blood 1983 (62):401-405
220 Catovsky D, Greaves MF, Rose M et al: Adult T-cell lymphoma-leukemia in blacks from West Indies. Lancet 1982 (1):6643
221 Hinuma Y, Nagata K, Hanaoka M et al: Adult T-cell leukemia antigen in ATL cell line and detection of antibodies to the antigen in human sera. Proc Natl Acad Sci USA 1981 (78):6476-6480
222 Tajima K and Kuroishi T: Estimation of rate of incidence of ATL among ATLV (HTLV-I) carriers in Kyushu, Japan. Jpn J Clin Oncol 1985 (15):423-430
223 Kikuchi M, Mitsui T, Matsui N et al: T-cell malignancies in adults: histopathological studies of lymph nodes in 110 patients. Jpn J Clin Oncol 1979 (9 suppl):407-422
224 Lennert K, Kikuchi M, Sato E et al: HTLV-positive and negative T-cell lymphomas. Morphological and immunohistochemical differences between European and HTLV-positive Japanese T-cell lymphomas. Int J Cancer 1985 (35):65-72
225 Griesser H, Tkachuk D, Reis MD, Mak TW: Gene rearrangements and translocations in lymphoproliferative diseases. Blood 1989 (73):1402-1415
226 Van Krieken JHJM, Andrade RE, Jaffe ES, Cossman J, Medeiros LJ: Rearrangement of the T-cell receptor delta chain gene in T-cell lymphomas

with a mature phenotype. Am J Pathol 1991 (139): 161-168
227 Isobe M, Sadamori N, Russo G et al: Rearrangements in the human T-cell receptor α-chain locus in patients with adult T-cell leukemia carrying translocations involving chromosome 14q11. Cancer Res 1990 (50):6171-6175
228 Suchi T, Lennert K, Tu LY et al: Histopathology and immunohistochemistry of peripheral T-cell lymphomas: a proposal for their classification. J Clin Pathol 1987 (40):995-1015
229 Stein H, Mason DY, Gerdes J et al: The expression of the Hodgkin's disease associated antigen Ki-1 in reactive and neoplastic lymphoid tissue: evidence that Reed-Sternberg cells and histiocytic malignancies are derived from activated lymphoid cells. Blood 1985 (66):848-858
230 Bitter MA, Franklin WA, Larsen RA et al: Morphology in Ki-1(CD30) positive non-Hodgkin's lymphoma is correlated with clinical features and the presence of a unique chromosomal abnormality, t(2;5) (p23:q35). Am J Surg Pathol 1990 (14):305-316
231 Chan JKC, Ng CS, Hui PK et al: Anaplastic large cell Ki-1 lymphoma. Delineation of two morphological types. Histopathology 1989 (15):11-34
232 Beljaards RC, Meijer CJLM, Sheffer E et al: Prognostic significance of CD30 (Ki-1/BerH2) expression in primary cutaneous large-cell lymphomas of T-cell origin. Am J Pathol 1989 (135):1169-1178
233 Chott A, Kaserer K, Augustin I et al: Ki-1-positive large cell lymphoma. A clinicopathologic study of 41 cases. Am J Pathol 1990 (114):439-448
234 Byrne E Jr and Rappaport H: Malignant histiocytosis. In: Akazaki K, Rappaport H, Berard CW, Bennett JM, Ishikawa E (eds) Malignant Diseases of the Hematopoietic System (Gann No. 15). University of Tokyo Press, Tokyo 1973 pp 145-162
235 Kadin ME: Primary Ki-1 positive anaplastic large cell lymphoma. A distinct clinicopathologic entity. Ann Oncol 1994 (5 suppl 1):25-30
236 Feller AC and Griesser H: DNA gene rearrangement studies in Hodgkin's disease and related lymphomas. A contribution to their cellular origin. Recent Results Cancer Res 1989 (117):27-34
237 Gustmann C, Altmannsberger M, Osborn M, Griesser H, Feller AC: Cytokeratin expression and vimentin content in large cell anaplastic lymphomas and other non-Hodgkin's lymphomas. Am J Pathol 1991 (138):1413-1422
238 Pallesen G and Hamilton-Dutoid SJ: Ki-1 (CD30) antigen is regularly expressed by tumor cells on embryonal carcinoma. Am J Pathol 1988 (33):446
239 Mason DY, Bastard C, Rimokh R et al: CD30-positive large cell lymphomas (Ki-1 lymphoma) are associated with a chromosomal translocation involving 5q35. Br J Haematol 1990 (74):161-168
240 Sainati L, Montaldi A, Stella M, Putti MC, Zanesco L, Basso G: A novel variant translocation t(2;13) (p23;q34) in Ki-1 large cell anaplastic lymphoma. Br J Haematol 1990 (75):621-622
241 Piris M, Brown DC, Gatter KC, Mason DY: CD30 expression in non-Hodgkin's lymphoma. Histopathology 1990 (17):211-218
242 Nakamura S, Takagi N, Kojima M et al: Clinicopathologic study of large cell anaplastic lymphoma (Ki-1 positive large cell lymphoma) among the Japanese. Cancer 1991 (68):118-129
243 Merz H, Houssiau FA, Orscheschek K et al: Interleukin-9 expression in human malignant lymphomas: Unique association with Hodgkin's disease and large cell anaplastic lymphoma. Blood 1991 (78):1311-1317
244 Myhre MJ and Isaacson PG: Primary B-cell gastric lymphoma. A reassessment of its histogenesis. J Pathol 1987 (152):1-11
245 Spencer J, Diss T, Isaacson P: A study of the properties of a low grade mucosal B-cell lymphoma using a monoclonal antibody specific for the tumor immunoglobulin. J Pathol 1990 (160):231-238
246 Piris M, Rivas C, Morente M, Cruz M, Rubio C, Oliva H: Monocytoid B-cell lymphoma, a tumour related to the marginal zone. Histopathology 1988 (12):383-392
247 Isaacson PG, Wright DH, Judd MA, Mephan BL: Primary gastrointestinal lymphomas: a classification of 66 cases. Cancer 1979 (44):1805-1819
248 Moller P, Eichelmann A et al: Expression of ß-1-integrins, H-CAM (CD44) and LECAM-1 in primary gastro-intestinal B-cell lymphomas as compared to the adhesion receptor profile of the gut-associated lymphoid system, tonsil and peripheral lymph node. Int J Cancer 1991 (49):846-855
249 Harris NL: Extranodal lymphomas and mucosa-associated lymphoid tissue (MALT): a unifying concept. Am J Surg Pathol 1991 (15):879-884
250 Isaacson PG, Androulakis-Papachristrou A, Diss TC, Pan L, Wright DH: Follicular colonization in thyroid lymphoma. Am J Pathol 1992 (41):43-52
251 Li G, Hansmann M, Zwingers T, Lennert K: Primary lymphomas of the lung: morphological, immunohistochemical and clinical features. Histopathology 1990 (16):519-531
252 Medeiros L and Harris NL: Lymphoid infiltrates of the orbit and conjunctiva: a morphologic and immunophenotypic study of 99 cases. Am J Surg Pathol 1989 (13):459-471
253 Zukerberg L, Ferry J, Southern J, Harris NL: Lymphoid infiltrates of the stomach: evaluation of histologic criteria for the diagnosis of low-grade gastric lymphoma on endoscopic biopsy specimens. Am J Surg Pathol 1990 (14):1087-1099
254 Hujek E, Smith WJ, Isaacson PG: Primary B-cell lymphoma of salivary gland and its relationship to myeloepithelial sialadenitis (MESA). Hum Pathol 1988 (19):766-769
255 Hujek E and Isaacson PG: Primary B cell lymphoma of the thyroid and its relationship to Hashimoto's thyroiditis. Hum Pathol 1988 (19):1315-1326
256 Li G, Hansmann M-L et al: Primary lymphomas of the lung: morphological, immunohistochemical and clinical features. Histopahtology 1990 (16):519-531
257 Wotherspoon AC, Diss TC, Pan LX et al: Primary low grade B-cell lymphoma of the conjuctiva: a mucosa-associated lymphoid tissue type lymphoma. Histopathology 1993 (23):414-427
258 Isaacson PR, Chan JKC, Tankg C, Addis BJ: Low-grade B-cell lymphoma of mucosa-associated lymphoid tissue arising in the thymus. A thymic lymphoma mimicking myoepithelial sialadenitis. Am J Surg Pathol 1990 (14):342-351

259 Wotherspoon AC, Doglioni C et al: Low-grade gastric-cell lymphoma of mucosa-associated lymphoid tissue (MALT): a multifocal disease. Histopathology 1992 (20):29-34
260 Arista-Nasr J, Jimenez A et al: The role of the endoscopic biopsy in the diagnosis of gastric lymphoma: a morphologic and immunohistochemical reappraisal. Hum Pathol 1991 (22):339-348
261 Fellbaum C, Strater J, Hansmann M-L: Follicular dendritic cells in extranodal non-Hodgkin lymphomas of MALT and non-MALT type. Virch Arch (A) 1993 (423):335-341
262 Bateman AC and Wright DH: Epitheliotropism in high-grade lymphomas of mucosa-associated lymphoid tissue. Histopathology 1993 (23):409-415
263 Zukerberg L, Ferry J, Southern J, Harris NL: Lymphoid infiltrates of the stomach: evaluation of histologic criteria for the diagnosis of low-grade gastric lymphoma on endoscopic biopsy specimens. Am J Surg Pathol 1990 (14):1087-1099
264 Mattia A, Ferry J, Harris NL: Breast lymphomas: a B-cell spectrum including the low grade B-cell lymphoma of mucosa-associated lymphoid tissue (MALT). Am J Surg Pathol 1993 (17):574-587
265 Ferry J, White W, Grove A, Harris NL: Malignant lymphoma of ocular adnexa. A spectrum of B-cell neoplasia including low grade B-cell lymphomas of MALT type. Lab Invest 1992 (66):77a (abstract)
266 Wotherspoon AC, Ortiz-Hidalgo C, Falzon MR, Isaacson PG: Helicobacter pylori-associated gastritis and primary B-cell gastric lymphoma. Lancet 1991 (338):1175-1176
267 Kim H, Dorfman RF, Rappaport H: Signet ring cell lymphoma. A rare morphologic and functional expression of nodular (follicular) lymphoma. Am J Surg Pathol 1978 (2):119-132
268 Weiss LM, Wood GS, Dorfman RF: T-cell signet-ring cell lymphoma: A histologic, ultrastructural and immunohistochemical study of two cases. Am J Surg Pathol 1985 (9):273-280
269 Stroup RM, Sheibani K, Moncada A, Purdy LJ, Battifora H: Angiotropic (intravascular) large cell lymphoma. A clinicopathologic study of seven cases with unique clinical presentations. Cancer 1990 (66):1781-1788
270 Wick MR, Mills SE, Schneithauer BW et al: Reassessment of malignant "angioendotheliomatosis". Evidence in favour of its reclassification as "intravascular lymphomatosis". Am J Surg Pathol 1986 (10):112-123
271 Abe S, Kumanishi T, Yoshida Y et al: Neoplastic angioendotheliosis: Demonstration of immunoglobulin gene rearrangements by the Southern blot hybridization technique. Virchows Arch B 1990 (58):241-244
272 Sepp N, Schuler G, Romani N et al: "Intravascular lymphomatosis" (angioendotheliomatosis): evidence for a T-cell origin in two cases. Hum Pathol 1990 (21):1051-1058
273 Katzenstein AA, Carrington CB, Liebow AA: Lymphomatoid granulomatosis: a clinicopathologic study of 152 cases. Cancer 1979 (43):360-373
274 DeRemee RA, Weiland LH, McDonald TJ: Polymorphic reticulosis, lymphomatoid granulomatosis: two diseases or one? Mayo Clinic Proceedings 1978 (53):634-640
275 Lipford EH, Margolick JB, Longo DL, Fauci AS, Jaffe ES: Angiocentric immunoproliferative lesions: a clinicopathologic spectrum of post-thymic T-cell proliferations. Blood 1988 (72):1674-1681
276 Medeiros LJ, Peiper SC et al: Angiocentric immunoproliferative lesions: a molecular analysis of eight cases. Hum Pathol 1991 (22):1150-1157
277 Donner LR, Robin S, Carrington D et al: Angiocentric immunoproliferative lesion (lymphoid granulomatosis). A cytogenetic, immunophenotypic and genotypic study. Cancer 1990 (65):249-254
278 Menestrina F, Chilosi M, Bonetti F et al: Mediastinal large-cell lymphoma of B-type with sclerosis: histopathological and immuno-histochemical study of eight cases. Histopathology 1986 (10):589-600
279 Moller P, Moldenhauer G, Momburg F et al: Mediastinal lymphoma of clear cell type is a tumor corresponding to terminal steps of B-cell differentiation. Blood 1987 (69):1087-1095
280 Perrone T, Frizzera G, Rosai J: Mediastinal diffuse large-cell lymphoma with sclerosis. A clinicopathologic study of 60 cases. Am J Surg Pathol 1986 (10):176-191
281 Addis BJ and Isaacson PG: Large cell lymphoma of the mediastium: a B-cell tumour of probable thymic origin. Histopathology 1986 (10):379-390
282 Bernier V and Azar HA: Filiform large cell lymphomas. An ultrastructural and immunohistochemical study. Am J Surg Pathol 1987 (11):387-396
283 Kinney MC, Click AD, Stein H, Collins RD: Comparison of anaplastic large-cell Ki-1 lymphomas and microvillous lymphomas in their immunologic and ultrastructural features. Am J Surg Pathol 1990 (14):1047-1060
284 Melo JV, Hedge V, Parreira A, Tompson T, Lampert TA, Catovsky D: Splenic B-cell lymphoma with circulating villous lymphocytes. Differential diagnosis of B-cell leukemias with large spleens. J Clin Pathol 1987 (40):642-651
285 Catovsky D and Foa R: The Lymphoid Leukaemias. Butterworth, London 1990
286 Neiman RS, Sullivan AL, Jaffe R: Malignant lymphoma simulating leukemic reticuloendotheliosis: a clinico-pathologic study of ten cases. Cancer 1979 (43):329-342
287 Oscier D, Matutes E, Gardiner A et al: Cytogenetic studies in splenic lymphoma with villous lymphocytes. Blood 1991 (78 suppl):113a
288 Brito-Babapulle V, Ellis J, Matutes E et al: Chromosome translocation t(11;14) (q13;q32) in chronic lymphoid disorders. Genes, Chromosomes and Cancer 1992 (5):158-165
289 Gossman J, Schnitzer B, Deegan MJ: Coexistence of two lymphomas with distinctive histologic, ultrastructural and immunologic features. Am J Clin Pathol 1978 (70):409-415
290 Hansmann ML, Fellbaum C et al: Morphological and immunohistochemical investigation of non-Hodgkin's lymphoma combined with Hodgkin's disease. Histopathology 1989 (15):35-48
291 Simrell CR, Balia KV, Long DL, Jaffe ES: Coexisting Hodgkin's disease and mycosis fungoides. Arch Pathol Lab Med 1986 (110):1029-1034

292 Slovak ML, Weiss LM, Natwani BN, Bernstein L, Levine AM: Cytogenetic studies of composite lymphomas: monocytoid B-cell lymphoma and other B-cell non-Hodgkin's lymphomas. Hum Pathol 1993 (24):1086-1094
293 Isaacson PG, O'Connor NTJ, Spencer J et al: Malignant histiocytosis of the intestine: a T-cell lymphoma. Lancet 1985 (11):688-691
294 Papadimitriou CS, Papacharalambous NX, Kittas C: Primary gastrointestinal malignant lymphomas. A morphologic and immunohistochemical study. Cancer 1985 (55):870-879
295 Salter DM, Krajewski AS, Dewar AE: Immunophenotype analysis of malignant histiocytosis of the intestine. J Clin Pathol 1986 (39):8-15
296 Guy-Grand D, Krajewski AS, Isaacson PG: Enteropathy-associated T cell lymphoma (malignant histiocytosis of the intestine) is recognized by a monoclonal antibody (HML-1) that defines a membrane molecule of human mucosal lymphocytes. Am J Pathol 1988 (132):1-5
297 Alfsen GC, Beiske K, Bell H, Marton PF: Low-grade intestinal lymphoma of intraepithelial T lymphocytes with concomitant enteropathy-associated T cell lymphoma: Case report suggesting a possible histogenetic relationship. Hum Pathol 1989 (20): 909-913
298 Spencer J, Certt-Benussam N, Jarry A et al: Enteropathy-associated T-cell lymphoma (malignant histiocytosis of the intestine) is recognized by a monoclonal antibody (HML-1) that defines a membrane molecule on human mucosal lymphocytes. Am J Pathol 1988 (132):1-5
299 Scheffer RW, Van Vloten WA, Meijer CJL: Lymphomatoid papulosis and Hodgkin's disease: are they related? Arch Dermatol Res 1988 (275):159-167
300 Kadin M, Nasu K, Said J, Vorderheid E: Lymphomatoid papulosis. A cutaneous proliferation of activated helper T-cells expressing Hodgkin's disease-associated antigens. Am J Pathol 1985 (119):315-325
301 Weiss LM, Wood GS, Treka MJ, Warnke RA, Sklar J: Clonal T cell populations in lymphomatoid papulosis: evidence for a lymphoproliferative origin for a clinically benign disease. N Engl J Med 1986 (315):475-479
302 Kadin ME, Vonderheid EC, Sako D, Clayton LK, Olbricht S: Clonal composition of T-cells in lymphomatoid papulosis. Am J Pathol 1987 (126):13-17
303 Kadin ME: Lymphomatoid papulosis and Ki1+ large cell lymphomas of the skin: pathology, immunology, natural history and relevance to Hodgkin's disease. In: Hanaoka M, Kadin ME, Mikata A, Watanabe S (eds) Lymphoid Malignancy: Immunocytology and Cytogenetics. Field and Wood, Philadelphia 1990 pp 189-195
304 Cattoretti G, Villa A et al: Malignant histiocytosis. A phenotypic and genotypic investigation. Am J Pathol 1990 (136):1005-1019
305 Carbone A, Gloghini A, Volpe R, Pinto A: KP1 (CD68)-positive large cell lymphomas: A histopathologic and immunophenotypic characterization of 12 cases. Hum Pathol 1993 (24):886-896
306 Macon WR, Williams ME et al: T-cell rich B-cell lymphomas. A clinicopathologic study of 19 cases. Am J Surg Pathol 1992 (16):351-363
307 Ng CS, Chan JKC et al: Large B-cell lymphomas with a high content of reactive T-cells. Hum Pathol 1989 (20):1145-1154
308 Miettinen M, Franssila KO, Saxen E: Hodgkin's disease lymphocytic predominance nodular-increased risk for subsequent non-Hogkin's lymphomas. Cancer 1983 (54):2293-2300
309 Sundeen JT, Cossman J, Jaffe ES: Lymphocyte predominant Hodgkin's disease nodular subtype with coexistent "large cell lymphoma". Histological progression or composite malignancy? Am J Surg Pathol 1988 (12):599-606
310 Papadimitriou CS and Bai MK: Primary non-Hodgkin's lymphomas of the nasal and mouth cavity and the Waldeyer's ring. A morphological and immunohistochemical study. Leukemia and Lymphoma 1991 (3):395-400
311 Ye Y-L, Zhou M-H et al: Nasopharyngeal and nasal malignant lymphoma: a clinicopathological study of 54 cases. Histopathology 1992 (20):511-516
312 Ferry JA, Sklar J, Zucerberg LR et al: Nasal lymphoma: A clinicopathologic study with immunophenotypic and genotypic analysis. Am J Surg Pathol 1991 (5):268-279
313 Kanavaros P, Lescs M-C, Briere J et al: Nasal T-cell lymphoma. A clinicopathologic entity associated with peculiar phenotype and with Epstein-Barr Virus. Blood 1993 (7):2689-2695
314 Pileri S, Falini B, Delsol G et al: Lymphohistiocytic T-cell lymphoma (anaplastic large cell lymphoma CD30+/Ki1+ with a high content of reactive histiocytes). Histopathology 1990 (16):383-391
315 Katzin WE, Linden MD et al: Immunophenotypic and genotypic characterization of diffuse mixed non-Hodgkin's lymphomas. Am J Pathol 1989 (135):615-621
316 Chittal SM, Caveriviere P, Schwarting R et al: Monoclonal antibodies in the diagnosis of Hodgkin's disease. The search for a rational panel. Am J Surg Pathol 1988 (12):9-21
317 Weiss LM, Strickler JG, Hu E, Warnke RA, Sklar J: Immunoglobulin gene rearrangements in Hodgkin's disease. Hum Pathol 1986 (17):1009-1014
318 Herbst H, Tippelman G, Anagnostopoulos I et al: Immunoglobulin and T-cell receptor gene rearrangements in Hodgkin's disease and Ki-1 positive anaplastic large cell lymphoma. Dissociation between phenotype and genotypes. Leuk Res 1989 (13): 103-116
319 Tesch H, May P et al: Analysis of immunoglobulin, T-cell receptor and bcr rearrangements in human malignant lymphoma and Hodgkin's disease. Oncology 1990 (47):215-223
320 Ross CW, Hanson CA et al: CD30 (Ki-1) positive anaplastic large cell lymphoma mimicking gastrointestinal carcinoma. Cancer 1992 (70):2517-2523
321 Chilosi M, Castelli P et al: Neoplastic epithelial cells in a subset of human thymomas express the B-cell-associated CD20 antigen. Am J Surg Pathol 1992 (16):988-997
322 Doglioni CD, Dell' Ort P et al: Cytokeratin-immunoreactive cells of human lymph nodes and spleen in

normal and pathological conditions. An immunohistochemical study. Virch Arch (A) 1990 (416): 479-490
323 Wotherspoon AC, Norton AJ et al: Immunoreactive cytokeratins in plasmacytomas. Histopathology 1989 (14):141-150
324 Kneba M, Bolz I et al: Clinical characteristics of high-grade lymphomas with immune genes in germline configuration. Cancer 1991 (67):603-609
325 Knowles DM, Jakobiec FA et al: Lymphoid hyperplasia and malignant lymphoma occurring in the ocular adnexa (orbit, conjuctiva, and eyelids): a prospective multiparametric analysis of 108 cases during 1977 to 1987. Hum Pathol 1990 (21):959-973
326 Osborne BM and Pugh WC: Practicality of molecular studies to evaluate small lymphocytic proliferations in endoscopic gastric biopsies. Am J Surg Pathol 1992 (16):838-844
327 Rubin A and Isaacson PG: Florid reactive lymphoid hyperplasia of the terminal ileum in adults: a condition bearing a close resemblance to low-grade malignant lymphoma. Histopathology 1991 (17):19-26
328 Shiota M, Kitamura K et al: Immunoglobulin idiotype expression in reactive lymphoid tissus and B-cell lymphomas. Virchows Archiv (A) 1992 (420):263-267
329 Scoazec JY, Brousse N, Potet F, Jeulain JF: Focal malignant lymphoma in gastric pseudolymphoma. Histologic and immunohistochemical study of a case. Cancer 1986 (57):1330-1336
330 Schmid V, Helbron D, Lennert K: Development of malignant lymphoma in myoepithelial sialadenitis (Sjogren's syndrome). Virchows Arch (A) 1982 (395):11-43
331 Addis BJ, Hujek E, Isaacson PG: Primary pulmonary lymphoma. A reappraisal of its histogenesis and its relationship to pseudolymphoma and interstitial pneumonia. Histopathology 1988 (13):1-17
332 Ohsaka A, Saito K et al: Clinicopathologic and therapeutic aspects of angioimmunoblastic lymphadenopathy-related lesions. Cancer 1992 (69): 1259-1267
333 Kruger GRF, Manak M et al: Persistent active herpes virus infection associated with atypical polyclonal lymphoproliferation (APL) and malignant lymphoma. Anticancer Res 1989 (9):1457-1476
334 Houmand A, Abrahamsen B et al: Relevance of Ki-67 expression in the classification of non-Hodgkin's lymphomas: a morphometric and double-immunostaining study. Histopathology 1992 (20): 13-20
335 Klemi PJ, Alanen K et al: Proliferating cell nuclear antigen (PCNA) as a prognostic factor in non-Hodgkin's lymphoma . Br J Cancer 1992 (66):739-743
336 Cattoretti G, Pileri S, Parravicini C et al: Antigen unmasking on formatin-fixed, paraffin-embedded tissue sections. J Pathol 1993 (171):83-98
337 McKee PH, Hobbs C, Hall PA: Antigen retrieval by microwave irradiation lowers immunohistological detection thresholds. Histopathology 1993 (23): 377-379
338 Fellbaum C, Radaszkiewicz T et al: C-myc mRNA expression in non-Hodgkin's lymphomas. Virch Arch (B) 1992 (62):61-68
339 Kittas C, Korkolopoulou P, Pangalis G, Tsenga A, Boussiotis VA, Spandidos DA: Expression of c-myc P62 oncoprotein in non-Hodgkin's lymphomas. Leukemia and Lymphoma 1990 (1):241-247
340 Reed SL, Kitada S, Takayama S, Miyashita T: Regulation of chemoresistance by the bcl2 oncoprotein in non-Hodgkin's lymphoma and lymphocytic leukemia cell lines. Ann Oncol 1994 (5 suppl):61-65
341 Swerdlow SH, Saboorian MH, Pelstring R, Williams ME: Centrocytic lymphoma: A morphometric study with comparison to other small cleaved follicular center cell lymphomas and gentoypic correlates. Am J Pathol 1993 (142):329-337
342 Swerdlow SH, Pelstring RJ et al: Morphometric analysis of follicular center cell lymphomas. Am J Pathol 1990 (137):953-963
343 Deverell M and Salisbury J: Nuclear morphometry of primary B cell thyroid lymphoma. Path Res Pract 1992 (188):500-503
344 Crocker J, MacCartney JC, Smith PJ: Correlation between DNA flow cytometric and nucleolar organizer region data in non-Hodgkin's lymphomas. J Pathol 1988 (154):151-156
345 Macon WR: Cytokine expression in malignant lymphomas. A complicated puzzle with many pieces to assemble (Editorial). Hum Pathol 1993 (24): 1039
346 Hsu S-M, Xie S-S, Waldron JA: Functional heterogeneity and pathogenic significance of interleukin-6 in B-cell lymphomas. Am J Pathol 1992 (141):915-923
347 Bennett WT, Pandolfi F et al: Dominant rearrangements among human tumor-infiltrating lymphocytes. Analysis of T-cells derived from 32 patients with melanoma, lung and renal cell carcinoma. Cancer 1992 (69): 2379-2384
348 Yoshimo I, Yano T et al: Oligoclonal T lymphocytes infiltrating human lung cancer tissues. Int J Cancer 1991 (47):654-658
349 Lorenzen J, Hansmann M-L et al: Expression of the bcl-2 oncogene product and chromosomal translocation t(14;18) in Hodgkin's disease. Hum Pathol 1992 (23):1205-1209
350 Ott MM, Muller-Hermelink HK et al: Chromosomal translocation detected by bcl-1 and bcl-2 rearrangement in low-grade B-cell lymphomas in a European population. Histopathology 1991 (19): 163-167
351 Ohshima K, Kikuchi M et al: Amplified bcl-2/JH rearrangements in reactive lymphadenopathy. Virch Arch (B) 1993 (63):197-199
352 Harris NL, Jagge ES, Stein H et al: A revised European-American classification of lymphoid neoplasms: a proposal from the International Lymphoma Study Group. Blood 1994 (84):1361-1392

Molecular Genetics and Oncogenes in Malignant Lymphomas

Paola Francia di Celle, Anna Carbone, Alessandro Cignetti, Gigliola Reato and Robin Foà

Dipartimento di Scienze Biomediche ed Oncologia Umana, Sezione Clinica, and Centro CNR "Immunogenetica ed Oncologia Sperimentale", University of Torino, via Genova 3, 10126 Torino, Italy

The application of molecular technologies to the study of lymphoid cells has led to the characterization of several molecular events which are associated with the normal differentiation pathway (i.e., immunoglobulin (Ig) and T-cell receptor (TCR) chain gene rearrangements), and to the identification of genes that may be activated during the process of malignant lymphoid transformation (i.e., oncogenes and tumour suppressor genes). Ig and TCR studies may help in the definition of clonality and lineage affiliation, as well as in the detection of minimal residual disease. Oncogene deregulation promotes cell growth and/or rescues the tumour population from programmed cell death. Tumour suppressor gene inactivation contributes to the abnormal growth typical of neoplastic cells. These molecular lesions are characteristically associated with a defined type of lymphoid leukaemia or lymphoma and represent useful tumour markers for early diagnosis, for monitoring the course of the disease or for the detection of the transformation of lymphoid neoplasms. In this review, we will summarize the most important results obtained with the utilization of DNA analysis in the study of malignant lymphoid leukaemias and lymphomas. In addition to the important clinico-diagnostic implications, we will underline the contribution of these studies to our understanding of the biological mechanisms of lymphomagenesis.

Gene Rearrangement Studies

Physiological rearrangements of the subunits of the Ig and TCR genes are early events which occur during the process of B and T lymphoid development, respectively [1,2]. The molecular juxtaposition (i.e., rearrangement) of gene segments that in the germ-line configuration are separated, results in the assembly of mature genes encoding a vast repertoire of Ig and TCR molecules responsible for antigen recognition. There is an orderly sequence of molecular events which occurs during the maturation of lymphoid cells. In B lymphocytes, the first rearrangement involves the Ig heavy (H) chain gene locus; next, there is an attempt to induce a light (L) chain gene rearrangement (κ and/or λ) [1]. In T lymphocytes, TCR δ and γ gene rearrangements precede that of TCR β, while TCR α is the last gene to rearrange [3].
The phenotypic and genotypic features of the various stages of lymphoid maturation are well represented by lymphoid leukaemias and lymphomas, which consist of clonally expanded lymphocytic populations [4,5]. Genotypic analyses at the Ig and TCR loci level may offer a valuable diagnostic tool and, in combination with morphological and immunocytochemical analysis, help in the classification of lymphoid neoplasms [4,5].
Southern blot analysis has been extensively performed in order to evaluate the Ig and/or TCR gene configurations in a large number and a high variety of cases. This modality of analysis has allowed the definition of the lineage and of the maturation level of acute and chronic lymphoproliferative disorders [4,5]. Ig and TCR gene rearrangements occur in B and T-cell neoplasms, respectively [6,7]. The differentiation level of the B-cell lymphoproliferative disorders is defined by the rearrangement of the IgL chain genes which occurs in the more ma-

ture forms [8]. T-cell malignancies of immature phenotype may present a rearrangement of the TCR δ gene as a unique lineage marker, while the TCR δ, γ and β genes are clonally rearranged in T-cell chronic lymphoid malignancies and in T-cell lymphomas [9,10]. The detection of inappropriate or cross-lineage (TCR δ and γ) rearrangements in a large proportion of B-cell leukaemias expressing an immature phenotype (i.e., common and "null" acute lymphoblastic leukaemias) has somewhat restricted the utilization of TCR analyses for lineage definition purposes [11]. Cross-lineage rearrangements very rarely emerge during Ig and TCR analysis of chronic B and T-cell neoplasms [5]. Nowadays, the genotypic definition of the different forms of lymphoproliferative disorders has been completed and associated with the immunological and cytochemical features for a better diagnostic classification. Some lymphoid neoplasms, for which the cellular origin cannot be unequivocally established by immunophenotyping, still benefit from a molecular-based lineage definition; this is, for example, the case for disorders in which the neoplastic cells apparently co-express different phenotypic markers [12]. Ig and TCR gene analyses offer other important diagnostic applications in given lymphoid conditions, for example 1) definition of clonality in the absence of other restriction markers (i.e., T-cell neoplasms), or when the distinction between the polyclonal or clonal nature of lymphoid cell proliferation may help to define the neoplastic or reactive origin of the disorder (e.g. large granular lymphocyte expansions of T-cell origin [13,14]); 2) the identification of molecular markers on the basis of the Ig or TCR rearrangement patterns which are characteristic of each B or T-cell clone. This approach may be useful in monitoring the disease during its clinical course (disappearance of the malignant clone [15,16], genotypic pattern variation [17,18], or emergence of new clones [19]); 3) the recognition of low numbers of clonal cells, useful for the long-term monitoring of minimal residual disease (MRD) [17]; 4) the definition of the Ig and TCR variable region repertoire, which may indicate a preferential region usage in lymphoid neoplasms, possibly associated with the mechanism of lymphomagenesis [20]. The main diagnostic applications of Ig and TCR gene analyses in leukaemias and lymphomas are summarized in Table 1.

Table 1. Usefulness of Ig and TCR gene rearrangement analysis in lymphoid malignancies

1) Definition of lineage and clonality:
   - Ig gene analysis in B-cell neoplasms
   - TCR gene analysis in T-cell neoplasms
   - Ig and TCR analyses in cases with unclear phenotypes
2) Definition of the level of maturation:
   - IgL chain gene rearrangement in B-cell neoplasms
   - TCR δ rearrangement or deletion in T-cell neoplasms
3) Distinction between polyclonal and monoclonal nature of lymphoproliferative disorders
4) Definition of molecular markers, specific for each patient, useful in monitoring the evolution of the disease
5) Recognition of very small numbers of clonal cells (MRD, early diagnosis and early relapse)

Recently, the sensitivity level of Southern blot analysis has been surpassed by the polymerase chain reaction (PCR) technique [21]. This approach has been proposed for a better and highly sensitive definition of the persistence of the clonal disease (i.e., MRD) [22], and for a rapid and simple diagnostic definition of clonal disorders (PCR screening prior to Southern blot analysis) [23]. The PCR amplification of Ig and TCR gene rearranged regions still requires some refinement in order to distinguish tumoral cells from surrounding normal lymphoid cells. Further studies will be necessary prior to the introduction of routine PCR determination of lymphoid gene rearrangements for diagnostic purposes.

Oncogenes in Human Lymphomas

Chromosome translocations have been associated with many types of human leukaemias and lymphomas, and genes located in these recurring breakpoints are involved in tumour pathogenesis [5,24]. These transforming genes are called oncogenes and their normal expression is important in regulating cell development and growth [25]. Some oncogenes encode growth factors or growth factor receptors. The proteins encoded by the oncogenes may also be intracellular signal transducers (e.g. RAS-related oncogenes) or nucleoproteins, important in regulating cellular gene expression (e.g. c-*myc*). Cellular oncogenes can be activated by insertional mutagenesis, point mutations, translocations, deletions or amplifications.

The identification of these specific molecular alterations in lymphoid neoplasms (predominantly in non-Hodgkin's lymphoma (NHL) of B-cell lineage) has important clinico-pathological implications: first of all, they represent genetic markers specific for the malignant clone and useful both for diagnosis and for monitoring of MRD (the PCR approach is the best technical choice for these purposes) [26]; secondly, they offer an approach to a better understanding of the complex mechanisms of lymphomagenesis [25].

The most common oncogene activation which occurs in B-NHL is the non-random chromosomal translocation of oncogenes to a transcriptionally active site [25]. This alteration may result in an increased expression and in changes in the stability of the corresponding mRNA and protein. Translocations involving the Ig loci on chromosome 2 (Igκ), 14 (IgH) and 22 (Igλ) and the c-*myc* oncogene on chromosome 8 are typical of Burkitt's leukaemias and lymphomas (BL) [27]. The precise breakpoint on chromosome 8 may be within the first exon or intron immediately 5' to the c-*myc* locus or at a considerable distance 5' to the gene; the molecular heterogeneity of the c-*myc* translocation reflects the geographic origin of the tumour (i.e., sporadic vs endemic BL) [28]. Due to the chromosomal translocation, c-*myc* comes under the influence of regulatory elements of the Ig genes, and this leads to an increased expression of the gene and to proliferation of the cells. The c-*myc* product has DNA binding properties and plays a role in the control of cell proliferation and differentiation [25]. *In vitro* transformation of human B cells may be induced by an abnormal c-*myc* expression, and an activated c-*myc* has been demonstrated to cause B-cell lymphoma in transgenic animals [29]. C-*myc* alone is probably insufficient to induce the lymphoma: in the endemic and in the AIDS-associated forms, the Epstein Barr virus (EBV) has been implicated as a cofactor [30].

A second non-random translocation associated with lymphoid tumours is the t(14;18), present in virtually all cases of low-grade follicular B-NHL and in some diffuse forms of intermediate grade [31]. This translocation directly involves the IgH locus and the *bcl*-2 gene on chromosomes 14 and 18, respectively; it results in high levels of expression of an apparently normal *bcl*-2 protein [25]. The 26 kDa product of the *bcl*-2 gene has been reported to be localized in the inner mitochondrial membrane [32]; its oncogenic role has been documented in transgenic mice bearing the *bcl*-2-Ig fusion gene which develop polyclonal lymphoid hyperplasia of small resting B cells [33]. The *bcl*-2 gene has recently been implicated as a component of the molecular processes that decide whether a cell lives or dies [32]. A deregulated *bcl*-2 expression confers a survival advantage of myeloid and lymphoid cells following growth factor deprivation, and interferes with programmed cell death (apoptosis). Although *bcl*-2 alone is insufficient to cause oncogenic transformation, the surviving cells bearing the t(14;18) translocation persist and could provide the substrate for further genetic changes to conventional oncogenes. It has recently been shown that c-*myc* is a potent inducer of apoptosis and that this effect can be reversed by *bcl*-2 overexpression. These findings suggest a complementary role for *bcl*-2 and c-*myc* in controlling cell survival and in inducing a transformed phenotype [34].

A large proportion (50%) of small lymphocytic mantle zone B-NHLs characteristically carry the t(11;14) translocation which juxtaposes the *bcl*-1 oncogene and the IgH locus from chromosomes 11 and 14, respectively [35]. The *bcl*-1 gene is a member of the cyclin gene family which encodes for proteins implicated in cell cycle progression [36]. This finding suggests that *bcl*-1 overexpression, which occurs after the translocation, plays a key role in the pathogenesis of this group of lymphomas, possibly leading to an abnormal cell proliferation.

Finally, B-NHLs show a high incidence of chromosomal translocations involving the 3q27 band [37]. This molecular alteration frequently occurs in diffuse large cells of intermediate-grade B-NHL (DLC-NHL) [37]. The junction region of a t(3;14)(q27;q32) translocation has been cloned from an NHL case and a new oncogene has been identified [38]. This gene has been called *bcl*-6 and encodes for a protein with homology with zinc-finger transcription factors (i.e., genes participating in the control of cell proliferation, differentiation and organ pattern formation). Thirty-three percent of DLC-

Table 2. Oncogene rearrangements in human B-NHL

Translocation	Oncogene	2nd gene	Pathology
t (8;14)	c-*myc*	IgH	Burkitt
t (2;8)	c-*myc*	Igκ	Burkitt
t (8;22)	c-*myc*	Igλ	Burkitt
t (14;18)	*bcl*-2	IgH	Follicular
t (11;14)	*bcl*-1	IgH	Mantle zone
t (3;...)*	*bcl*-6	.....*	Diffuse large cell

* Several different chromosome partners have been identified in B-cell neoplasms

NHL cases show a monoallelic rearrangement of *bcl*-6, while the other NHL subtypes maintain a germ-line configuration [38]. The identification of a specific molecular alteration in highly aggressive forms of NHL bears important diagnostic and pathogenetic implications.

The most frequent oncogene rearrangements which occur in B-NHL are reported in Table 2.

Tumour Suppressor Genes

A second class of oncogenes, known as "tumour suppressor genes", whose normal cellular functions seem to be related to growth or cell cycle control, has been identified [39]. These genes appear to be constitutively expressed in differentiated tissues and the loss of their normal function is associated with tumour development [39]. The general model for suppressor genes is the inactivation of both normal autosomal alleles: while the first inactivation event may occur with no apparent phenotypic consequences at the cellular level, the second mutation represents an important step towards cellular transformation to a malignant phenotype (the mutant allele is recessive to the normal allele) [39].

The first tumour suppressor gene to be identified has been the retinoblastoma (RB) gene: mutations of the RB gene have been found in a variety of tumour types in addition to retinoblastoma, including carcinomas of the bladder, breast and prostate, small cell carcinoma of the lung, osteosarcoma and various soft tissue sarcomas [40]. Cytogenetic findings and loss of heterozygosity analyses have suggested a possible association of RB gene inactivation and lymphoid neoplasms [41]. Southern blot analyses have detected deletions at the RB locus level only in a minority of B and T-cell lymphomas, while *in situ* hybridization has revealed RB inactivation in 30% of B-cell chronic lymphocytic leukaemias (B-CLL) [42]. RB mutations appear to be prevalent in high-grade neoplasms, suggesting a role of RB gene alterations during the progression of the disease.

Another gene involved in the negative regulation of cell growth, named *p53*, has been identified on chromosome 17 [39]. Several types of human tumours may display the monoallelic loss of the *p53* locus (colon, breast, lung, brain malignancies) and normal *p53* can reverse the malignant phenotype of tumour cells *in vitro* [39]. With regard to lymphoid leukaemias and lymphomas, the best correlation between *p53* inactivation and tumour development has been found in BL and B-CLL (particularly in the more malignant Richter's transformation form) [43]. More recently, single-strand conformational polymorphism analysis of the *p53* locus has revealed the appearance of a mutated pattern in 4 of 5 B-NHLs displaying histological transformation from the follicular (carrying wild-type alleles) to the diffuse type [44]. These findings may have relevant clinical implications and *p53* mutations may be a useful marker for the early detection of malignant lymphomatous transformation.

AIDS-Related Lymphomas

BL and other B-NHLs represent frequent clinical manifestations of AIDS [45]. The majority (70%) of reported cases are high-grade lymphomas (small non-cleaved cell and large cell immunoblastic-plasmacytoid forms) and the remaining 30% are intermediate-grade lymphomas of the large non-cleaved cell type [45]. Multiple monoclonal B-cell expansions have been detected in lymph nodes from patients with lymphadenopathy syndrome (benign follicular hyperplasia), which may predispose to the development of B-NHL [46]. Cytogenetic and molecular studies of AIDS-associated NHL have shown that, despite the different prognostic features, they exhibit the same spectrum of alterations previously described (e.g. t(8;14) and variants in BL) [47]. In addition, approximately 30-40% of these tumours contain the EBV genome and an aetiopathogenetic role of EBV infection in malignant clonal B-cell expansions has been suggested [45]. A lymphomagenetic model has been proposed in which EBV infection and immunosuppression may favour the expansion of immortalised B cells and increase the target-cell population where the occurrence of an additional genetic alteration (i.e., c-*myc* translocation) could lead to malignant transformation [46]. In the majority of cases of AIDS-related B-NHL, EBV infection precedes the clonal expansion (monomorphic EBV-fused termini), suggesting a contributory role to the process of clonal expansion in these malignancies [48]. EBV sequences are, however, absent in a significant proportion of AIDS-NHL cases and in these cases a different pathogenetic mechanism is probably involved [48].

Recently, the role of several oncogenes and tumour suppressor genes relevant to B-cell lymphomagenesis has been investigated in a large series of AIDS-related B-NHLs. *C-myc* translocation and *p53* mutations are the most frequent molecular lesions occurring in the small non-cleaved cell lymphoma subtype, and in 80% and 40%, respectively, of the total series of AIDS-NHL analysed [49]. RB gene inactivation does not seem to be involved in this group of neoplasms. These data indicate that AIDS-NHL may be characterized by the accumulation of multiple distinct genetic lesions (c-*myc* activation and *p53* mutation) that may differ in the various histological subtypes, suggesting that alternative molecular pathways may be associated with AIDS lymphomagenesis.

Conclusions

The analysis of the Ig and TCR chain gene configuration and the identification of molecular lesions involving oncogenes and tumour suppressor genes has enabled the clinical utilization of sensitive and specific early diagnostic procedures, and has opened the way to monitoring the clinical course of human leukaemias and lymphomas. Indeed, the heterogeneous molecular features make it possible to distinguish different lymphoid neoplastic forms which are phenotypically identical, and to recognize forms that have a poor prognosis. Multiple molecular lesions have been associated in the same neoplastic clone, suggesting that tumour development is sustained by additional mechanisms. It is likely that in the near future the extended use of molecular technologies will allow an increasingly refined characterization of lymphoid neoplasms both at diagnosis and at relapse, as well as a better understanding of the complex and as yet unknown mechanisms of lymphomagenesis.

Acknowledgements

This work was supported by the Consiglio Nazionale delle Ricerche (CNR) Finalized Project "Applicazioni Cliniche della Ricerca Oncologica" and by the Ministero dell'Università e della Ricerca Scientifica, Roma, Italy. Paola Francia di Celle and Gigliola Reato received a fellowship from the Comitato "G. Ghirotti" (Torino), Anna Carbone from the Istituto Superiore di Sanità (Roma) and Alessandro Cignetti from the Associazione Italiana per la Ricerca sul Cancro (AIRC, Milano).

REFERENCES

1 Alt FW, Blackwell TK, Yancopoulos GD: Development of the primary antibody repertoire. Science 1987 (38):1079-1087

2 Davis MM and Bjorkman PJ: T-cell antigen receptor genes and T-cell recognition. Nature 1988 (334): 395-402

3 Havran WL and Allison JP: Developmentally ordered appearance of thymocytes expressing different T-cell antigen receptors. Nature 1988 (335):443-445

4 Waldmann TA: The arrangement of immunoglobulin and T-cell receptor genes in human lymphoproliferative disorders. In: Dixon FJ (ed) Advances in Immunology. Academic Press, San Diego 1987 pp 247-321

5 Griesser H, Tkachuk D, Reis MD, Mak TW: Gene rearrangements and translocations in lymphoproliferative diseases. Blood 1989 (73):1402-1415

6 Arnold A, Cossman J, Bakhshi A, Jaffe ES, Waldmann TA, Korsmeyer SJ: Immunoglobulin-gene rearrangements as unique clonal markers in human lymphoid neoplasms. N Engl J Med 1983 (309): 1593-1599

7 Waldmann TA, Davis MM, Bongiovanni KF, Korsmeyer SJ: Rearrangements of genes for the antigen receptor on T cells as markers of lineage and clonality in human lymphoid neoplasms. N Engl J Med 1985 (313):776-783

8 Korsmeyer SJ, Hieter PA, Ravetch JV, Poplack DG, Waldmann TA, Leder P: Developmental hierarchy of immunoglobulin gene rearrangements in human leukemic pre-B-cells. Proc Natl Acad Sci USA 1981 (78):7096-7100

9 Foroni L, Foldi J, Matutes E, Catovsky D, O'Connor NJ, Baer R, Forster A, Rabbitts TH, Luzzatto L: α, β and γ T-cell receptor genes: rearrangements correlate with haematological phenotype in T cell leukaemias. Br J Haematol 1987 (67):307-318

10 Foroni L, Laffan M, Boehm T, Rabbitts TH, Catovsky D, Luzzatto L: Rearrangement of the T-cell receptor δ genes in human T-cell leukemias. Blood 1989 (73):559-566

11 Biondi A, Francia di Celle P, Rossi V, Casorati G, Matullo G, Giudici G, Foa R, Migone N: High prevalence of T-cell receptor Vδ2-(D)-Dδ3 or Dδ 1/2-Dδ3 rearrangements in B-precursor acute lymphoblastic leukemias. Blood 1990 (75):1834-1840

12 Callea V, Morabito F, Lista P et al: Multilineage cell involvement in Ph1-negative, bcr-negative chronic myeloid leukemia. Leuk Res 1988 (12):637-645

13 Foa R, Pelicci PG, Migone N, Lauria F, Pizzolo G, Flug F, Knowles II DM, Dalla-Favera R: Analysis of T-cell receptor beta chain (Tβ) gene rearrangements demonstrates the monoclonal nature of T-cell chronic lymphoproliferative disorders. Blood 1986 (67):247-250

14 Francia di Celle P, Migone N, Carbone A et al: Polyclonal nature of some granular T-cell expansions (CD3+, CD8+) based on the configuration of the T-cell receptor β and γ chain gene regions. J Immunol Res 1990 (2):144-150

15 Zehnbauer BA, Pardoll DM, Burke PJ, Graham ML, Vogelstein B: Immunoglobulin gene rearrangements in remission bone marrow specimens from patients with acute lymphoblastic leukemia. Blood 1986 (67):835-838

16 Brugiatelli M, Callea V, Morabito F et al: Immunological and molecular evaluation of residual disease in B-cell chronic lymphocytic leukemia patients in clinical remission phase. Cancer 1989 (63):1979-1984

17 Wright JJ, Poplack DG, Bakhshi A et al: Gene rearrangements as markers of clonal variation and minimal residual disease in acute lymphoblastic leukemia. J Clin Oncol 1987 (5):735-741

18 Ciolli S, Leoni F, Caporale A et al: Mixed acute leukemia with genotypic lineage switch: a case report. Leukemia 1993 (7):1061-1065

19 Kerim S, Geuna M, Francia di Celle P et al: Heterogeneous immunoglobulin gene rearrangements in a B-chronic lymphocytic leukemia progressing into non-Hodgkin lymphoma (Richter syndrome). Cancer 1993 (71):359-363

20 Kipps TJ, Tomhave E, Pratt LF, Duffy S, Chen PP, Carson DA: Developmentally restricted immunoglobulin heavy chain variable region gene expressed at high frequency in chronic lymphocytic leukemia. Proc Natl Acad Sci USA 1989 (86):5913-5917

21 Saiki RK, Gelfand DH, Stoffel S et al: Primer-directed enzymatic amplification of DNA with a thermostable DNA polymerase. Science 1988 (239): 487-494

22 Negrin RS and Blume KG: The use of the polymerase chain reaction for the detection of minimal residual malignant disease. Blood 1991 (78):255-258

23 Deane M and Norton JD: Detection of immunoglobulin gene rearrangement in B cell neoplasias by polymerase chain reaction gene amplification. Leukemia and Lymphoma 1991 (5):9-22

24 Leder P, Battey J, Lenoir G et al: Translocations among antibody genes in human cancer. Science 1983 (222):765-771

25 Sawyers CL, Denny CT, Witte ON: Leukemia and the disruption of normal hematopoiesis. Cell 1991 (64): 337-350

26 Lee M, Chang K, Cabanillas F, Freireich EJ, Trujillo JM, Stass SA: Detection of minimal residual cells carrying the t(14;18) by DNA sequence amplification. Science 1987 (237):175-178

27 Dalla-Favera R, Bregni M, Erickson J, Patterson D, Gallo RC, Croce CM: Human c-myc oncogene is located on the region of chromosome 8 that is translocated in Burkitt lymphoma cells. Proc Natl Acad Sci USA 1982 (79):7824-7827

28 Pelicci PG, Knowles DK, Magrath I, Dalla-Favera R: Chromosomal breakpoints and structural alterations of the c-myc locus differ in endemic and sporadic forms of Burkitt lymphoma. Proc Natl Acad Sci USA 1986 (83):2984-2988

29 Adams JM, Harris AW, Pinkert CA et al: The c-myc oncogene driven by immunoglobulin enhancers induces lymphoid malignancy in transgenic mice. Nature 1985 (318): 533-538

30 Lombardi L, Newcomb EW, Dalla-Favera R: Pathogenesis of Burkitt lymphoma: expression of an activated c-myc oncogene causes the tumori-

genic conversion of EBV-infected human B lymphoblasts. Cell 1987 (49):161-170
31 Tsujimoto Y, Cossman J, Croce CM: Involvement of the bcl-2 gene in human follicular lymphoma. Science 1985 (228):1440-1443
32 Hockenbery D, Nunez G, Milliman C, Schreiber RD, Korsmeyer SJ: Bcl-2 is an inner mitochondrial membrane protein that blocks programmed cell death. Nature 1990 (348):334-336
33 McDonnel TJ, Deane N, Platt FM et al: Bcl-2-immunoglobulin transgenic mice demonstrate extended B cell survival and follicular lymphoproliferation. Cell 1989 (57):79-88
34 Fanidi A, Harrington EA, Evan GI: Cooperative interaction between c-myc and bcl-2 proto-oncogenes. Nature 1992 (359):554-556
35 Williams ME, Meeker TC, Swerdlow SH: Rearrangement of the chromosome 11 bcl-1 locus in centrocytic lymphoma: analysis with multiple breakpoint probes. Blood 1991 (78):493-498
36 Rosenberg CL, Wong E, Petty EM, Bale AE, Tsujimoto Y, Harris NL and Arnold A: PRAD1, a candidate BCL-1 oncogene: mapping and expression in centrocytic lymphoma. Proc Natl Acad Sci USA 1991 (88):9638-9642
37 Bastard C, Tilly H, Lenormand B et al: Translocations involving band 3q27 and Ig gene regions in non-Hodgkin's lymphoma. Blood 1992 (79):2527-2531
38 Ye BH, Lista F, Lo Coco F et al: Alterations of a zinc finger-encoding gene, BCL-6, in diffuse large-cell lymphoma. Science 1993 (262):747-749
39 Marshall CJ: Tumor suppressor genes. Cell 1991 (64):313-326
40 Benedict WF, Xu H-J, Hu S-X, Takahashi R: Role of the retinoblastoma gene in the initiation and progression of human cancer. J Clin Invest 1990 (85): 988-993
41 Ginsberg AM, Raffeld M, Cossman J: Mutations of the retinoblastoma gene in human lymphoid neoplasms. Leukemia and Lymphoma 1992 (7):359-362
42 Stilgenbauer S, Dohner H, Bulgay-Morschel M, Weitz S, Bentz M and Lichter P: High frequency of monoallelic retinoblastoma gene deletion in B-cell chronic lymphoid leukemia shown by interphase cytogenetics. Blood 1993 (81):2118-2124
43 Gaidano GL, Ballerini P, Gong JZ et al: p53 mutations in human lymphoid malignancies: association with Burkitt lymphoma and chronic lymphocytic leukemia. Proc Natl Acad Sci USA 1991 (88):5413-5417
44 Lo Coco F, Gaidano GL, Louie DC, Offit K, Chaganti RSK and Dalla-Favera R: p53 mutations are associated with histologic transformation of follicular lymphoma. Blood 1993 (82):2289-2295
45 Karp JE and Broder S: Acquired immunodeficiency syndrome and non-Hodgkin's lymphomas. Cancer Res 1991 (51):4743-4756
46 Pelicci PG, Knowles DM, Arlin ZA et al: Multiple monoclonal B cell expansions and c-myc oncogene rearrangements in acquired immune deficiency syndrome-related lymphoproliferative disorders. J Exp Med 1986 (164):2049-2076
47 Haluska FG, Russo G, Kant J, Andreef M, Croce CM: Molecular resemblance of an AIDS-associated lymphoma and endemic Burkitt lymphomas: implications for their pathogenesis. Proc Natl Acad Sci USA 1989 (86):8907-8911
48 Neri A, Barriga F, Inghirami G et al: Epstein-barr virus infection precedes clonal expansion in Burkitt's and acquired immunodeficiency syndrome-associated lymphoma. Blood 1991 (77):1092-1095
49 Ballerini P, Gaidano GL, Gong JZ et al: Multiple genetic lesions in acquired immunodeficiency syndrome-related non-Hodgkin's lymphoma. Blood 1993 (81): 166-176

Lymphokines in Malignant Lymphomas

Panayiotis Panayiotidis

Department of Haematology, Royal Free Hospital and School of Medicine, Pond Street, London NW3 2QG, United Kingdom

The lymphokines are glycoproteins (approx. 70-550 amino acids long) produced by a variety of cell types (haematopoietic and non-haematopoietic) regulating the generation and function of haematopoietic and immune cells (Table 1). Lymphokines are subdivided into interleukins, interferons, growth factors, cytotoxic factors, etc. These molecules exert their biological actions via specific, high/intermediate affinity receptors expressed on the surface of target cells.

Pleiotropy and Redundancy

In vitro studies with recombinant lymphokines have shown that most lymphokines have pleiotropic and redundant actions. Interleukin-6 (IL-6) is a typical example of a pleiotropic lymphokine. It was originally identified as a B cell differentiating factor inducing the maturation of B cells to antibody producing cells. Subsequent studies have, however, established its role in the haematopoietic, endocrine, hepatic and neural systems. The redundancy in lymphokine function is illustrated by the finding that not only IL-6, but IL-2, IL-4, IL-5, and gamma interferon (IFN-γ) can induce antibody production in B cells *in vitro*.

Although the *in vitro* data are always valuable, *in vivo* animal models are more informative. The multiple functions of a given lymphokine are better analysed in transgenic animals overexpressing this lymphokine, while the contribution of each lymphokine in the morphogenesis/functions of various organs/systems is studied in lymphokine gene "knockout" animals. For example transgenic mice overexpressing IL-6 exhibit dramatic changes, including generation of plasmatocytomas, mesangial proliferative glomerulonephritis, cachexia, hypercalcaemia and thrombocytosis [40]. IL-6 knockout mice, however, appear almost normal, showing the *in vivo* functional redundancy of multifunctional lymphokines [41].

The need for *in vivo* models was emphasized by the discrepancy between the *in vitro* and *in vivo* actions of IL-2. IL-2 was originally identified as a T-cell growth factor and is thought to play a key role in the thymic and post-thymic T-cell development and regulation of T-cell immune responses. IL-2 transgenic mice have increased numbers of T cells infiltrating various organs, including the CNS, lungs, testes, etc.

In contrast to the concept of the unique role of IL-2 in T cells, IL-2 knockout mice were normal with regard to thymocyte and peripheral T-cell subsets, indicating that IL-2 was not essential for the *in vivo* development and function of T cells [42].

Lymphokine Receptors

The majority of lymphokine receptors belong to a large family characterized by an extracellular ~200 amino-acid region of structural homology. The homologous region contains 4 conserved cysteine residues and a Tryptophane-Serine-X-Tryptophane-Serine motif (X is a non-conserved amino acid). Members of this family are IL-2R (ß and γ-chains), IL-3R, IL-4R, IL-5R, IL-6R, IL-7R, IL-9R, erythropoietin-R, G-CSF-R, GM-CSF-R and LIF-R [43]. The receptors for growth hormone and prolactin are also members of this family.

A number of lymphokine receptors belong to the TNF-R/NGF-R family (tumour necrosis

Table 1. Characteristics and functions of the lymphokines

Name	Size (AA)	Chrom.	Functions	Ref.
IL-1α IL-1ß	159 153	2q13 2q13-q21	Fever, ↑ acute phase proteins, costimulation of B + T lymphocytes, stimulation of endothelial cells. Inhibition of apoptosis in AL cells.	1,2
IL-2	133	4q26-q27	Proliferation + differentiation of T, NK, B lymphocytes in some NHLs and in CLL cases.	3,4
IL-3	134-140	5q23-q31	Multipotent CSF.	5,6
IL-4	120	5q23-q31	Proliferation of B + T lymphocytes. ↑ in IgG_1/IgE synthesis. ↑ or ↓ of DNA synthesis in CLL.↓ of apoptosis of CLL, follicular NHL. IL-4 + anti-CD40 → long-term culture of normal B-cells.	7,8
IL-5	115	5q23-q31	Differentiation of basophils. B-cell growth factor in mice.	9,10
IL-6	189	7p15-q21	Growth factor for B, T, myeloma cells, hepatocytes. ↑ acute phase protein synthesis. ↓ of apoptosis in AL cells.	11,12
IL-7	152	?	Proliferation of thymocytes, pre-B cells.	13
IL-8	72	4q13-q21	Chemotaxis/activation of neutrophils.	14,15
IL-9	126	5q23-q31	Stimulation of $CD4^+$ ly, BFU-E.	16
IL-10	160	?	↓ IFN-γ, IL-2 synthesis by T (TH1) lymphocytes.	17,18
IL-11	180	?	↑ growth of CFU-megakaryocyte.	19
IL-12	306 + 197*	?	*Disulphide bond heterodimer. ↑ in NK activity, proliferation of T-cells.	20,21
TNF-α TNF-ß	157 171	6p21 6p21	Cytotoxic for tumour cells. Induction of fever, septic shock, expression of adhesion molecules. Growth factor for T, B, CLL and HCL cells. Activation of endothelial cells.	22-24
IFN-γ	146	12q24	Antiviral and ↓ proliferation in various cells.↑ in NK activity, HLA II expression. ↓ in apoptosis of CLL cells.	25,26
Rantes	60	?	↑ chemotaxis of monocytes, memory T cells.	27
LIF/HILDA	170	?	↓ in growth of some AL cell lines. ↑ acute phase protein synthesis, hepatocyte proliferation.	28,29
SCF	248	?	Stem cell and mast cell growth factor.	30,31
BCGF-12kDa	124	?	↑ in growth of B-cells and CLL cells (?).	32
TGF-ß	112	19q3	↓ functions of B and T cells. Stimulation/chemotaxis of inflammatory cells	33,34
G-CSF	177	17q11-q21	Granulocyte progenitor growth factor. Activation of granulocytes.	35,36
GM-CSF	127	5q21-q32	Growth factor for monocyte/granulocyte progenitors. Activation of endothelial cells, granulocytes, monocytes. ↓ of apoptosis of myeloid cells, AML cells.	37,38
M-CSF	522, 224**	5q31-q37	**Multiple forms due to post-translational modification. Proliferation/differentiation of monocyte progenitors.	39

factor/nerve growth factor receptor). These include the TNF-R type I and II, NGF-R, the apoptosis-related molecule FAS, the CD40 antigen, and others [44]. A limited number of receptors (including IL-1R and IL-8R) belong to the immunoglobulin supergene family.

The functional pleiotropy and redundancy of lymphokines is explained by the structure of their receptors. Most of them consist of a multichain complex, (a) unique ligand-specific receptor(s) and a signal transducer protein shared with a number of other receptor complexes. Characteristic examples are the IL-6R and the IL-2R.

The IL-6R comprises a ligand binding chain (80 kDa IL-6R) and a non-binding but signal transducing chain (130 kDa, gp130). The gp130, however, is also used as a signal transducing chain in a variety of other receptors, e.g. LIF-R, IL-11R, ciliary neurotrophic factor-R and oncostatin M-R. As expected, these factors share some of the effects of IL-6 (e.g. acute phase protein synthesis, megakaryocytes and plasmatocytoma growth) via interaction with the common gp130 molecule [41,45].

The IL-2R has 3 polypeptide chains, α, β and γ, and the heterodimer of the β and γ-chains is responsible for the IL-2 signal transduction [46]. Recently the γ-chain was found to participate in the formation of IL-4R, IL-7R, IL-9R and IL-13R [45,47,48]. This observation explains the overlapping activities of these lymphokines on T lymphocytes *in vitro*. It also offers an explanation to the puzzling observation of normal T-lymphocyte development in IL-2 knockout mice, and even in IL-2 and IL-4 double knockout mice [49].

The complex structure and interactions of the lymphokines with their receptors are further complicated by the presence of soluble forms of the lymphokine receptors. Many of these soluble receptors can bind to their ligands and therefore interfere with their actions not only *in vitro* but also in *in vivo* models. These receptors are soluble because they lack their transmembrane region, either due to proteolytic cleavage of the cell-bound receptor, or to alternative splicing of the receptor mRNA.

These soluble receptors can exert an antagonistic or even agonistic action on lymphokine effects. Soluble IL-6Rs bind IL-6, and associate with cell-bound gp130, thus having an agonistic effect. In contrast, soluble gp130 molecules are bound to IL-6/IL-6R complexes and no signal transduction occurs (antagonistic effect) [41]. Soluble IL-2 and IL-4 receptors bind IL-2 and IL-4, respectively, and have an antagonistic effect [45]. It has also been proposed that some soluble receptors (e.g. sTNF-R) bind and stabilize their ligand; the ligand dissociates slowly from the complex and its biological activity is enhanced.

Lymphokines in Lymphomas

The potential role of lymphokines in lymphomas covers many areas including:

1. The pathogenesis of lymphomas.
2. Use of exogenous lymphokines for therapy or acceleration of haematopoietic recovery in treated lymphoma patients.
3. Secondary effects of lymphoma cell-derived lymphokines on the haematopoiesis, metabolism, immune and endocrine systems in lymphoma patients.

Pathogenesis

Are lymphokines involved in the generation of lymphomas?

It is tempting to hypothesize that constitutive expresssion of lymphokine receptors and/or production of lymphokines may be responsible for the generation of lymphomas or leukaemias. Freshly isolated lymphoma or leukaemia cells express a variety of lymphokine receptors. The IL-2 receptor α-chain (55 kDa) is expressed in ATL, HCL, CLL, and some NHL and RS cells; the β-chain of the IL-2 receptor is expressed in AL, T-lymphoblastic lymphomas, peripheral T-lymphomas, CLL and small lymphocytic lymphoma cells [50]. Some malignant T cells expressing biologically active IL-2R can produce IL-2, and they may use normal T-cell derived IL-2 as a paracrine growth factor [51]. In the case of ATL, the transcriptional activation of the IL-2Rα gene by the $p40^{tax}$ gene product of the HTLV-1 virus, is considered to contribute to the pathogenesis of this disease. The TNF receptor (type I and/or type II) is expressed on HCL and CLL cells, IL-6R is found on plasmatocytomas, myelomas, CLL, and Hodgkin cells. The expression of lymphokine receptors in lymphoma cells is thought to correspond to the stage of differentiation of the malignant cell and not to be linked to the pathogenesis of these malignancies. Furthermore, not all expressed receptors are biologically active.

Lymphoma cells, like their normal cellular counterparts (when they can be identified), can produce either spontaneously or after stimulation various lymphokines: CLL and HCL cells produce IL-1, IL-6, TGF-ß and TNF-α [52,53]; Hodgkin cells and cell lines can produce IL-1α, IL-4, IL-5, IL-6, IL8, IL-9, and TNFα and ß [54]. The hypothesis that hyperexpression of lymphokine genes is not responsible for the generation of leukaemias/lymphomas is further supported by *in vivo* data with transgenic animals. Transgenic mice aberrantly expressing a lymphokine gene do not develop haematopoietic malignancies, but have a variety of other disorders. IL-2 transgenic mice showed motor ataxia, alopecia, pneumonia and atrophic testes, associated with infiltration of these tissues by lymphocytes [55]. These lymphocytes are NK-like cells, and the mice die by 4 weeks of age [56]. GM-CSF transgenic mice develop an unusual syndrome of blindness, tissue damage and wasting, associated with accumulation of haematopoietic cells and high expression of the TNF-α, IL-1α and basic fibroblast growth factor m-RNA in their macrophages and granulocytes. IL-6 transgenic mice develop plasmacytomas, but these are of polyclonal origin and are not transplantable to syngeneic animals [41]. The only exception may be the IL-9 transgenic mice, in which thymic lymphomas develop in approximately 5% of the animals [57] .

Growth/survival of lymphoma cells

Due to the difficulties in identifying lymphoma "clonogenic" cells, the *in vitro* experimental approach to evaluate the effects of lymphokines on the growth of lymphoma cells is usually based on the induction of DNA synthesis on 10^4-10^5 lymphoma cells. These experiments, however, provide limited, if any, information about the growth regulation of the lymphoma "progenitor" cells.

Many lymphokines have been shown to induce DNA synhesis in lymphoma cells; IL-2 in ATL, CLL and large cell lymphoma (LCL) cells; IL-6 in myeloma cells; IL-9 in Hodgkin cells and LCL; the 12 kDa-BCGF in Burkitt and LCL cells. It should be noted, however, that depending on the co-stimulus used, lymphokines may enhance or inhibit DNA synthesis in lymphoma cells. For example, IL-4 inhibits the spontaneous DNA synthesis in CLL and follicular lymphoma cells, but when the CD40 molecule is ligated by anti-CD40 antibodies or CD-40 ligand, IL-4 increases DNA synthesis [58].

As is the case in all malignancies, the lymphoma cell numbers in a patient are regulated by a) the rate of proliferation of the "progenitor" lymphoma cells, and b) the rate of lymphoma cell death by apoptosis. For example, Burkitt's lymphomas have a high rate of proliferation and apoptosis while low-grade lymphomas have a low proliferative and apoptotic rate.

It is very interesting that all lymphoma cells are factor dependent for their survival *in vitro*. Folicullar lymphoma (FL) cells carrying the 14;18 translocation constitutively express high levels of the *bcl*-2 protein, which is able to suppress the apoptotic cell death in a variety of *in vitro* and *in vivo* systems. *In vitro*, however, FL cells die rapidly and only stimulation with IL-4 and ligation of the CD40 surface antigen extends their survival.

Lymphokines are used as "survival" factors by lymphoma cells (maintenance of cell viability in the absence of cell proliferation) in a paracrine or even autocrine fashion. IL-4, IFN-α and IFN-γ inhibit the apoptotic cell death of CLL cells *in vitro*. These lymphokines inhibit the *in vitro* cytotoxic effects of corticosteroids on CLL cells and may contribute to the resistance to corticosteroids *in vivo* [59,60]. IFN-α also prevents the apoptosis of Burkitt cells.

Therapy

Lymphokines as therapeutic agents in lymphomas

Lymphokines have been given to lymphoma/AL patients in order to induce/boost antitumour responses by activated lymphocytes/monocytes. IL-2 has been used in several studies, based on the *in vitro* finding that LAK cells (lymphokine activated killer cells, generated after culture of lymphocytes with IL-2) are cytotoxic against leukaemia/lymphoma cells. In a phase II study disappointing results were reported in HD and NHL patients with advanced disease treated with high-dose continuous i.v. IL-2 [61]. Another study reported partial responses (reduction in blood lymphocytes, decrease in lymph node and spleen size) in 2/12 CLL patients treated with IL-2 i.v. infusion [62]. Partial responses to IL-2 therapy of CLL patients were achieved also in another study [63]. In a recent phase II multicentre study IL-2 was administered as a continuous i.v. infusion for 3 cycles in 61 radiotherapy-resistant patients (low and high-grade NHL, HD and Sezary's syndrome). No response was observed in HD, there was 1 CR in the 24 low-grade NHL, and 3 CRs and 2 PRs in the 23 high-grade NHL. Interestingly, 1 CR and 4 PRs were obtained in the 7 mycosis fungoides cases [64]. The systemic toxicity of IL-2, however, is a limiting factor in designing similar studies. The availability of IL-12, a lymphokine that increases NK activity, with limited toxicity *in vivo*, may offer a new therapeutic approach. G-CSF and GM-CSF have been used to minimize haematological toxicity after chemotherapy/transplantation, to intensify chemotherapy regimens and to mobilize haematopoietic progenitor cells to the periphery, in numbers sufficient to reconstitute transplanted patients [65, 66]. It is worrying, however, that certain lymphokines are actually either growth or "survival" factors for leukaemia/lymphoma cells [67, 68].

Targeting lymphokine receptors

The most commonly found lymphokine receptor on lymphoma/leukaemia cells, the α-chain of the IL-2 receptor, has been the target of immunotherapy. A variety of approaches have been used. Patients were given unconjugated monoclonals, murine or humanized, and monoclonals conjugated with toxins or isotopes (^{212}Bi, or ^{90}Y). Other investigators have administered IL-2 labelled with toxins or isotopes to target and destroy IL-2 receptor+ lymphoma cells [69,70]. Although encouraging results have been reported, most patients develop anti-monoclonal or anti-IL-2/toxin antibodies.
Some *in vitro* studies have suggested the use of antibodies against the apoptosis-related surface antigen FAS/APO-1 [44]. ATL cells are FAS+ and they are killed efficiently *in vitro* in the presence of anti-FAS antibodies. The efficiency of killing is higher than when anti-IL-2R antibodies were used. These studies are hampered by the finding that normal tissues (hepatocytes, heart, lungs, etc.) express high levels of FAS antigen. Indeed, mice administered anti-mouse FAS antibodies die rapidly due to massive hepatocyte death [71].

Secondary Effects of Lymphoma-Derived Lymphokines

Hypercalcaemia

Hypercalcaemia associated with malignancies is caused by factors having either systemic (humoural hypercalcaemia) or local effects (local osteolytic hypercalcaemia). Two factors are mainly implicated in the systemic humoural hypercalcaemia: the parathyroid hormone-related peptide (PTHrP) and the metabolically active form of vitamin D 1,25-$(OH)_2$-D_3 (calcitriol). A number of lymphokines are involved in development of local osteolytic lesions, including IL-1, TNF-α/ß, IL-6, LIF, TGF-α and prostaglandins [72].
PTHrP has been implicated in the hypercalcaemia associated with epidermoid, renal and breast cancers. In the haematopoietic malignancies it is thought to play a central role in the hypercalcaemia of ATLL and very rarely in NHL.
In the majority of HD and NHL cases with hypercalcaemia, the elevated calcium levels are due to high calcitriol levels, which stimulate both intestinal absorption of calcium and osteoclast activity [72]. In patients with HD hypercalcaemia is not often found, and mainly in advanced stages. Canellos has reported a 0.9% incidence of hypercalcaemia in stage IV HD patients [73]. In the reported series 74% of hypercalcaemic patients were stage III/IV, 68% had B symptoms, but in very few there was evidence of lytic bone lesions [72]. Hypercalcaemia is very uncommon in low-grade lymphomas, but its incidence is higher in intermediate and high-grade NHL [74].

B symptoms

The constitutional symptoms associated with lymphomas (fever, weight loss, pruritus, profuse sweating) are due to the production of soluble factor(s) either by the malignant cells or by adjacent reactive normal cells. Despite the efforts to identify these factor(s), there is no convincing evidence that any of the known lymphokines are responsible for any of the B symptoms. Most of the studies deal with measurements of lymphokines (e.g. IL-1, TNF) in plasma/serum of patients with/without B symptoms [75]. The existence, however, of unknown levels of binding soluble receptors for these lymphokines in plasma/biological fluids, is a parameter that may interfere with their *in vivo* biological activities.

Eosinophilia and leukocytosis

Eosinophilia is most commonly encountered in HD and in a minority of NHL patients. Recent reports suggest that IL-5 produced by the malignant cells is responsible for this finding; IL-5 mRNA has been detected by *in situ* hybridisation in RS cells of lymph node biopsies from patients with eosinophilia. In patients without eosinophilia no IL-5 mRNA was detected [76]. Leukocytosis (due to a neutrophil increase) is a frequent finding in HD, and CSFs produced either by RS cells or by infiltrating inflammatory cells may be responsible.

Conclusions

The *in vitro* studies on the role of lymphokines/lymphokine receptors in the biology of lymphomas are often difficult to interpret and sometimes contradictory. Preparations of freshly isolated lymphoma cells may contain residual numbers of normal cells that interfere with the experimental results. The cells are cultured in the presence of serum (animal or human) which contains soluble interleukin receptors that may again interact with the lymphokines under study. The sensitivity of the methods used is a crucial factor, too; many of the early reports on the expression of lymphokine receptors were based on immunocytochemistry or Northern blots, which are less sensitive than fluorescence-activated sorter analysis (FACS) and polymerase chain reaction (PCR), respectively. The availability of very sensitive methods that allow the study of single cells and not cell populations (e.g. *in situ* hybridization, single cell PCR amplification) will allow the precise analysis of the role of lymphokines and their receptors in all haematopoietic malignancies [77]. Although there is little evidence that lymphokines are involved in the pathogenesis of lymphomas, there are many studies indicating that lymphoma cells are growth factor dependent for their survival and proliferation. The recent findings that lymphokines a) increase the survival of leukaemia/lymphoma cells by inhibiting apoptosis and b) protect these cells from the cytotoxic effects of various chemotherapeutic agents [67,68,78] indicate that studies involving lymphokine therapy must be very carefully planned and monitored.

REFERENCES

1 Dinarello CA: Interleukin-1. Rev Infect Dis 1984 (6): 51-95
2 March CJ, Mosley B, Larsen A et al: Cloning, sequence and expression of two distinct human interleukin-1 complementary DNAs. Nature 1985 (315):641-647
3 Taniguchi T, Matsui H, Fujita T et al: Structure and expression of a cloned cDNA for human interleukin-2. Nature 1983 (302):305-310
4 Smith KA: Interleukin-2: inception, impact, and implications. Science 1988 (240):1169-1176
5 Yang YC, Ciarletta AB, Temple PA et al: Human IL-3 (multi-CSF): identification by expression cloning of a novel hematopoietic growth factor related to murine IL-3. Cell 1986 (47):3-10
6 Clark SC and Kamen R: The human hematopoietic colony-stimulating factors. Science 1987 (236): 1229-1237
7 Yokota T, Otsuka T, Mosmann T et al: Isolation and characterization of a human interleukin cDNA clone, homologous to mouse B-cell stimulatory factor 1, that expresses B-cell-and T-cell-stimulating activities. PNAS 1986 (83):5894-5898
8 Paul WE and Ohara J: B-cell stimulatory factor-1/interleukin-4. Ann Rev Immunol 1987 (5): 429-459
9 Azuma C, Tanabe T, Konishi M et al: Cloning of cDNA for human T-cell replacing factor (interleukin-5) and comparison with the murine homologue. Nucl Acid Res 1986 (22):9149-9158
10 Yokota T, Arai N, de Vries J et al: Molecular biology of interleukin 4 and interleukin 5 genes and biology of their products that stimulate B cells, T cells and hemopoietic cells. Immunol Rev 1988 (102):137-187
11 Hirano T, Yasukawa K, Harada H et al: Complementary DNA for a novel human interleukin (BSF-2) that induces B lymphocytes to produce immunoglobulin. Nature 1986 (324):73-76
12 Ishibashi T, Kimura H, Shikama Y et al: Interleukin-6 is a potent thrombopoietic factor in vivo in mice. Blood 1989 (74):1241-1244
13 Goodwin RG, Lupton S, Schmierer A et al: Human interleukin 7: molecular cloning and growth factor activity on human and murine B-lineage cells. PNAS 1989 (8):302-306
14 Matsushima K, Morishita K, Yoshimura T et al: Molecular cloning of a human monocyte-derived neutrophil chemotactic factor (MDNCF) and the induction of MDNCF mRNA by interleukin 1 and tumor necrosis factor. J Exper Med 1988 (167): 1883-1893
15 Matsushima K and Oppenheim JJ: Interleukin 8 and MCAF: novel inflammatory cytokines inducible by IL 1 and TNF. Cytokine 1989 (1):2-13
16 Yang YC, Ricciardi S, Ciarletta A, Calvetti J, Kelleher K, Clark SC: Expression cloning of cDNA encoding a novel human hematopoietic growth factor: human homologue of murine T-cell growth factor P40. Blood 1989 (74):1880-1884
17 Moore KW, Vieira P, Fiorentino DF, Trounstine ML, Khan TA, Mosmann TR: Homology of cytokine synthesis inhibitory factor (IL-10) to the Epstein-Barr virus gene BCRFI. Science 1990 (248):1230-1234
18 Vieira P, de Waal-Malefyt R, Dang MN et al: Isolation and expression of human cytokine synthesis inhibitory factor cDNA clones: homology to Epstein-Barr virus open reading frame BCRFI. PNAS 1991 (88):1172-1176
19 Paul SR, Bennett F, Calvetti JA et al: Molecular cloning of a cDNA encoding interleukin 11, a stromal cell-derived lymphopoietic and hematopoietic cytokine. PNAS 1990 (87):7512-7516
20 Stern AS, Podlaski FJ, Hulmes JD et al: Purification to homogeneity and partial characterization of cytotoxic lymphocyte maturation factor from human B-lymphoblastoid cells. PNAS 1990 (87):6808-6812
21 Gubler U, Chua AO, Schoenhaut DS et al: Coexpression of two distinct genes is required to generate secreted bioactive cytotoxic lymphocyte maturation factor. PNAS 1991 (88):4143-4147
22 Pennica D, Nedwin GE, Hayflick JS et al: Human tumour necrosis factor: precursor structure, expression and homology to lymphotoxin. Nature 1984 (312):724-729
23 Beutler B and Cerami A: Tumor necrosis, cachexia, shock, and inflammation: a common mediator. Ann Rev Biochem 1988 (57):505-518
24 Gray PW, Aggarwal BB, Benton CV et al: Cloning and expression of cDNA for human lymphotoxin, a lymphokine with tumour necrosis activity. Nature (312):721-724
25 Devos R, Cheroutre H, Taya Y, Degrave W, Van Heuverswyn H, Fiers W: Molecular cloning of human immune interferon cDNA and its expression in eukaryotic cells. Nucl Acid Res 1982 (10):2487-2501
26 Pestka S, Langer JA, Zoon KC, Samuel CE: Interferons and their actions. Ann Rev Biochem 1987 (56):727-777
27 Schall TJ, Bacon K, Toy KJ, Goeddel DV: Selective attraction of monocytes and T lymphocytes of the memory phenotype by cytokine RANTES. Nature 1990 (347):669-671
28 Moreau JF, Donaldson DD, Bennett F, Witek-Giannotti J, Clark SC, Wong GG: Leukaemia inhibitory factor is identical to the myeloid growth factor human interleukin for DA cells. Nature 1988 (336):690-692
29 Gearing DP, Gough NM, King JA et al: Molecular cloning and expression of cDNA encoding a murine myeloid leukaemia inhibitory factor (LIF). EMBO J 1987 (6):3995-4002
30 Martin FH, Suggs SV, Langley KE et al: Primary structure and functional expression of rat and human stem cell factor DNAs. Cell 1990 (63):203-211
31 Anderson DM, Lyman SD, Baird A et al: Molecular cloning of mast cell growth factor, a hematopoietin that is active in both membrane bound and soluble forms. Cell 1990 (63):235-243
32 Sharma S, Mehta S, Morgan J, Maizel A: Molecular cloning and expression of a human B-cell growth factor gene in Escherichia coli. Science 1987 (235): 1489-1492
33 Derynck R, Jarrett JA, Chen EY et al: Human transforming growth factor-beta complementary

DNA sequence and expression in normal and transformed cells. Nature (316):701-705
34 Barnard JA, Lyons RM, Moses HL: The cell biology of transforming growth factor beta. Biochim Biophys Acta 1990 (1032):79-87
35 Nagata S, Tsuchiya M, Asano S et al: Molecular cloning and expression of cDNA for human granulocyte colony-stimulating factor. Nature 1986 (319): 415-418
36 Nicola NA: Hemopoietic cell growth factors and their receptors. Ann Rev Biochem 1989 (58):45-77
37 Wong GG, Witek JS, Temple PA et al: Human GM-CSF: molecular cloning of the complementary DNA and purification of the natural and recombinant proteins. Science 1985 (228):810-815
38 Metcalf D: The molecular biology and functions of the granulocyte-macrophage colony-stimulating factors. Blood 1986 (67):257-267
39 Wong GG, Temple PA, Leary AC et al: Human CSF-1: molecular cloning and expression of 4-kb cDNA encoding the human urinary protein. Science 1987 (235):1504-1508
40 Suematsu S, Matsusaka T, Matsuda T et al: Generation of plasmatocytomas with the chromosomal translocation s t(12;15) in IL-6 transgenic mice. PNAS 1992 (69):232-235
41 Akira S, Taga T, Kishimoto T: Interleukin-6 in biology and medicine. Adv Immunol 1993 (54):51-77
42 Schorle H, Hotltschke T, Hunig T, Shimle A, Horak I: Development and function of T cells in mice rendered interleukin-2 deficient by gene targeting. Nature 1991 (352):621-624
43 Bazan JF: Structural design and molecular evolution of a cytokine receptor superfamily. PNAS 1990 (87): 6934-6938
44 Itoh N and Nagata SA: Novel protein domain required for apoptosis. Mutational analysis of the human FAS antigen. J Biol Chem 1993 (268):10932-10937
45 Kishimoto T, Taga T, Akira S: Cytokine signal transduction. Cell 1994 (76):253-262
46 Takeshita T, Asao H, Ohtani K et al: Cloning of the γ chain of the human IL-2 receptor. Science 1992 (257):379-382
47 Kondo K, Takeshita T, Ishii N et al: Sharing of the IL-2 receptor γ chain between receptors for IL-2 and IL-4. Science 1993 (262):1874-1877
48 Noguchi M, Nakamura Y, Russel SM et al: Interleukin-2 receptor γ chain; a functional component of the interleukin-7 receptor. Science 1993 (262):1877-1880
49 Sadlack B, Kuhn R, Schorle H, Rajeewsky K, Muller W, Horak I: Development and proliferation of lymphocytes in mice deficient for both interleukins-2 and 4. Eur J Immunol 1994 (24):281-284
50 Rosolen A, Nakanishi M, Poplack DG et al: Expression of interleukin-2 receptor beta subunit in hematopoietic malignancies. Blood 1989 (73):1968-1972
51 Peuchmaur M, Emilie D, Crevon MC et al: IL-2 mRNA expression in Tac-positive malignant lymphomas. Am J Pathol 1990 (136):383-390
52 Cordingley FT, Hoffbrand AV, Heslop HE et al: Tumor necrosis factor as an autocrine growth factor for chronic B cell malignancies. Lancet 1988 (i):969-971
53 Foa R, Massaia M, Cardona S et al: Production of tumor necrosis factor alpha by B-cell chronic lymphocytic leukemia cells: a possible regulatory role of TNF in the progression of the disease. Blood 1990 (76):393-400
54 Gruss H-J, Brach MA, Drexler HG, Bonifer R, Mertelsmann R, Herrmann F: Expression of cytokine genes, cytokine receptor genes and transcription factors in cultured Hodgkin and Reed-Sternberg cells. Cancer Res 1992 (52):3353-3360
55 Ishida Y, Nishi M, Taguchi O et al: Effects of the deregulated expression of human interleukin-2 in transgenic mice. Internat Immunol 1989 (1):113-120
56 Ishida Y, Nishi M, Taguchi O et al: Expansion of natural killer cells but not T cells in human interleukin 2/interleukin 2 receptor (Tac) transgenic mice. J Exper Med 1989 (170):1103-1115
57 Renauld J-C, Houssiau F, Louahed J, Vink A, Van Snick J, Uyttenhove C: Interleukin 9. Adv Immunol 1993 (54):79-97
58 Fluckiger AC, Rossi JF, Bussel A, Bryon P, Banechareau J, Defrance T: Responsiveness of chronic lymphocytic leukemia B cells activated via surface Igs or CD40 to B-cell trophic factors. Blood 1993 (80):3173-3181
59 Panayiotidis P, Ganeshaguru K, Jabbar SAB et al: Interleukin-4 inhibits apoptotic cell death and loss of the bcl-2 protein in B-chronic lymphocytic leukaemia cells in vitro. Br J Haematol 1993 (85):439-445
60 Panayiotidis P, Ganeshaguru K, Jabbar SAB et al: Alpha-interferon protects B-chronic lymphocytic leukemia cells from apoptotic cell death in vitro. Br J Haematol 1994 (86):169-173
61 Lim SH, Worman CP, Callaghan T, Jewell A, Smith MP, Goldstone H: Continuous intravenous infusion of high dose recombinant IL-2 for advanced lymphomas. A phase II study. Leuk Res 1991 (15): 435-439
62 Kay NE, Oken MM, Mazza JJ, Bradley EC: Evidence for tumor reduction in refractory or relapsed B-CLL patients with infusional interleukin-2. Nouv Rev Fr Hematol 1988 (30):475-478
63 Allison MA, Jones SE, McGuffey P: Phase II trial of outpatient interleukin-2 in malignant lymphoma, chronic lymphocytic leukemia, and selected solid tumors. J Clin Oncol 1989 (7):75-80
64 Gisselbrecht C, Marachini D, Pico JL et al: Interleukin-2 treatment in lymphoma: a phase II multicenter study. Blood 1994 (83):2081-2085
65 Visani G, Gamberi B Greenberg P et al: The use of GM-CSF as an adjunct to autologous/syngeneic bone marrow transplantation: a prospective randomized controlled trial. Bone Marrow Transplantation 1991 (7 suppl 2):81-85
66 Armitage JO: The use of granulocyte-macrophage colony-stimulating factor in bone marrow transplantation. Sem Hematol 1992 (29 suppl 3):14-18
67 Sachs L and Lotem J: Control of programmed cell death in normal and leukemic cells: new implications for therapy. Blood 1993 (82):15-21
68 Lotem J and Sachs L: Hematopoietic cytokines inhibit apoptosis induced by transforming growth factor beta 1 and cancer chemotherapy compounds in myeloid leukemic cells. Blood 1992 (80):1750-1757

69 LeMaistre CF, Meneghetti C, Rosenblum M et al: Phase I trial of an interleukin-2 (IL-2) fusion toxin (DAB486IL-2) in hematologic malignancies expressing the IL-2 receptor. Blood 1992 (79):2547-2554
70 Higuchi CM, Thompson JA, Petersen FB, Buckner CD, Fefer A: Toxicity and immunomodulatory effects of interleukin-2 after autologous bone marrow transplantation for hematologic malignancies. Blood 1991 (77):2561-2568
71 Ogasawara J, Watanabe-Fukunaga R, Adachi M et al: Lethal effects of the anti-FAS antibody in mice. Nature 1993 (364):806-809
72 Seymour JF and Gagel RF: Calcitriol: the major humoral mediator of hypercalcemia in Hodgkin's disease and non-Hodgkin's lymphomas. Blood 1993 (82):1383-1394
73 Canellos GP: Hypercalcemia in malignant lymphoma and leukemia. Ann NY Acad Sci 1974 (230):240-247
74 Burt ME and Brennan MF: Incidence of hypercalcemia and malignant neoplasm. Arch Surg 1980 (115): 705-709
75 Ishii E, Ogha S, Ueda K: Tumor necrosis factor and fever at diagnosis in children with solid tumors. Ped Hematol Oncol 1990 (3):253-257
76 Samoszuk M and Nansen L: Detection of interleukin-5 mRNA in Reed-Sternberg cells of Hodgkin's disease with eosinophilia. Blood 1990 (75):13-16
77 Trumper LH, Brady G, Bagg A et al: Single-cell analysis of Hodgkin and Reed-Sternberg cells: molecular heterogeneity of gene expression and p53 mutations. Blood 1993 (81):3097-3115
78 Hoffbrand AV, Panayiotidis P, Reittie J, Ganeshaguru K: Autocrine and paracrine growth loops in chronic lymphocytic leukemia. Sem Haematol 1993 (30):306-317

Biology, Staging and Treatment of Hodgkin's Disease

Ulrich Rüffer, Markus Sieber, Hans Tesch, Andreas Engert and Volker Diehl

Klinik I für Innere Medizin, Universität zu Köln, Joseph-Stelzmann-Straße 9, 5000 Köln 41, Germany

Definition and Epidemiology

Hodgkin's disease, first described by Thomas Hodgkin (1798-1866), is a malignant disease characterized by the presence of Hodgkin and Reed-Sternberg giant cells (H-RS). In the tissues involved, H-RS cells are usually sparse and surrounded by a variety of reactive "bystander" cells.

The incidence of Hodgkin's disease is 2-3/ 100,000 per year. There is a bimodal distribution of Hodgkin's disease in western countries with two peaks, at 26 years and at 60 years of age. Epidemiologic studies show an increased incidence of Hodgkin's disease in affluent settings. The incidence pattern of Hodgkin's disease therefore resembles that of virally transmitted diseases like infectious mononucleosis or paralytic polio [1].

Hodgkin and Reed-Sternberg Cells (H-RS)

The origin of the mononuclear Hodgkin cell and the polynuclear Reed-Sternberg cell has been enigmatic for many years. The low number of H-RS cells in involved tissues and the fragility of these cells contributed to the difficulty in obtaining reproducible data on the cellular origin of Hodgkin's disease. H-RS cells share features with most nucleated mononuclear cells like histiocytes, macrophages, interdigitating reticulum cells and lymphocytes [2].

Biochemical and immunological insight was gained by the isolation of HD-derived cell lines [3]. Monoclonal antibodies were isolated in mice against two of these lines (L428 and L540). One of these antibodies (Ki-1) detects an antigen which is regularly expressed on H-SR cells and on activated normal B and T lymphocytes; the antigen was subsequently classified as CD30 [4]. Based on biochemical characterization and molecular cloning, the CD30 antigen is a new member of the nerve growth factor superfamily. Growth of H-RS cells might depend on specific stimulation via the recently cloned and sequenced CD30 ligand [5].

Immune electron microscopy and cytocentrifuge preparation in recent studies revealed antigens such as CD2, CD3, CD4, CD5, CD6, CD25, and CD30 on H-RS cells in the majority of cases, suggesting a close relationship to T lymphocytes [6]. However, the expression of T-cell antigens varies considerably from case to case and from site to site [7]. Markers of B-lineage cells, like immunoglobulin, gene-rearrangement and positive staining for IgG-κ and IgG-λ in paraffin sections, are also a common finding among H-RS cells. It has therefore been postulated that H-RS cells might arise from peripheral lymphoid cells which are further transformed depending on the microenvironment and location within the lymph node.

Cytokines secreted from H-SR cells or from reactive bystander cells might be involved in the perpetuation of the malignant phenotype. Both Hodgkin cell lines and H-RS cells from fresh tissue biopsies express an abundance of high-affinity interleukin-2 (IL-2) receptors. However, no direct stimulation of H-RS cells via IL-2 has been demonstrated yet. A candidate cytokine for growth stimulation of H-SR cells is interleukin-9 [8]. After transplantation into mice, IL-2-stimulated T cells which had been transfected with the IL-9 gene grow as lymphomas resembling Hodgkin's disease (lymphocyte depletion subtype) or large cell anaplastic lymphoma. Multiple other cytokines such as IL-1, IL-4,

IL-6, M-CSF, GM-CSF and TNF-α have been reported as possible mediators between H-RS cells and the surrounding bystander cells. TGF-ß may be responsible for the fibrosis in nodular sclerosis (NS) type Hodgkin's disease. Interleukin-5 has been associated with eosinophilia, which is frequently observed in Hodgkin's disease. Interleukin-6 was identified on cell lines and fresh H-RS cells, suggesting a possible paracrine stimulation. The reactive bystander cells are part of the unique histomorphological picture in Hodgkin's disease. These bystander cells might be attracted by cytokines secreted from the H-RS cells. In addition, bystander cells themselves might promote the growth of H-RS cells via different cytokines. Interaction between H-RS cells and surrounding bystander cells probably involves cellular adhesion and receptor molecules, like the beta-1 integrins, beta-2 integrins, selectins, immunoglobulins, and T-cell receptors (CD3, CD28).

New theories regarding the role of bystander cells in the pathogenesis of Hodgkin's disease suggest that these cells might serve as precursors for the malignant cell population. This hypothesis is based on transplantation experiments of primary Hodgkin tissues into SCID mice [9]. Epidemiological studies had demonstrated a significant correlation of Hodgkin's disease and infectious mononucleosis [10]. More sensitive techniques such as the polymerase chain reaction demonstrated the EBV genome in 40-80% of the Hodgkin's tissues investigated [11]. Additional technical progress in the generation of single-cell cDNA libraries from H-RS cells will allow further insight into the genetic regulation of Hodgkin's disease [12]. The biological heterogeneity in Hodgkin's disease might be a result of a gradual transformation of different EBV-infected bystander cells into H-RS cells. Recent methodical improvements have identified EBV genome and EBV gene products in up to 50% of H-RS cells from patients with Hodgkin's disease.

Laboratory Features

There is no laboratory test available which is specific for Hodgkin's disease. However, a number of unspecific parameters indicate disease activity. The erythrocyte sedimentation rate (ESR) and serum lactate dehydrogenase (LDH) are elevated in up to 50% of patients at presentation and are frequently associated with B symptoms and advanced disease. These unspecific changes may provide helpful activity parameters indicating an imminent relapse. Other laboratory features on HD are elevated levels of alkaline phosphatase, ferritin, granulocytes, platelets or lymphocytopenia, anaemia, and thrombocytopenia. Patients with Hodgkin's disease have a defect in cell-mediated immunity because the number of circulating T lymphocytes and, in particular, CD4-positive T-helper cells, is diminished. The cell defect puts patients with Hodgkin's disease at an increased risk for infections with opportunistic organisms such as mycobacteria, fungi and viruses. In contrast, the humoural immune defence is normal in most cases.

In recent studies, the excretion of cytokines and soluble antigens shed from the surface of H-RS cells in the serum has become increasingly interesting. sCD25 and CD30 seem to be correlated with disease activity in Hodgkin's disease [13].

Histology

There are 4 main histological subtypes in Hodgkin's disease according to the Rye classification: lymphocyte predominance (LP), nodular sclerosis (NS), mixed-cellularity (MC), and lymphocyte depletion (LD).

Lymphocyte Predominance

Histologically and in its clinical course LP Hodgkin's disease resembles indolent B-cell non-Hodgkin's lymphoma. This type has therefore been established as a separate entity [14]. There are two major subtypes: the nodular paragranuloma is characterized by a nodular distribution pattern of H-RS cells surrounded by multiple small lymphocytes and histiocytes [15]. In contrast, the diffuse paragranuloma has a random distribution of H-RS cells between lymphocytes and histiocytes without any nodular structure [16]. Lymphocyte-predominance Hodgkin's disease constitutes about 3% of all cases.

Nodular Sclerosis

NS Hodgkin's disease is characterized by a nodular infiltration of lymphatic cells surrounded by collagen fibres. The H-RS cells are located within these nodular structures. Recently, two subtypes of nodular sclerosis have been described [17]: nodular sclerosis type II, in contrast to type I, is characterized by areas of lymphocyte depletion and numerous H-RS cells. Clinically, nodular sclerosis type II is more often correlated with B symptoms, elevated ESR and anaemia. The prognosis of NS type II is significantly worse than that of type I.

Mixed Cellularity

The mixed cellularity subtype of Hodgkin's disease presents histologically as a polymorphic pattern with eosinophils, histiocytes and variable numbers of plasma cells. Mononuclear Hodgkin cells and polynuclear RS cells are frequently found.

Lymphocyte Depletion

The lymphocyte depletion subtype is characterized by a large proportion of H-RS cells and few reactive inflammatory cells. This subtype often presents with advanced stages and B symptoms.

Diagnostic Features

The diagnosis of Hodgkin's disease is based on the histological assessment of typical H-RS cells. Since H-RS cells can be very sparse in the tissues involved (<0.1%), a lymph node biopsy and histological examination are essential for diagnosis. After histological verification of the diagnosis, thorough staging has to be performed, possibly including laparotomy and splenectomy, to precisely define the extent of disease. A clinical staging procedure (CS) is recommended including history (B symptoms?), physical examination, laboratory tests, chest X-ray and CT-scan, abdominal ultrasound and CT scan, bone marrow scintigraphy and bone marrow trepanation. After these clinical procedures, the patient is classified according to the Ann Arbor criteria. Based on recent data from a meta-analysis of risk factors [18], patients can be divided into 3 different subgroups (localized stages, intermediate stages and advanced stages). Further diagnostics and the choice of treatment depend on the initial classification into these 3 groups. Inclusion criteria vary among different study groups. The following criteria are based on the guidelines of the German Hodgkin Study Group (GHSG).

Group 1: Patients in localized stages CS I and II without risk factors (mediastinal bulk, extranodal disease, ESR >50 in A stages or >30 in B stages, massive spleen involvement and 3 or more involved lymph node areas).

Group 2: The intermediate stage includes patients in clinical stages CS I and IIA with one or more of the following risk factors: mediastinal bulky disease, extranodal disease, diffuse or massive splenic involvement, ESR >50 in A stages or >30 in B stages, 3 or more involved lymph node areas. Patients in stage CS IIB with ESR 30 and/or 3 or more involved lymph node areas and patients staged as CS IIIA without risk factors are also included in the intermediate-risk group.

Group 3: This group includes all patients in stages IIIB and IV, patients in clinical stages CS IIIA with all risk factors, and patients staged as CS IIB with mediastinal bulky disease, extranodal disease and/or massive splenic involvement.

Prognostic Factors

The stratification of clinical trials on Hodgkin's disease is strongly influenced by the identification of prognostic factors. The most important prognostic factor remains the stage of the disease at first presentation. For example, the long-term relapse-free survival in histologically verified stages PS I and PS IIA is greater than 90% after radiation therapy. By contrast, the relapse-free survival is only about 50% in ad-

Table 1. Summary of prognostic factors

	Reproducible, shown in large cohorts	To be reproduced
Constitution	Age Gender	
Extent of disease	Stage Number of LN areas Bulk (MMT)	Tumour burden
Localization	Infradiaphragmatic E disease Splenic involvement	Bone marrow
Histology	LD, MC histology	Tumour cell concentration NS histology
Biology	B symptoms ESR, albumin	IL-2R, CD30, CD 8 Hb, LDH, AP, Lymphocyte count

vanced stages IIIB and IV despite intensive combined modality treatment. A meta-analysis of more than 14,000 patients with Hodgkin's disease [18] defined the risk factors associated with a poor prognosis.
Table 1 gives a summary of prognostic factors grouped into accepted and estimated factors.

Treatment of Localized Stages

Radiotherapy is still considered as the treatment of choice for localized stages [19]. Patients with PS/CS I-IIA are treated with 35-44 Gy in extended field technique. The optimal dose of treatment still remains to be defined. In the recently closed HD-4 trial of the GHSG a standard therapy consisting of 40 Gy extended field was compared to a treatment with 30 Gy extended field and 10 Gy involved field in pathologically staged patients with PS I/II without risk factors. A current interim analysis of 171 patients shows a complete remission rate of 98% with a freedom from treatment failure (FFTF) of 88% at 22 months of median observation time (Fig. 1). Although the survival is 95% after 5 years in this group, important questions still remain to be solved. Current studies evaluate the addition of chemotherapy to the treatment of localized stages [20] to avoid the invasive diagnostic procedures, i.e., laparotomy and splenectomy, which are associated with a mortality of 0.5% and a morbidity of 3% [21], and to improve the FFTF rate (FFTF expected after radiotherapy alone is 75% at 5 years). However, the potential toxicity of chemotherapy in addition to radiotherapy should be taken into consideration. Therefore, one major goal of future studies will be the identification of prognostic factors that allow the exact definition of subgroups of patients at particularly low risk in whom invasive staging procedures can be avoided without reducing the long-term prospects. This concept was adapted by the ongoing EORTC study. In this trial, patients with defined prognostic factors such as favourable histology (NS, LP), female sex, age younger than 40 years are treated with radiotherapy without the initial diagnostic laparotomy. Unfortunately this group of patients represents only 1-2 % of all cases.

Intermediate Stages

Intermediate stages are treated with a combined modality approach of chemotherapy and radiation. Radiotherapy alone is not sufficient to control disease activity in this group. Most studies use a combination therapy consisting of 4 cycles of MOPP, COPP, and/or ABVD, and additional radiotherapy.
Patients with intermediate disease stages are defined by stage and risk factors. In the GHSG these risk factors include bulky mediastinal tumour, B symptoms, extranodal disease, 3 or more involved lymph node areas and ESR. Currently, the outcome of combined modality treatment in intermediate stages is about 90% CR with survival rates of about 80% after 5 years (Diehl et al., unpublished data). The major obstacle of combined modality treatment is the increasing number of second neoplasms, like solid tumours (15%), non-Hodgkin's lymphomas (3%), and acute leukaemias (2%) [22]. Current strategies in intermediate stages therefore evaluate a possible reduction of the toxicity. One approach would be the identification of patients with a particularly good prognosis prior to the initiation of treatment, which would permit a reduction of treatment intensity in this group. The recently performed analysis of the GHSG shows that patients in clinical

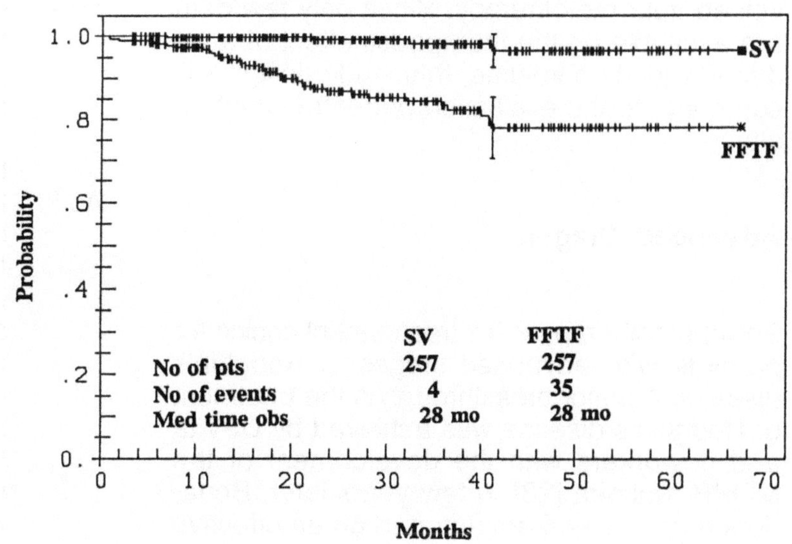

Fig. 1. PS I,II without risk factors (HD4 trial 1988-93). Survival and freedom from treatment failure

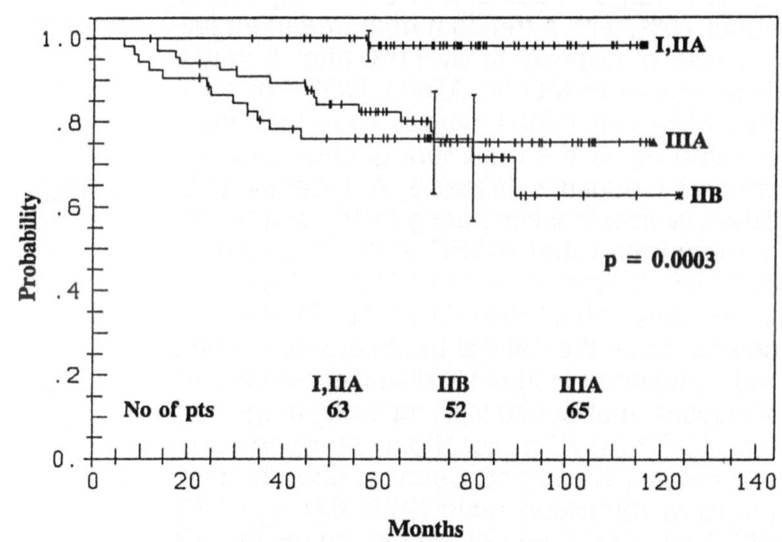

Fig. 2. CS/PS I,II,IIIA with large MT, E or massive splenic involvement (HD1 trial 1983-88). Survival by stage I,IIA vs IIB vs IIIA

stages I-IIA with risk factors (bulky tumour, extranodal disease, massive spleen involvement) have a good prognosis with a freedom from treatment failure (FFTF) rate of 85% after 4 years (Fig. 2). These patients were treated with 2 cycles of COPP/ABVD and additional radiation therapy of either 40 Gy EF or 20 Gy EF + 20 Gy to tumour bulk. Thus, a reduction of treatment intensity might be possible for this group of patients. In contrast, patients at clinical stages IIB and IIIA treated accordingly had FFTF values of 70% after 4 years.

A reduction in the intensity of therapy can be considered for both chemotherapy and radiotherapy. Reducing the toxicity of chemotherapy can be achieved by 1) fewer chemotherapy cycles; 2) the use of fewer cytostatic drugs, and 3) a reduced dose of certain drugs. Ongoing clinical trials at Stanford University evaluate the possibility of a reduced number of cytostatic drugs within the VBM regimen (vinblastine, bleomycin, methotrexate). An interim analysis of this ongoing trial suggests that this regimen can be administered with low-dose bleomycin, resulting in reduced toxicity and comparable efficacy. Another possible reduction in toxicity might be achieved by a reduced radiation volume. In an ongoing trial of the GHSG (HD8), patients with intermediate-stage disease are randomly assigned to two cycles of COPP-ABVD plus 30 Gy extended field radiotherapy or 2 x COPP-ABVD + 30 Gy involved field radiotherapy. Since only few data are available on the therapeutic effect of a reduced radiation volume, this study design will contribute to the evaluation of treatment intensity.

Advanced Stages

Polychemotherapy is the treatment of choice for patients with advanced stages of Hodgkin's disease. A major breakthrough in the treatment of Hodgkin's disease was achieved by DeVita and coworkers with the development of the MOPP regimen [23]. A few years later, Bonadonna and coworkers reported on an effective non-cross-resistant regimen (ABVD) [24]. The complete remission rate in patients with advanced stages treated with either regimen is about 75%, with a freedom from treatment failure rate of approximately 50% after 5 years. Eight cycles of MOPP, ABVD, COPP or 4 cycles of MOPP-ABVD hybrids have long been considered as the treatment of choice for advanced Hodgkin's disease. A recently published clinical trial comparing ABVD and MOPP demonstrated that MOPP alone is inferior to both ABVD and MOPP-ABVD [25]. Based on these data, MOPP/ABVD or ABVD are considered to be the optimal treatment for patients with advanced Hodgkin's disease. Several international multicentre trials replacing drugs from the MOPP-ABVD protocol did not report superior results. Klimo and Connors published impressive remission rates (97% CR and 77% FFTF after 7 years) with an alternating MOPP/ABV hybrid of the third generation based on rapid alternation of cytostatic drugs [26]. These data from a non-randomized pilot study were not reproduced in a randomized multicentre trial comparing MOPP/ABVD with the MOPP/ABV hybrid [27]. Treatment-related toxicity was more severe in the group treated with the MOPP-ABV hybrid protocol.

In conclusion, the treatment results in advanced stages are not yet satisfactory. Current and future studies will try to improve remission rates by: 1) the use of new chemotherapeutic drugs; 2) intensification of currently available regimens; 3) the evaluation of high-dose chemotherapy (HDC) with subsequent stem cell transplantation (ABMT) in previously untreated patients.

Ad 1: Etoposide (VP16) has been demonstrated to be a new potent cytostatic drug in the treatment of Hodgkin's disease. The drug has been used mostly in relapse regimens and is currently being tested as first-line therapy.

Ad 2: Intensification of the current regimens can be achieved by shorter duration of treatment or by a dose intensification of certain drugs. The use of growth factors such as G-CSF might facilitate dose intensification by reducing the time of granulocytopenia after chemotherapy. An example of this type of clinical trial is the HD9 study of the GHSG [28] which compares a standard chemotherapy regimen with a dose escalated protocol.

Ad 3: ABMT has been accepted as standard therapy for patients with sensitive (good partial or complete remission after HDC) relapses. However, no firm data are available yet regarding the superiority of HDC+ABMT as primary treatment for relapsed patients because randomized studies comparing HDC + ABMT and conventional second-line treatment are lacking. Recently the GHSG started a European multicentre trial comparing HDC + ABMT with a standard salvage regimen in first relapse (HD-R1). The use of HDC + ABMT in the frontline treatment of high-risk patients with advanced Hodgkin's disease is currently being investigated by an Italian study group (Carella et al.), but is hampered by the lack of reproducible prognostic factors in this group of patients.

A summary of the study family of the GSHG is given in Table 2.

Second-Line Treatment

Several regimens have been used in the treatment of relapsed Hodgkin's patients, producing response rates ranging from 50% to 70%. The duration of a second remission is generally short. Patients with sensitive relapses have therefore been treated with HDC + ABMT, resulting in approximately 50% complete remissions, of long duration in 30-50% of

Table 2. German Hodgkin Study Group trials (first-line therapy)

Generation	Time	Trial	Target group	Trial design	Question
			HD0 CS/PS I, II without RF		No trial only documentation
I	1984-1988	**HD1-3** (500 pts.)	**HD1** CS/PS I, II A/B, IIIA with RF	R: 2 x COPP/ABVD + 40 Gy EF 2 x COPP/ABVD + 20 Gy EF	Reduction of radiotherapy after standard chemo-therapy
			HD3 CS/PS IIIB, IV	3 x COPP/ABVD -> CR -> R: 1 x COPP/ABVD 20 Gy IF	Comparison between chemo- and radiotherapy as consolidation
			HD4 PS I, II A/B without RF	R: 40 Gy EF 30 Gy EF + 10 Gy IF	Reduction of radiation dose in the extended field
II	1988-1993	**HD4-6** (1900 pts.)	**HD5** CS/PS I, II A/B with RF, IIIA	R: 2 x COPP/ABVD + 30 Gy EF + 10 Gy bulk 2 x COPP/ABV/IMEP + 30 Gy EF + 10 Gy bulk	Comparison between a standard chemotherapy regimen and a rapidly alternating hybrid regimen (Goldie-Coltman)
			HD6 CS/PS IIIB, IV	R: 4 x COPP/ABVD ± RT 4 x COPP/ABV/IMEP ± RT	
			HD7 CS I, II A/B without RF	R: 2 x ABVD + 30 Gy EF + 10 Gy IF 30 Gy EF + 10 Gy IF	Prevention of relapse after EF-radiotherapy by use of mild chemotherapy
III	1993-1997	**HD7-9**	**HD8** CS/PS I A/B, IIA with RF, IIB with RF d/e, IIIA without RF	R: 2 x COPP/ABVD + 30 Gy EF + 10 Gy bulk 2 x COPP/ABVD + 30 Gy IF + 10 Gy bulk	Reduction of acute and long-term toxicity
			HD9 CS/PS IIB with RF a-c, IIIA with RF, IIIB, IIIAS, IV	R: 4 x COPP/ABVD ± RT 8 x BEACOPP ± RT 8 x BEACOPP ± RT	Improvement of treatment results by intensification of chemotherapy

CS = clinical stage; PS = pathological stage: RF = risk factors; EF = extended field; IF = involved field
E, C: escalated according to the BEACOPP escalation study; A: escalated to a fixed dosage

Explanation of chemotherapy regimens mentioned in Table 2.

COPP + ABVD

Cyclophosphamide	650 mg/m ^{2}	i.v.	Day 1 + 8
Vincristine	1.4 mg/m ^{2}	i.v. (max. 2 mg)	Day 1 + 8
Procarbazine	100 mg/m ^{2}	p.o.	Day 1-14
Prednisone	40 mg/m ^{2}	p.o.	Day 1-14
Doxorubicin	25 mg/m ^{2}	i.v.	Day 29 + 43
Bleomycin	10 mg/m ^{2}	i.v.	Day 29 + 43
Vinblastine	6 mg/m ^{2}	i.v.	Day 29 + 43
DTIC	375 mg/m ^{2}	i.v.	Day 29 + 43

Repeat on day 57

COPP + ABV + IMEP

Cyclophosphamide	800 mg/m ^{2}	i.v.	Day 1
Vincristine	1.4 mg/m ^{2}	i.v. (max. 2 mg)	Day 1
Procarbazine	100 mg/m ^{2}	p.o.	Day 1-10
Prednisone	40 mg/m ^{2}	p.o.	Day 1-15
Doxorubicin	40 mg/m ^{2}	i.v.	Day 15
Bleomycin	10 mg/m ^{2}	i.v.	Day 15
Vinblastine	6 mg/m ^{2}	i.v.	Day 15
Ifosfamide	1000 mg/m ^{2}	i.v.	Day 29-33
Methotrexate	30 mg/m ^{2}	i.v.	Day 31
Etoposide	100 mg/m ^{2}	i.v.	Day 29-31
Prednisone	40 mg/m ^{2}	p.o.	Day 29-35

Repeat on day 43

BEACOPP

Cyclophosphamide	650 mg/m ^{2}	i.v.	Day 1
Doxorubicin	25 mg/m ^{2}	i.v.	Day 1
Procarbazine	100 mg/m ^{2}	p.o.	Day 1-7
Etoposide	100 mg/m ^{2}	i.v.	Day 1-3
Vincristine	1.4 mg/m ^{2}	i.v. (max 2 mg)	Day 8
Bleomycin	10 mg/m ^{2}	i.v.	Day 8
Prednisone	40 mg/m ^{2}	p.o.	Day 1-14

Repeat on day 22

BEACOPP escalated

Cyclophosphamide	1250 mg/m ^{2}	i.v.
Etoposide	200 mg/m ^{2}	i.v.
Doxorubicin	35 mg/m ^{2}	i.v.

Dosage given according to the BEACOPP escalation study (data in press)

cases. Therefore, HDC+ABMT might be the treatment of choice for sensitive patients.

Sequelae of Treatment

Investigation of an international database covering 12,411 patients calculated a cumulative incidence rate of second tumours of 11.2% after 15 years [22], comprising 2.2% acute leukaemias, 1.8% non-Hodgkin's lymphomas, and 7.5% solid tumours. Most acute leukaemias are probably related to the use of alkylating agents. Acute myeloid leukaemias develop between 3 and 10 years after treatment for Hodgkin's disease. The prognosis of this type of acute leukaemia, which frequently involves translocation of chromosome 5, is poor, with remission rates of 30-40% and survival rates of less than 5%. The incidence of solid tumours is particularly alarming since there is a continuous increase in incidence rates. Risk factors for the development of solid tumours are age and radiotherapy.

Non-malignant sequelae of chemotherapy and radiotherapy in Hodgkin's disease patients are gonadal dysfunction observed in up to 86% of men and 77% of women treated with COPP-ABVD [29]. Other sequelae are thyroidal dysfunction, interstitial fibrosis, radiation-induced pneumocytis, cardiomyopathia and ischaemic coronary heart disease [30].

Experimental Treatment of Hodgkin's Disease

Hodgkin's disease may be an ideal target for immunotherapy for several reasons: the malignant Hodgkin and Reed-Sternberg cells (H-RS) express large quantities of antigens on the cell surface, like CD25 and CD30 which can be selectively recognized and destroyed by monoclonal antibody-based immunotoxins. In addition, Hodgkin's disease lymph nodes are well vascularized, which suggests that the access of antibodies or immunotoxins to the target antigens is easier than in solid tumours. The majority of cells in Hodgkin's tissue are reactive bystander cells. Therefore, the number of H-RS cells that have to be destroyed is relatively small. Thus a combined modality treatment might be feasible, consisting of standard chemotherapy or radiotherapy to reduce bulky disease, followed by administration of antibody-based immunotoxins to destroy residual tumour cells. Current experimental strategies involve bispecific monoclonal antibodies, anti-idiotypic antibodies and prodrugs which are activated by site-directed antibody-enzyme conjugates [31]. Ongoing clinical studies in patients with resistant Hodgkin's disease evaluate the use of ricin A-chain immunotoxins [32] or Saporin-6 immunotoxins [33]. These so-called magic bullets consist of potent toxins chemically linked to an antibody [31-33]. After binding to the cell surface, the immunotoxin is endocytosed. Intracellularly the toxin is released from the antibody and katalytically inhibits protein synthesis, resulting in cell death. Preliminary results seem to indicate a therapeutic effect of this approach in heavily pretreated patients.

REFERENCES

1 Glaser SL: Hodgkin's disease in black populations: A review of the epidemiologic literature. Sem Oncol 1990 (6):643-659
2 Diehl V, von Kalle C, Fonatsch C, Tesch H, Jücker M, Schaadt M: The cell of origin of Hodgkin's disease. Sem Oncol 1991 (17):660-672
3 Diehl V, Kirchner HH, Schaadt H et al: Hodgkin`s disease: establishment and characterization of four in vitro cell lines. J Cancer Res Clin Oncol 1981 (101):111-124
4 Stein H, Mason DY, Gerdes J et al: The expression of the Hodgkin's disease associated antigen Ki-1 in reactive and neoplastic lymphoid tissue: Evidence that Reed-Sternberg cells and histiocytic malignancies are derived from activated lymphoid cells. Blood 1985 (4):848-856
5 Dürkop H, Latza U, Hummel M et al: Molecular cloning and expression of a new member of the nerve growth factor receptor family that is characteristic for Hodgkin's disease. Cell 1992 (68):421-427
6 Kadin M: The Reed-Sternberg cell, an activated T-cell? The evidence has come full circle. Leukemia and Lymphoma Reviews 1992 (1):281-288
7 Poppema S, van Imhoff G, Torensma R et al: Lymphadenopathy morphologically consistent with Hodgkin's disease associated with EBV infection. Am J Clin Pathol 1985 (84):385-390
8 Gruss HJ, Brach MA, Drexler HG et al: Interleukin 9 Is expressed by primary and cultured Hodgkin and Reed-Sternberg cells. Cancer Res 1992 (52):1026-1031
9 Kapp U, Wolf J, von Kalle C et al: Growth of Hodgkin's lymphoma derived cell lines in immune compromised mice. Ann Oncol 1992 (3 suppl 4):21-24
10 Mueller N, Evans A, Harris NL et al: Hodgkin's disease and Epstein-Barr virus. N Engl J Med 1989 (320):689-692
11 Herbst H, Steinbrecher E, Nidobitek G et al: Distribution and phenotype of EBV-harboring cells in Hodgkin´s disease. Blood 1992 (80): in press
12 Trümper LH, Brady G, Vicini S, Cossman J, Mak TW: Gene expression in single Reed Sternberg cells of Hodgkin's disease: Results from PCR generated single cell cDNA libraries. Ann Oncol 1992 (3 suppl 4):25-26
13 Gause A, Jung W, Schmits R et al: Soluble CD8, CD25 and CD30 antigen as prognostic markers in patients with untreated Hodgkin's lymphoma. Ann Oncol 1992 (3 suppl 4): 49-52
14 Stein H, Schwarting R, Dallenbach F, Dienemann D: Immunology of Hodgkin and Reed-Sternberg cells. Rec Res Cancer Res 1989 (117):14-27
15 Lukes RJ, Butler JJ, Hicks EB: Natural history of Hodgkin's disease is related to its pathologic picture. Cancer 1966 (19):317-344
16 Hansmann ML, Wacker HH, Radzun HJ: Paragranuloma is a variant of Hodgkin's disease with predominance of B-cells. Virchows Arch A 1986 (409):171-181
17 MacLennan K A, Bennet MH, Ru A et al: Relationship of histopathologic features to survival and relapse in nodular sclerosing Hodgkin's disease. Cancer 1989 (64):1686-1693
18 Loeffler M, Mauch P, MacLennan K, Specht L, Henry-Amar M: Review on prognostic factors. Ann Oncol 1992 (3 suppl 4): 63-66
19 Kaplan HS: Hodgkin's disease: Unfolding concepts concerning its nature, management and prognosis. Cancer 1980 (45):2439-1474
20 Horning SJ, Hoppe RT, Hancock SL et al. Vinblastine, bleomycin and methotrexate: an effective adjuvant in favorable Hodgkin's disease. J Clin Oncol 1988 (6):1822-1831
21 Mauch P, Larson D, Osteen R et al: Prognostic factors for positive surgical staging in patients with Hodgkin's disease. J Clin Oncol 1990 (2):257-265
22 Henry-Amar M: Second cancer after the treatment for Hodgkin's disease: A report from the International Database on Hodgkin´s disease. Ann Oncol 1992 (3 suppl 4):117-128
23 Hellman S, Jaffe ES, DeVita VT: Hodgkin's Disease. Lippincott Company, Philadelphia 1989 pp 1696-1740
24 Bonadonna G and Santoro A: ABVD chemotherapy in the treatment of Hodgkin's disease. Cancer Treat Rev 1982 (9):21-35
25 Bonadonna G, Valagussa P, Santorano A: Alternating non-cross-resistant combination or MOPP in stage IV Hodgkin's disease. A report of 8-year results. Ann Intern Med 1986 (104):739-746
26 Klimo P and Connors JM: An update on the Vancouver experience in the management of advanced Hodgkin's disease treated with the MOPP/ABV hybrid program. Sem Hematol 1988 (25):34-40
27 Connors JM: MOPP/ABV hybrid versus alternating MOPP/ABVD for advanced Hodgkin's disease. Proc ASCO 1992 (11):1073a
28 Diehl V: Dose escalation study for the treatment of Hodgkin's disease. Ann Hematol 1992 (66):139-140
29 Kreuser ED, Felsenberg D, Behles C et al: Long-term gonadal dysfunction and its impact on bone mineralization in patients following COPP/ABVD chemotherapy for Hodgkin's disease. Ann Oncol 1992 (3 suppl 4):105-110
30 Valagussa P, Santoro A, Bonadonna G: Thyroid, pulmonary, and cardiac sequelae after treatment for Hodgkin's disease. Ann Oncol 1992 (3 suppl 4):111-116
31 Engert A, Pohl C, Diehl V: Experimental therapy in Hodgkin's disease. Ann Oncol 1992 (3 suppl 4):97-100
32 Engert A, Burrows F, Jung W et. al: Evaluation of ricin A-chain containing immunotoxins directed against CD30 as potential reagents for the treatment of Hodgkin's disease. Cancer Res 1990 (50): 84-88
33 Falini B, Bolognesi A, Flenghi L et al: Response of refractory Hodgkin's disease to monoclonal anti-CD30 immunotoxin. Lancet 1992 (339):1195

Normal B-Cell Ontogeny and B-Cell Malignancies: Biology of Low Grade Non-Hodgkin's Lymphomas

Vassiliki A. Boussiotis [1] and Gerassimos A. Pangalis [2]

1 Harvard Medical School, Division of Hematologic Malignancies, Dana-Farber Cancer Institute, Boston, MA 02115, U.S.A.
2 Leukaemia and Lymphoma Clinic, National and Kapodistrian University of Greece, School of Medicine, 1st Department of Medicine, Laikon General Hospital, Athens 11527, Greece

The non-Hodgkin's lymphomas (NHLs) are neoplasms of the immune system. Lymphomas retain the characteristics of their monoclonal counterparts to a greater or lesser extent and can be classified on this basis. The major advances in the understanding of the functional characteristics of normal lymphocytes have led to similar progress in our ability to characterize the neoplasms of lymphoid cells. B cells are traditionally defined as cells which express surface immunoglobulin (sIg) or could be induced to secrete immunoglobulin. T cells, although morphologically indistinguishable from B cells, have been classically defined by expression of sheep red blood cell receptors (E rosette receptor).

Thanks to the development of vast numbers of monoclonal antibodies (MoAbs) in the last decade, cell surface lymphoid differentiation Ags have been characterized. The identification of lineage-restricted markers for B and T cells has permitted the assignment of a lineage derivation for virtually all NHLs. Several studies report that over 80% of all cases of non-Hodgkin's lymphomas are of B-cell origin. This observation is based upon the expression of B-lineage restricted antigens and rearrangements of immunoglobulin heavy and light chain genes. The B-cell NHLs correspond to normal cells in the mid stages of normal differentiation [1,2]. The majority of lymphoblastic lymphomas correspond to stages of intrathymic differentiation whereas the peripheral T-cell NHLs generally resemble subsets of normal activated CD4+ T cells. A large number of studies have examined the relationship between surface marker expression and prognosis in NHL; however, their results remain controversial.

Ontogeny of Normal B Lymphocytes and B-Cell Malignancies

The main function of B lymphocytes is antigen recognition, which is facilitated by surface immunoglobulin molecules. This procedure activates the B lymphocyte and transforms it into an antibody secreting cell. B lymphocytes originate from the committed stem cell, which is produced in bone marrow and in fetal liver. This cell expresses only surface MHC class II antigens. In the next stage of differentiation pre-B lymphocytes acquire B-cell line characteristics (heavy-chain gene rearrangement) detectable at the molecular level. No surface immunoglobulin is yet detectable and the cell is not capable of recognizing antigens and secreting antibodies. At the next stage of maturation CD34 and CD19 appear on the cell surface. CD19 is a 95 kDa glycoprotein which appears to be involved in B cell growth and may play a role in the regulation of Ca^{++} levels. CD19 is the most reliable cell surface marker of B lineage at the pre-B cell level. CD34, a 115 kDa glycoprotein, is also present on myeloid progenitor cells. In addition to these cell surface proteins, a B-cell restricted Ag, CD22, is present in the cytoplasm (cCD22) at the earliest stages of pre-B differentiation and exported to the cell surface at the mature resting B-cell stage when IgD is first expressed. CD22 has homologies to myelin-associated glycoprotein and the neural adhesion molecule NCAM. CD22 may be involved in transducing signals via surface Ig.

Following the appearance of CD19 and cytoplasmic CD22, cells express CD10 (CALLA).

CD10 is a zinc metalloprotease which is identical to neural endopeptidase and encephalinase. This enzyme is capable of inactivating a variety of peptide hormones including glucagon, encephalin, atrial natriuretic peptide, substance P, oxytokin, bradykinin, neutrotensin and angiotensins I and II. However, to date its precise function on lymphoid cells is unknown. Pre-B cells next express the pan-B cell restricted Ag CD20. CD20 is a non-glycosylated phosphoprotein which probably functions as an ion channel. At the last stage of pre-B cell ontogeny after the completion of heavy chain immunoglobulin gene rearrangements, cytoplasmic μ Ig heavy chain appears without the expression of light chains. After the completion of light chain immunoglobulin gene rearrangements (κ,λ), IgM with or without IgD is expressed on the cell surface. This immature B lymphocyte (early and intermediate) expresses also CD21 (receptor for mouse erythrocytes) and is the normal counterpart of chronic lymphocytic leukaemia and small lymphocytic lymphoma. As the cells mature, the CD21 antigen is lost, surface IgM increases and cells acquire the ability of responding to antigens. Mature B cells are exported to the peripheral blood and secondary lymphoid organs, where they reside until activated by Ag. Mature B cells express sIgM/D and HLA-DR, CD19, CD20, CD24, CD22 but not CD10. Coincident with the maturation to the sIg+ stage, cells express CD11a/18 (LFA-1), a member of the integrin family of adhesion molecules. CD11a/18 mediates a variety of cell-cell interactions of B cells including homotypic (B-B) adhesion as well as adhesion of B cells to T lymphocytes, monocytes and endothelium. Resting B cells also express a 90 kDa glycoprotein, CD44, and LAM-1 (Leu 8), which have recently been shown to be involved in lymphocyte recirculation and homing, including the adhesion of lymphocytes to endothelial venules. Two complement receptors, CD21 and CD35, are also present on resting B cells. Following triggering with Ag or various polyclonal mitogens, resting B cells are activated and subsequently proliferate. Within 24 hours of activation resting B cells begin to lose sIgD, CD21 and CD22 and this process is completed by 72 to 96 hrs. As these Ags are lost, a number of B restricted and associated Ags sequentially appear. Antigen-stimulated mature B lymphocyte becomes activated and expresses activation antigens (CD71 (transferrin receptor), CD54 (ICAM-1) Blast-1, CD25, CD5, CD23, B5, B7 and T9). These activation Ags include growth factor receptors, which regulate proliferation and differentiation and structures involved in cell-cell interaction and molecules which play a role in the localization and binding of activated B cells within a microenvironment. Some of the activated B lymphocytes retain their surface Ig and become memory cells and others undergo heavy chain class switch and become antibody secreting cells, capable of responding to antigens by secreting immunoglobulin (IgM, IgD, IgG, IgA, IgE) [2]. Normal activated B cells bind to germinal centres (GC) by adhesive interactions mediated by the receptor-ligand pair VLA-4 (expressed on B cells): VCAM-1 (expressed on follicular dendritic cells) [3]. Neoplastic counterparts of mature B cells are follicular lymphoma, prolymphocytic leukaemia, chronic lymphocytic leukaemia, hairy cell leukaemia and Waldenström's macroglobulinaemia. The final stage of B-cell differentiation is the plasma cell. These mature cells, which are able to synthesize and secrete immunoglobulins, lack all the B-cell specific markers and express only cytoplasmic immunoglobulin and the new surface antigens PC-1 and PA-1.

One typical biological characteristic of lymphomas is the escape from the normal regulation of cellular proliferation. Escape from normal growth control results from a defect in the external regulatory mechanism itself or from an intrinsic defect in a cell's ability to respond to regulatory signals. These two very different types of derangements provide a convenient and logical means of defining neoplastic and non-neoplastic lymphoproliferation.

Determining the presence of cytogenetic abnormalities and, at another level, molecular genetic abnormalities, may be a particularly valuable method of classifying lymphomas, since their genetic changes are critical to the pathogenesis. The most accurate definition of lymphoma type is one which includes all of these characteristics. In the case of molecular abnormalities, which are unique to the malignant clone, the methods of detection have become so sensitive that the presence of neoplastic cells in some tissues can be detected in the absence of morphological evidence. The classification of low-grade lymphomas, including

Table 1. Classification of Low Grade Non-Hodgkin's Lymphomas

Working Formulation	Rappaport	Cellular origin B	T (%)	Chromosomal abnormalities
Small Lymphocytic	Diffuse well differentiated lymphocytic	98	2	Trisomy 12 t(11;14)* t(14;19)
Follicular predominantly small cleaved	Nodular poorly differentiated lymphocytic	100		t(14;18)
Follicular mixed, small cleaved and large cell	Nodular mixed lymphocytic histiocytic	100		t(14;18) Trisomy 8

* This chromosomal aberration is very frequently found in mantle cell lymphoma so it is currently considered as a specific marker for this type of lymphoma

their histological and immunological characteristics and chromosomal abnormalities, is shown in Table 1.

Classification and Biology of Low Grade Lymphomas

Small Lymphocytic Lymphoma (SLL)

Although on lymph node tissue sections SLL is morphologically indistinguishable from chronic lymphocytic leukaemia (CLL), it differs from the latter in the absence of absolute blood lymphocytosis, the rare complication of anaemia, autoimmune haemolysis and hypo-gammaglobulinaemia, and the expression of adhesion molecules [4]. The vast majority of SLLs express B-cell markers including sIg, usually of IgM type with or without IgD, although of low intensity compared to that of follicular lymphomas. SLL may have plasmatocytoid features with amphophilic cytoplasm or intracellular inclusion of immunoglobulin and may be accompanied by a monoclonal, usually IgM, component. Although this latter entity has been classified as a separate category by the Kiel classification, the biology, immunological findings and natural history of the disease do not differ significantly from that of other SLLs [4]. Other surface markers include complement receptors for the Fc portion of IgG; in addition, the cells express CD5, a pan-T-cell antigen with unique expression in CLL and small lymphocytic lymphoma [4]. Trisomy 12 is common in CLL. It is speculated that neoplastic transformation or abnormal proliferation in these cases may be related to the cellular ki-*ras*-2 oncogene present on chromosome 12 [5].

Follicular Cell Lymphoma (FCL)

Based on their morphologic and phenotypic characteristics, FCL cells are thought to be the neoplastic counterparts of germinal centre (GC) B cells. Furthermore, the architecture of these tumours reproduces the structure and cellular composition of normal secondary follicles as evidenced by the presence of follicular dendritic cells (FDCs) and CD4+ T cells [6]. It is unknown what makes FCL reproduce the structure of normal GCs. A possible explanation could be that neoplastic B cells use similar mechanisms of localization and adhesion as normal B cells in binding to GCs. FCLs are characteristically diseases that are widely disseminated at diagnosis with infiltration of peripheral and mesenteric lymphoid tissue, bone marrow and peripheral blood. The hypothesis that FCLs are neoplastic counterparts of GC B cells may explain the pattern of spread. A subset of normal GC B cells leave the GC microenvironment to become terminally differentiated B cells in the bone marrow, circulating memory B cells or mucosa-associated plasma cells. FCLs reflect the migration pattern of normal GC cells, with some neoplastic cells remaining in the follicles and others having the capacity to migrate to the bone marrow, gut-associated lymphoid tissue and mesenteric nodes, common sites of disease involvement. Neoplastic and normal GCs are composed of similar types of non-neoplastic cells [6]. In particular the FDCs in FCL are reported to be phenotypically similar to normal FDCs. Although VCAM-1 is expressed in malignant GCs, its ability to function as a ligand for VLA-4 is abnormal. The disseminated nature of FCL may reflect the fact that adhesive interactions via VLA-4:VCAM-1 on FDCs in multiple secondary lymphoid tissue contribute to the tropism for these sites seen in follicular NHLs [7]. Recent studies have indicated that lymphoma cells might determine and direct the architecture of the tumour. Moreover, a *de novo* appearance of numerous FDCs in the paratrabecular bone marrow infiltrates has been reported in FCL. This suggests that cells of two different lineages, lymphoid neoplastic B cells and non-lymphoid FDCs, are proliferating in this neoplasm. The cellular interaction of follicular NHL cells and their microenvironment may not only be of biological significance but also of prognostic importance.

Approximately 85% of FCLs bear the translocation t(14;18) (q32;q21) [8]. The *bcl*-2 oncogene was discovered in the t(14;18) (q32;q21) breakpoint [9]. The *bcl*-2 translocation comprises 2 exons transcribed into 3 messages of 8, 5 and 3.2 kb which arise by differential splicing and polyadenylation. These transcripts encode two proteins, *bcl*-2a (239 amino acids) and *bcl*-2b (205 amino acids), which differ at their carboxy termini. *Bcl*-2 is novel among the proto-oncogenes in that it localizes in mitochondria [10]. In addition, it appears to be a member of a new category of oncogenes named "regulators of programmed cell death". Programmed cell death represents an autonomous suicidal pathway that helps restrict cell numbers. *Bcl*-2 displays a unique functional role of blocking programmed cell death independent of affecting proliferation. The restricted topographic distribution of the *bcl*-2 protein has provided useful information regarding its physiological role. One of the most striking examples was provided by study of the secondary germinal centres. *Bcl*-2 was absent from the zone of rapidly proliferating cells and from the area in which centrocytes die by apoptosis. In contrast, it was present in the area of long-lived recirculating B cells and the zone in which a subset of B cells is thought to be selected for survival by their affinity for residual antigen, present on follicular dendritic cells. Furthermore, in an *in vivo* murine model it has been shown that the physiological role of *bcl*-2 involves generation and maintenance of B-cell memory.

All haematopoietic cell lineages that derive from a renewing stem cell display high levels of *bcl*-2. It has also been found in plasma cell dyscrasias, chronic myelogenous leukaemia and T-cell neoplasms of mature phenotype. It is present in the surviving mature thymocytes of the thymic medulla, and in several other normal tissues in which apoptosis moulds developing structures or helps maintain tissue homeostasis. The increased cell numbers in neoplastic tissue can be a result of dysregulation of normal homeostasis. The maintenance of remarkably stable cell numbers must reflect tightly regulated death pathways as well as controlled proliferation. The expression of *bcl*-2, which prevents cell death, can be a potential mechanism involved in the development of neoplasia. The detection of t(14;18) breakpoints allows the identification of a single clonogenic cell population. Polymerase chain reaction (PCR) enables the detection of one malignant cell within 10^5 normal cells [11] and can be helpful in diagnosis, follow-up and detection of minimal residual disease.

Mantle Cell Lymphoma

Mantle cell lymphomas (MCL) belong to the category of "intermediate differentiated" lymphomas as their morphology is similar both to small cleaved cell and small lymphocytic lymphoma [12]. The phenotypic characteristics of these lymphomas are those of the cells in the normal mantle surrounding germinal centres [12]. These lymphomas, in contrast to other B-cell malignancies, are more likely to express the λ light chain. They are CD5 positive like B chronic lymphocytic leukaemia but CD23 and CD10 negative. In addition to morphology and immunophenotyping, cytogenetic similarities among these lymphomas support their common cell origin and their distinction from SLL and FCL. The most common cytogenetic marker in MCL is the t(11;14) (q13;q32) translocation, in which the rearranged *bcl*-1 (also called PRAD1) gene from chromosome 11 is juxtaposed to the IgH enhancer locus on chromosome 14 [13]. The *bcl*-1/PRAD1 gene encodes for cyclin D, which was found to be abnormally expressed in all *bcl*-1-positive MCL [13-15]. The deregulation of the normal control of the cell cycle which is the consequence of cyclin D overexpression, appears to be associated with the malignant aberration. Although the t(11;14) has also been detected in other B-cell malignancies, it has a significantly higher incidence in mantle cell lymphomas [16]. The significance of this translocation appears to be analogous to that of *bcl*-2 or c-*myc* translocation and dysregulation, which are associated with the malignant transformation in follicular lymphomas and Burkitt's lymphoma, respectively.

REFERENCES

1 Foon KA: Laboratory and clinical applications of monoclonal antibodies for leukemias and non-Hodgkin's lymphoma. Curr Probl Cancer 1989 (13):57-128

2 Freedman AS and Nadler LM: Immunologic markers in non-Hodgkin's lymphoma. Hematol/Oncol Clin North Am 1991(5):871-889

3 Freedman AS, Munro MJ, Rice GE et al: Adhesion of human B cells to germinal centers in vitro involves VLA-4 and INCAM-110. Science 1990 (249):1030-1033

4 Pangalis GA, Boussiotis VA, Kittas Ch: Malignant disorders of small lymphocytes. Small lymphocytic lymphoma, lymphoplasmacytic lymphoma and chronic lymphocytic leukemia: Their clinical and laboratory relationship. Am J Clin Pathol 1993 (99): 402-408

5 Jhanwar SC, Neel BG, Hayward WS, Chaganti RS: Localization of c-ras oncogene family on human germ line chromosomes. Proc Natl Acad Sci 1983 (80):4794-4797

6 Stein H, Gerdes J, Mason DY: The normal and malignant germinal center. Clin Hematol 1982 (11):531-559

7 Freedman AS, Munro MJ, Morimoto C, McIntyre BW, Rhynhart K, Lee N, Nadler LM: Follicular non-Hodgkin's lymphoma cell adhesion to normal germinal centers and neoplastic follicles involves very late antigen-4 and vascular adhesion molecule-1. Blood 1992 (79):206-212

8 Yunis JJ, Frizzera G, Oken MM, McKenna J, Theologides A, Arnesen M: Multiple recurrent genomic defects in follicular lymphoma. N Engl J Med 1987 (316):79-84

9 Cleary ML and Sklar J: Nucleoside sequence of a t(14;18) chromosomal breakpoint in follicular lymphoma and demonstration of a breakpoint cluster region near a transcriptionally active locus on chromosome 18. Proc Natl Acad Sci USA 1985 (81): 593-597

10 Korsmeyer SJ: Bcl-2 initiates a new category of oncogenes: Regulators of cell death. Blood 1992 (80):879-886

11 Gribben JG, Neuberg D, Freedman AS et al: Detection by polymerase chain reaction of residual cells with the bcl-2 translocation is associated with increased risk of relapse after autologous bone marrow transplantation for B-cell lymphoma. Blood 1993 (81):3449-3457

12 Weisenburger DD: Mantle cell lymphoma. In: Knowles DM (ed) Neoplastic Hematopathology. Williams and Wilkins, Baltimore 1992 pp 617-628

13 Rosenberg CL, Wong E, Petty EM, Bale AE, Tsujimoto Y, Harris NL, Arnold A: PRAD-1, a candidate BCL1 oncogene: Mapping and expression in centrocytic lymphoma. Proc Natl Acad Sci 1991 (88):9638-9642

14 Motokura T, Bloom T, Kim HG et al: A novel cyclin encoded by a bcl-1 linked candidate oncogene. Nature 1991 (359):512-515

15 Raffeld M, Sander CA, Yano T, Jaffe E: Mantle cell lymphoma: An update. Leukemia and Lymphoma 1992 (8):161-166

16 De Wolf-Peeters and Pittalega S: Mantle cell lymphoma. Ann Oncology 1994 (5 suppl 1):35-37

Treatment of Low-Grade Non-Hodgkin's Lymphomas

Maria K. Angelopoulou and Gerassimos A. Pangalis

Leukaemia and Lymphoma Clinic, 1st Department of Internal Medicine, National and Kapodistrian University of Greece, School of Medicine, Laikon General Hospital, Athens 11527, Greece

Low-grade non-Hodgkin's lymphomas (LGNHL) are characterized by a rather indolent clinical course, in contrast to the intermediate and high-grade lymphomas. To this category belong diffuse well differentiated lymphocytic lymphoma (DLWD), nodular lymphocytic poorly differentiated lymphoma (NLPD), nodular mixed lymphocytic-histiocytic lymphoma (NM) and nodular histiocytic lymphoma (NH) according to the Rappaport classification; small lymphocytic lymphoma (SLL), lymphoplasmacytic lymphoma (LPL), follicular small cleaved-cell lymphoma (FSCL) and follicular mixed small cleaved and large cell lymphoma (FML) according to the Working Formulation. These two classifications have been extensively used in clinical trials and their clinical value has been acknowledged. In addition to the above categories new histological entities have recently been recognised in the group of LGNHLs which deserve special mention. These are the nodular form of mantle cell lymphoma, the monocytoid B-cell lymphoma and some forms of the mucosa-associated lymphoid tissue (MALT) lymphomas. Most patients (~75-80%) with LGNHL present with advanced disease (stage III or IV) which proves to be incurable although many new drugs and combinations have been added to the therapeutic armamentarium [1-3]. In spite of the fact that the median survival of some of these lymphoma types has reached 9 years [2], their natural history seems only modestly affected by the available therapeutic manoeuvres.

Newly diagnosed LGNHL patients respond adequately to treatment, but afterwards relapses are the rule, even many years after the documentation of complete remission [4]. When relapses occur, refractoriness to conventional chemotherapy usually develops so that desperate salvage treatment is needed. Furthermore, 15-50% of these patients develop histological transformation to intermediate-grade NHL [5-7] with a poor prognosis (median survival < 1 year) [5-7]. In this chapter we will discuss the different therapeutic approaches to these undefeatable categories of lymphomas.

Single-Agent Chemotherapy

Chlorambucil and Cyclophosphamide

Chemotherapy with oral alkylating agents and prednisone is the most frequently used treatment for LGNHL, producing a response rate of approximately 65-80% in newly diagnosed patients [3,8-11]. The standard therapy is chlorambucil 10 mg orally per day for 10-14 days every month for 4-24 months in different studies [1,8,12]. Prednisone may be added if blood counts are low due to bone marrow infiltration, or when B symptoms are prominent [13].

The ECOG [1,14] used alkylators in randomized studies: either daily cyclophosphamide or chlorambucil, or pulse chlorambucil or cyclophosphamide. The duration of treatment to achieve a response is quite long [1] (longer than with combined modality treatment), therefore single agents should not be selected when urgent reduction of the disease is required, for example in the case of compressive phenomena or bulky tumour. In addition, patients with discordant histology at diagnosis, displaying a large cell component, should receive more intensive therapy than alkylators alone. In our Unit [15] 25 patients with FSCL were randomly assigned to receive either chlorambucil plus prednisone or the CVP regimen. Fourteen of them were treated with chlorambucil at a dose of 10 mg/day for 10 days and prednisone at a dose of 60 mg/day for 10 days orally every month for 2 years. The response rate was 64% [15]. In a later report from our Unit 53 patients with LGNHL were treated either with chlorambucil only or chlorambucil plus interferon α-2b [12]. Nineteen of them were treated with chlorambucil only at a dose of 10 mg/day orally for 10 days every month for at least 6 months and prolonged to 9, 12, 15 or 18 months if a consistent response was evident. The overall response rate was 79% with 31.5% complete remission (CR). The median duration of CR was 16 months. The median time to achieve maximum response was 7.6 months [12].

In a large randomized study Hoppe et al. compared single-agent chemotherapy, combination chemotherapy (CVP) and whole body irradiation [1]. Oral chlorambucil or cyclophosphamide was administered as a single agent for 2 years. CR was achieved in 64% of the patients who received single-agent therapy. The median time to achieve a CR was 12 months [1].

During the last decade many trials have been published, some of them randomized, with similar results. CR rates range between 45% and 65% with an overall response rate (including PR) up to 90% [3,11,14,16,17].

Ezdinli et al. made some important observations on the response to single agents in relation to the different histological subtypes [17]. It seems that alkylators are more effective in diffuse well differentiated lymphocytic lymphoma than combined chemotherapy, with a CR rate of 60% vs 51% with COPP and 40% with BCVP; however, DLWD patients had the lowest 1-year survival compared to NM or NLPD. By contrast in NLPD, which is the most favourable subtype, single-agent chemotherapy achieved the lowest CR rate (48% vs 65% with COPP and 69% with BCVP) [17].

In conclusion, monotherapy with alkylating agents (chlorambucil or cyclophosphamide) seems to be the standard approach for patients with LGNHL. In many randomized trials no benefit was proved for more aggressive regimens over single-agent therapy. The higher response rate that may be achieved by combination chemotherapy does not reflect a better disease-free survival (DFS) or a better overall survival [18,19]. The milder toxicity of single-agent therapy shoud also be taken into consideration.

Mitoxanthrone

Mitoxanthrone is an anthracycline derivative. It causes cell death by intercalating DNA and inducing single strand and double strand breaks. It inhibits DNA and RNA synthesis [20]. It induces a block in the G_2 phase of the cell cycle [20]. Cells are more sensitive in the S phase. The drug is not cell cycle-specific and is also effective in non dividing lymphocytes [20]. Mitoxanthrone accumulates at high quantities in bone marrow, white blood cells and lymph node malignant cells [20]. The most important route of elimination is faecal [21].

In recent studies mitoxanthrone has been used as monotherapy for LGNHL [22-24] (Table 1). Gams et al. used mitoxanthrone in pretreated patients with refractory non-Hodgkin's lymphoma. This study was not restricted to low-grade histology [22]. Two different schedules were used: a) a dose of 5 mg/m^2/day every week for a total of 6 courses, and b) a dose of 14 mg/m^2 once every 4 weeks for a total of 2 courses. With the first schedule they achieved a 13% response rate but no responses in the LGNHL category. The high-dose intermittent schedule proved to be significantly more effective, with a 63% response rate and most of the responses occurring in the low-grade group [22]. Nissen and Hansen studied a group of 21 untreated patients with advanced-stage LGNHL [23]. They administered mitoxanthrone at a dose of 5 mg/m^2/day for 3 consecutive days every 3 weeks for a minimum of 8 cycles. They obtained a 100% response rate with 43% CR. The best response was observed in follicular histology [23].

In our Unit we used mitoxanthrone monotherapy as salvage treatment for relapsed LGNHL patients who were refractory to conventional chemotherapy [24]. All 14 patients were pretreated with 2-6 prior regimens. We administered mitoxanthrone at a dose of 6 mg/m^2/day for 3 consecutive days every 3 or 4 weeks. The median number of treatment cycles was 4. We observed an overall response rate of 54% with 7.7% CR. Response to treatment was significantly better in less pretreated patients. We also observed a trend towards a better

Table 1. Mitoxanthrone in LGNHL

Author	No. of pts.	Schedule	Response	Duration of response Survival
Gams 1983 [22]	a. 6	a. 5 mg/m2/week	CR + PR: 0%, SD: 50%	NG
	b. 5, pretreated intermediate also included	b. 14 mg/m2/3 weeks	PR: 80%	
Coltman 1983 [22a]	37, pretreated low-intermediate and high-grade also included	12 mg/m2/3 weeks	CR: 6% PR: 18%	NG
Nissen 1990 [23]	21, untreated	5 mg/m2/day for 3 days/3 weeks	CR: 43% PR: 57%	5-yr FFS: 48% 5-yr overall survival: 90%
Angelopoulou 1994 [24]	14, pretreated	6 mg/m2/day for 3 days/3-4 weeks	CR: 8% PR: 46%	med. dur. CR: 3 mo med. dur. PR: 3.5 mo med. over. surv.: 7 mo

CR: complete remission; PR: partial response; SD: stable disease; FFS: failure-free survival; NG: not given

outcome in follicular histology. The median survival after mitoxanthrone administration was 7 months. We concluded that mitoxanthrone is quite effective as salvage treatment in relapsed LGNHL, considering the limited therapeutic alternatives for these patients [24].

Combination Chemotherapy

Many different regimens have been used for the treatment of LGNHL in an effort to obtain not only higher remission rates but also, and most importantly, a cure for these diseases, which proved to be incurable with single agents: the overall and disease-free survival curves showed no plateau even at 10 years, despite the high response rates with chlorambucil or cyclophosphamide [25-27]. Relapses, even late ones, are the rule [27]. After relapse the outcome is bad, as in most cases refractoriness develops.

The initial trials used CVP (cyclophosphamide, vincristine and prednisone) as combined modality treatment. Different schedules were employed, e.g. every other week for a minimum of 6 cycles [28], weekly for 6 weeks [29], or oral cyclophosphamide and prednisone 5 days a week and vincristine on day 1, to be repeated every 3 weeks for a minimum of 6 cycles [14]. In all these studies the CR rates ranged from 30% to 57% [6,28,29]. The overall response rate was also very high (up to 90%). In later studies with CVP, higher complete response rates were achieved due to prolongation of treatment, with a CR ranging between 62% and 81% and a median duration of CR between 17 and 40 months [30-33].

In our Unit patients with FSCL were randomized to receive either chlorambucil and prednisone or CVP (cyclophosphamide 600 mg/m2/week x 6 weeks i.v., vincristine 1.4 mg/m2/week x 6 weeks i.v. and prednisone 60 mg/day x 28 days orally) [15]. The complete remission rate was almost identical in the two groups (64% vs 63%) and so was the relapse rate (42%) [15].

Kennedy et al. studied a series of 53 patients with LGNHL who were randomly assigned to receive either cyclophosphamide orally or CVP [14]. They obtained a CR rate of 68% with CVP vs 48% with the single agent [14]. The duration of response was 37+ months for the CVP group vs 25+ months for the other group, but this difference and the median survival were not statistically significant [14]. On further analysis of their results they found that CVP was highly effective in nodular lymphomas when compared to cyclophosphamide alone, with an almost double CR rate. The duration of CR and survival were also better in the CVP-treated group, and the majority of patients who were alive at the time of publication received the CVP regimen [14].

Hoppe et al. studied 51 patients randomized to receive either chlorambucil or cyclophosphamide as a single agent, or CVP or whole body irradiation (WBI) [1]. Higher CR rates were observed also in this study with CVP vs the single agent (88% vs 64%) [1]. The time required for CR achievement was shorter for CVP-treated patients (5 vs 12 months). In this study and in all others no significant differences could be found in overall and disease-free survival between single agent therapy and CVP. The actuarial survival at 4 years was 84%, with 25% being free of relapse [1]. In most of the patients the natural history of the disease does not change with the CVP regimen. Higher response rates can be achieved with longer administration of either single-agent or combined therapy.

Other groups have used more aggressive chemotherapy in an effort to cure. The NCI group investigated the ProMACE/MOPP regimen vs watchful waiting for LGNHL patients [34]. Eighty-nine patients were randomized to receive ProMACE/MOPP+TNI or no treatment. Of the 43 patients in the former group, 78% achieved a CR with a median duration of response >45 months. After 4 years >70% of the patients were in CR. In the "watch-and-wait" group 56% were still under observation and 44% had to cross over to ProMACE/MOPP due to disease progression, with a lower response rate (43%). The overall survival was similar (83% vs 84%), but a significantly larger number of patients treated with the combined modality are alive without disease (51% vs 12%) and alive continuously free of disease (51% vs 0%). Although the CR rates are similar in different aggressive chemotherapeutic regimens, ProMACE/MOPP produced longer CR (45+ months vs 12-26 months) and better DFS (51% vs 24%) [34].

McLaughlin et al. administered CHOP-Bleo to 96 patients with stage IV disease, obtaining a CR rate of 77% and a PR of 20% [35]. Failure-free survival (FFS) at 5 years was 29% for all patients and 37% for CRs. Survival and FFS curves did not reach a plateau. The median FFS was 30 months, while the median survival was 102 months. Only 30% survived at 10 years, mostly with disease. From the analysis of the above data it seems that patients who achieved a CR had a better outcome (40 months FFS vs 8 months for PRs and 100 months overall survival vs 37 months) [35,36].

In many studies the 5-year DFS is significantly better, especially in follicular mixed lymphoma in which a survival advantage has even been documented with the CHOP-Bleo regimen. This has been confirmed by the CALGB group, which compared CHOP-Bleo with cyclophosphamide in the mixed and small cleaved-cell lymphomas [37-39]. The SWOG studied follicular lymphoma and found no significant differences with COP-Bleo, CHOP-Bleo or CHOP-BCG [40]. The NCI group investigated the effect of C-MOPP on the follicular mixed variety. The CR rate was 76%, and 52% of the patients were still in CR at 7 years [41]. The median survival was estimated to be 13 years for CRs vs 19 months for non-CRs [41]. In a study by Ezdinli et al. patients randomly received COPP, BCVP or CP (cyclophosphamide plus prednisone). No statistically significant differences were found between the 3 groups. The toxicity, however, was higher with the aggressive regimen [17]. The same observations were made by Jones et al. comparing CHOP with COP-Bleo. In another study by ECOG, cyclophosphamide, vincristine and adriamycin were administered on day 1 and prednisone on days 1-5 every 4 weeks, with a CR rate of 29% and a PR rate of 57% [42]. The GELF group has used the CAP-VM26 combination which consists of cyclophosphamide, VM26 and adriamycin on day 1 and prednisone on days 1-5 with CR 13% and PR 45% [43]. In another ECOG study BCNU plus prednisone gave poorer results than cyclophosphamide [44].

In follicular mixed lymphoma survival depends strongly upon the achievement of CR (median survival for CRs 13 years vs 19 months for non-CRs) [41]. Therefore it is essential in FML that CR be obtained with any type of treatment. Initially follicular mixed lymphoma seemed to be a curable subtype, but late relapses occur also in this category [18,41].

New combinations are currently being tried for newly diagnosed and refractory patients with LGNHL, for example BP-VACOP plus RT [45], mitoxanthrone-etoposide and prednisone (MEP) [46], bleomycin, vincristine and methyloprednisone [47], or oral etoposide, chlorambucil, procarbazine and prednisone [48]. McLaughlin et al. have introduced a new intensive regimen for stage IV LGNHL consisting of

3 alternating combinations [49]: a) CHOP-Bleo (based on cyclophosphamide, doxorubicin), b) ESHAP (with VP16, ara-C, platinum) and c) NOPP (based on mitoxanthrone, procarbazine). The CR rate was 81%. The overal survival was 94% at 4 years and the FFS 52%. No plateau in the FFS curve was observed here either.

As can be seen little improvement has been made with this variety of combination regimens as far as overall survival is concerned, except for the follicular mixed lymphoma [37-39,41]. Benefits which are not confirmed by all studies might be a higher CR rate, a longer CR rate, a longer duration of response and a better DFS.

Interferon-alpha

Many different mechanisms of action have been postulated for its efficacy such as modulation of oncogenes (e.g. c-*myc*), cell cycle arrest and others [50]. Especially for lymphoid malignancies the following actions have been presumed. IFN-α induces the enzyme 2-5 oligoadenylate-synthetase which leads, through RNA degrading, to activation of growth promoting oncogenes or genes responsible for growth factors such as TNF-α and interleukins [50]. The immunoregulatory effects of INF-α play a certain role too. It upregulates specific cell surface antigens such as MHC, and therefore application of IFN-α with monoclonal antibodies may be a valid approach for treating lymphoid malignancies [51].

Interferon-α has been given to LGNHL patients in several phase I and II randomized trials and it has been shown to be mostly effective in LGNHL. Many forms of application have been investigated: a) as a single agent, b) in combination with single-agent chemotherapy, c) in combination with more aggressive chemotherapy, and d) together with other biological agents (on the basis of its upregulation of cell surface antigens).

Interferon-alpha as a Single Agent

Interferon-α has been used in LGNHL at a dose of 3-50 MU/m^2 as monotherapy, in different schedules, with a modest effect [52,53-66] (Table 2). In phase I and II trials a response rate of 40-50% with 5-33% CRs was observed [52,53-66]. The response to IFN-α is very slow and therefore it is not an appropriate treatment for patients with bulky or symptomatic disease, in whom immediate disease regression is needed. Between 1978 and 1990 19 studies reported in the literature used IFN-α as monotherapy in pretreated patients with LGNHL. Response rates (CR+PR) ranged from 11% to 100% [19,53-66]. The 100% rate was achieved in the study of Merigan et al. which inlcuded only 3 patients [53]. The mean response rate in these studies was 40%. One should bear in mind that the patients included were pretreated patients who had relapsed after other treatments.

Interferon-alpha in Combination with Alkylating Agents

In order to obtain higher response rates in LGNHL IFN-α was combined with single-agent or combination chemotherapy. In many published trials IFN-α was used either in the induction phase or as maintenance therapy in patients with minimal residual disease or in both.

Response rates up to 85% have been reported (Table 3) [12,67-74]. Chisesi et al. compared the effect of chlorambucil alone vs chlorambucil plus IFN-α. Chlorambucil was administered orally at 5 mg/day on days 1-21 and IFN-α2b at a dose of 3 MU/m^2 subcutaneously 3 times/week for 6 months. In the other group, patients received chlorambucil 10 mg/day orally on days 1-21 as monotherapy. No significant difference in response was observed [72]. On the other hand results from our Unit show an advantage in the group of patients who had been treated with chlorambucil plus IFN-α2b versus chlorambucil alone [12]. With our schedule patients received IFN-α2b at a dose of 3 MU/day for 5 days and subsequently chlorambucil 10 mg/day for 10 days or chlorambucil only for at least 6 months up to 18 months, depending on the response. A significant difference was observed as far as CR was concerned with an advantage for the group that received IFN-α2b (CR rate: 47.5% vs 31.5%). In addition, responders (CR+PR) received or did not receive IFN-α2b as maintenance therapy. No statistically significant differences were observed in relapse rate or duration

Table 2. Interferon-α in LGNHL as monotherapy

Author	No. of pts.	Schedule	Response	Duration of response Survival
Gutterman 1980 [54]	7 (6 LGNHL)	$3x10^6$ IU/m^2/d IFN partially purified	CR: 33% PR: 17%	Duration of response: 4-11 mo
Louie 1981 [55]	11 (8 LGNHL)	Partially purified human leukocyte IFN $5x10^6$ IU/m^2 twice daily for 1 month	CR: 12.5% PR: 37.5%	Duration of response: 6-12 mo
Foon 1984 [64]	37 (24 LGNHL)	Recombinant α-2a-IFN $50x10^6$ IU/m^2 3x/w, mostly reduced to $5x10^6$/m^2 i.m. for 3 mo+	CR: 17% PR: 37.5%	Median duration of response: 8 months
Gams 1984 [58]	17 follicular pretreated	Polyclonal lymphoblastoid IFN a. $5x10^6$ IU/m^2 3x/week x 8 weeks b. if failure to a. $30x10^6$ IU/m^2/dx10 days	CR+PR: 23% with a. PR: 33% with b.	NG
Quesada 1984 [59]	17	Recombinant α-2a-IFN $3\text{-}50x10^6$ IU/m^2/d for 8 weeks i.m.	CR: 12% PR: 24%	Duration of response: 2-12 mo
Horning 1985 [60]	18 follicular	Partially purified human IFN 1,3,$9x10^6$ IU/d in x30 d	PR: 17% MR: 17%	Duration of response: 4-8 mo
Wagstaff 1986 [62]	34 pretreated (intermediate also included)	Recombinant α-2a-IFN $2x10^6$ IU/m^2 3x/week x 12 mo	CR: 6% PR: 44%	NG
O'Connell 1986 [63]	16	Recombinant α-2a-IFN $12x10^6$ IU/m^2 3x/week then once a week for 1 month	CR: 6% PR:37.5%	Median duration of response: 6 months
Leavitt 1987 [65]	46 (21 LGNHL)	Recombinant α-2b-IFN $10x10^6$ IU/m^2 3x/week	CR: 14% PR: 14%	Median duration of response for all responders 3.5 mo (intermediate, high included)
Foon 1987 [57]	24	Recombinant α-2a-IFN $50x10^6$ IU/m^2 3x/week	CR+PR: 54%	Median duration of response: 8 mo
Mantovani 1989 [66]	27 pretreated	Monotherapy	CR+PR: 45%	

CR: complete remission; PR: partial response; MR: mixed response; NG: not given

Table 3. Interferon-α in LGNHL in combination with single-agent chemotherapy

Author	No. of pts.	Schedule	Response	Duration of response Survival
Karanes 1986 [67]	25	Chlorambucil 16 mg/m²/dx5d IFN 2x10⁶ IU/m², d 8, every other day for a total of 10 doses	CR: 24% PR: 40%	NG
Ozer 1987 [68]	60	CTX: 100 mg/m²/d p.o. IFN: 2x10⁶ IU/m² on alternate days	CR+PR: 72%	NG
Rohatiner 1987 [69]	22	Chlorambucil 10 mg/day IFN 2x10⁶ IU/m² 3x/week	CR: 4.5% PR: 59%	Duration of response: 3-17+ mo
Chisesi 1988 [70]	22, intermediate also included	Chlorambucil 10 mg/day IFN 3x10⁶ IU 3x/week	CR: 9% PR: 54.5%	Duration of response: 3-17+ mo
Clark 1989 [71]	13, intermediate also included	Chlorambucil 16 mg/m²/d days 5-9/mo IFN-α 6x10⁹ IU days 1-5/mo	CR: 38% PR: 8%	Mean duration of response: 456+ days
Chisesi 1991 [72]	34	Chlorambucil 5 mg/d 3x/w monthly IFN 5x10⁶ IU/m² 3x/w x 3w monthly	CR: 23.5% PR: 41.2%	Predicted overall survival at 10 years: 70%
Price1991 [73]	108	Chlorambucil 10 mg/d) intermittently } x 4 mo IFN 2x10⁶ IU/m² 3x/w)	CR: 16% PR: 39%	--
Peterson1993 [74]	531 follicular (pts in the other arm of the study included)	CTX: 100 mg/m²/day p.o IFN α-2b 12x10⁶ IU/m² 3x/week	CR: 45% PR: 39%	3-year duration of response: 37% 3-year survival (overall): 78%
Pangalis 1993 [12]	34	IFN α-2b 3x10⁶ IU/d x 5d followed by Chlorambucil 10 mg/d for 10d/mo x 6-18 mo	CR: 53% PR: 32%	Duration of CR: 20+ mo Relapse rate in maintenance group: 41%

CR: complete remission; PR: partial response; NG: not given

of response. Peterson et al. published completely opposite results in a phase III trial including patients with FSCL with stage III and IV disease [74]. Addition of IFN-α to cyclophosphamide as induction treatment did not improve the response rates [74].
In conclusion, no important advantage of alkylators combined with IFN-α over alkylators as single agents has been proved. Of course, a longer follow-up is needed.

Interferon-alpha in Combination with More Aggressive Chemotherapy

Several trials have been based on this approach (Table 4) [35,42,75-77]. The earliest trial using this modality with the longest follow-up is the one of M.D. Anderson Cancer Center [35,75]. Patients with LGNHL histology and stage IV disease were included, and the median follow-up was 55 months. Patients re-

Table 4. Interferon-α in LGNHL with combination chemotherapy

Author	No. of pts.	Schedule	Results	Survival
McLaughlin 1992 [35]	127 49 as induction (good-risk pts)	IFN $3x10^6$ IU/m^2/d for 8w followed by CHOP-Bleo x 12-18 mo	CR: 73% PR: 23%	FFS at 5y for all pts: 47% FFS at 5 y for CRs: 60% overall survival at 5y for all pts: 74%
Smalley 1992 [42]	122 (pts with diffuse small cleaved cell and nodular histiocytic also included)	I-COPA CTX: 600 mg/m^2 Vincristine: 1.2 mg/m^2 Doxorubicin: 50 mg/m^2 i.v. on day 1 Prednisone: 100 mg/m^2 p.o. days 1-5 IFN α-2a: $6x10^6$ IU/m^2 on days 22-26 every 38 days for at least 8 cycles	CR: 32% PR: 54%	Time to treatment failure at 4y: 35% Overall survival at 4y: 70%
Solal-Celigny 1993 [43]	123 follicular	CHPV+IFN CTX: 600 mg/m^2 Vincristine: 1.2 mg/m^2 VM-26: 60 mg/m^2 i.v. on day 1 Prednisone: 40 mg/m^2 p.o. days 1-5 every month x 6 cycles, then every 2 mo for 1 year IFN α-2b: $5x10^6$ U 3xweek for 18 mo	CR+PR: 76% at 6 mo CR+PR: 85% at 18 mo	Event-free survival at 3y: 45 ± 5% Median event-free survival: 34 mo Overall survival at 3y: 86 ± 3%

CR: complete remission; PR: partial response; FFS: failure-free survival

ceived IFN-α x 8 weeks (only good-risk patients) and subsequently CHOP-Bleo x 12-18 months and responders (CRs) continued with IFN-α at a dose of 3 x 10^6/m^2/day x 8 weeks as maintenance. The control group was treated with CHOP-Bleo alone. Patients receiving IFN-α had a statistically significant longer FFS (47% vs 29% at 5 years) and showed a trend towards longer overall survival at 5 years (60% vs 37%). The SWOG investigated Pro-MACE/MOPP + IFN-α as maintenance, but it is too early for meaningful conclusions [52]. In another randomized study from the GELF higher response rates were observed in patients receiving combined chemotherapy plus IFN-α [43]. In this study CAP-VM26 was administered every 4 weeks. Patients were randomly assigned to additional treatment with IFN-α2b for 18 months or chemotherapy alone. A statistically significant benefit was seen for the IFN-α arm of the study (overall response rate 86% vs 69%) [43].

The ECOG designed a randomized study in which patients received COPA with or without IFN-α as induction therapy [42]. An advantage concerning duration of CR, disease-free survival and overall survival was observed in the group of patients who received IFN-α (DFS at 2 years 71% vs 46%, overall survival at 2 years 87% vs 79%) [42].

Interferon-alpha Maintenance

The utilization of interferon-α as maintenance treatment for LGNHL responders after remission induction with chemotherapy with or without interferon-α, seems a reasonable approach; firstly because at the time of minimal residual disease, biological response modifiers such as IFN-α may have a more potent action, and secondly there may be a benefit in using IFN after immunosuppressive therapy owing to the immunomodulatory properties of IFN, so

that the immune response against tumour antigens may be improved in such patients.
In our Unit, complete responders with LGNHL were randomized, after induction treatment with chlorambucil + interferon-α2b, to receive IFN-α2b at a dose of 3 x 10^6 IU/week for one year or no treatment [12]. The addition of IFN did not improve the relapse rate (41% in both groups). This may be due to the low dose we used in this study. In a trial by Peterson et al. interferon-α was administered to complete responders at a dose of 2 x 10^6 IU/m^2 3 times a week for 2 years as maintenance after induction with cyclophosphamide + IFN-α, but the results regarding maintenance cannot be assessed [74]. Price et al. demonstrated a prolongation of response duration with IFN maintenance after remission induction with chlorambucil alone or combined with interferon-α [73]. No significant differences in relapse incidence between patients who received maintenance with IFN-α and patients who did not receive further treatment were observed by Chisesi et al., although they found a lower relapse rate in patients who were treated with IFN in the induction phase [72].
Hagenbeek et al. in a large randomized phase II trial including 331 patients observed that IFN-α maintenance prolongs progression-free survival (PFS) in patients with LGNHL [77]. Patients were treated with CVP chemotherapy and iceberg radiotherapy and subsequently responders and patients with stable disease were randomized to receive IFN-α at a dose of 3 x 10^6 IU 3 times a week for 12 months, or no further treatment. With a median follow-up of 2 years PFS was significantly longer in the interferon arm (135 weeks vs 86 weeks). McLaughlin et al. administered IFN-α at a dose of 3 x 10^6 IU/m^2 3 times a week for 1 year as maintenance treatment for CRs after CHOP-Bleo chemotherapy, with a RFS at 3 years of 83% [75]. They compared these results with 91 controls who received CHOP-Bleo alone and demonstrated a trend towards a better RFS for patients receiving maintenance therapy.
In a trial by Solal-Celigny and colleagues, patients were treated with a regimen containing cyclophosphamide, adriamycin, VM26 and prednisone with or without IFN-α for 6 months [43]. Subsequently, the patients in the IFN arm received further IFN-α at a dose of 5 x 10^6 IU 3 times a week for 12 additional months. Not only the response rates were higher in the IFN arm, but event-free and overall survival at 3 years were also superior.
Considering the promising results of the above-mentioned studies it can be concluded that IFN-α may contribute to the treatment of LGNHL in combination with more aggressive chemotherapy either as induction or as maintenance. In particular its role as maintenance treatment when minimal residual disease is present needs further investigation in order to estimate its effect on DFS and overall survival.

Purine Analogues

Fludarabine Monophosphate

Fludarabine is a nucleoside analogue derived from structure modification of vidarabine (ara-A) [78]. It is the adenosine deaminase-resistant fluorinated purine analogue F-ara-A monophosphate (9-β-D-arabinosyl-2-fluoroadenosine) [79]. Its major mechanism of action is inhibition of DNA synthesis by direct competition with dATP for utilization by DNA polymerases [79] and secondly by incorporation into DNA [80]. Termination of RNA synthesis may contribute to its cytotoxic activity, especially in malignancies with low proliferation rates such as LGNHLs. Inhibition of DNA repair, depletion of NAD pools, inhibition of enzymes which interfere with RNA and DNA synthesis, are other possible mechanisms of action [81]. The usual dose and schedule of fludarabine for LGNHL treatment is 25 mg/m^2 i.v./day on days 1-5 repeated every 4 to 5 weeks. Six cycles are usually needed for maximal response with 3 more cycles for responders [82]. Other treatment schedules have also been proposed. Dose reduction is needed if renal insufficiency or bone marrow toxicity is present.
Most studies with fludarabine include pretreated patients refractory to conventional treatment approaches. The response rates for these patients range from 30-50%, with the duration of response ranging from 2 to 27 months (Table 5) [83-88].
In a study by Leiby et al. fludarabine was administered at a loading dose of 20 mg/m^2 followed by a continuous infusion of 30 mg/m^2/day for 48 hours [84]. The response rate was 32% [84]. Hochster et al. studied 22

Table 5. Fludarabine in LGNHL

Author	No. of pts.	Schedule	Results	Duration of response Survival
Leiby 1987 [84]	25 (pts with DLPD also included)	20 mg/m^2/d loading dose 30 mg/m^2/d x 2 days i.v.	CR: 4% PR: 28%	Duration of CR: >9 mo Duration of PR: 2-20 mo
Hochster 1990 [88]	22	18 mg/m^2/d x 5 days i.v.	CR: 18% PR: 27%	NG
Hochster 1992 [83]	25 pretreated	18 mg/m^2/d x 5 days i.v.	CR: 20% PR: 32%	Overall: 9.3 mo For CRs: >20.8 mo
Redman 1992 [85]	38 pretreated	25 mg/m^2/d x 5 days i.v.	CR: 13% PR: 42%	Duration of CR: 8->27 mo
Whelan 1993 [89]	25 pretreated (1 pt with diffuse centrocytic centroblastic NHL)	25 mg/m^2/d x 5 days i.v.	CR+PR: 68%	NG

CR: complete remission; PR: partial response; NG: not given

patients with LGNHL histology, stage III or IV, who had been pretreated with two other regimens (alkylators and combination chemotherapy) and had subsequently relapsed [88]. The response rate was found to be 45% [88]. With regard to the histological subtypes, FSCL seemed to respond better, with a rate of 72%. In this study fludarabine was administered at a dose of 18 mg/m^2/day for 5 days every 25 days for a minimum of 6 months for responders [88]. Whelan et al. used fludarabine in pretreated patients with refractory advanced LGNHL at a dose of 25 mg/m^2/day i.v. for 5 days every 21 days for a maximum of 6 cycles, with an overall response rate of 68% [89]. They also observed a better outcome in patients with follicular lymphoma, with an overall response rate of up to 75% [89]. The ECOG studied the efficacy of fludarabine with the same schedule as in the study by Hochster in 64 patients with non-Hodgkin's lymphomas [83]. Of these patients 27 had low-grade histology and 25 were evaluable for response [83]. They observed an overall response rate of 52% with a 64% response among patients with FSCL [83]. In a phase II trial by Redman et al. fludarabine was administered at a dose of 25 mg/m^2 for 5 days and the results seemed very promising [85]. Seventy-six patients were evaluable. Of the 38 patients with low-grade histology 21 responded (55%) [85]. The highest response rates were observed in the FSCL histology (62%) and in FML (89%) [85]. Waldenström's macroglobulinaemia resistant to conventional treatment also responded to fludarabine with a rate of 45% [90].

The toxicity of fludarabine in conventional doses is mainly restricted to myelosuppression. There is a report about the accumulation of this suppression [83,87]. Fludarabine causes a depletion of helper lymphocytes (CD4) leading to susceptibility to opportunistic and other infections [83,87]. Fever, nausea/vomiting, interstitial pneumonitis, severe autoimmune haemolytic anaemia and tumour lysis syndrome have been reported. Severe neurological complications have been observed with doses >90 mg/m^2/day for 5 days, but these events could be avoided with dose reduction [83].

Overall, fludarabine seems to be a promising new agent in the treatment of LGNHL and indeed in refractory, pretreated patients who need salvage therapy. A longer follow-up is needed to determine its effect on DFS and overall survival. In addition, new studies have been started in which fludarabine is used in newly diagnosed patients.

2-Chlorodeoxyadenosine and Deoxycoformycin

The idea of investigating new purine analogues as possible therapeutic agents for lymphoid malignancies has originated from the observation of lymphocyte depletion or immunologic incompetence in children with adenosine deaminase (ADA) deficiency [91]. The degradation of purine deoxyribonucleotides is fully dependent on ADA. Therefore, in case of ADA inhibition, the subsequent accumulation of deoxyribonucleotides in lymphocytes might lead to cell death. Lymphocytes have a high deoxycytidine kinase activity, which phosphorylates deoxyadenosine to deoxyadenosine monophosphate, whereas the activity of 5-nucleotidase that dephosphorylates dAMP to deoxyadenosine is low. In the absence of ADA, dAMP and dATP would accumulate in lymphocytes and provoke cell death, but not in cells with low deoxyadenosine kinase and high 5-nucleotidase activity. Furthermore, there are two ways to reach a lethal concentration of deoxyribonucleotides in lymphocytes: 1) by using an ADA inhibitor such as 2-deoxycoformycin (2-DcF), and 2) by administering a purine nucleoside analogue resistant to ADA so that its derivatives, e.g. 2-chlorodeoxyadenosine (2-CdA) concentrate in the lymphocyte and produce cell death [92]. Deoxypurine nucleosides such as 2-CdA and 2-DcF are phosphorylated by deoxycytidine kinase to their mononucleotides after entering the cells. The 2-CdA and 2-DcF induced accumulation of deoxynucleotides takes place in cells with a high deoxycytidine kinase activity and a low 5-nucleotidase activity such as lymphocytes [83]. These two purine analogues are thus lymphocyte specific.

Mechanism of action

2-CdA: 2-CdA is resistant to ADA. It is directly incorporated into DNA, but this is not the major mechanism. The above-mentioned accumulation of deoxynucleotides triggers the phenomenon of apoptosis by causing DNA strand breaks and disturbance of DNA repair [93]. Depletion of NAD pools is another possible mechanism [93].
2-DcF: As already mentioned, 2-DcF is an ADA inhibitor. Inhibition of DNA and RNA synthesis, depletion of NAD pools, disturbance of procedures dependent on ATP and accumulation of deoxynucleotides are the most prominent mechanisms [94].

Efficacy of 2-CdA and 2-DcF

2-CdA: Kay et al. investigated the efficacy of 2-CdA in 40 patients with LGNHL who were refractory to conventional treatment after a median of 3 prior therapies [95]. 2-CdA was given at a dose of 0.1 mg/kg/day as a 7-day continuous i.v. infusion every 5 weeks. Patients received 2-CdA until maximal response or prohibitive toxicity, if they responded after the second cycle. Otherwise treatment was discontinued. The median number of cycles in this study was 3 (range 1-6). Responses were observed in 43%, with 20% CRs. Duration of CR and PR ranged between 1 and 33+ months (median 6 months) and 3-6 months, respectively. Follicular histology seemed to respond better. The significant CR rate which was achieved, especially in these multirelapsed patients, should be mentioned. It was surprising that histological progression to more aggressive types of lymphoma did not result in poorer response (Table 6) [95]. 2-CdA seems to be an effective agent in LGNHL perhaps because its killing is independent of cell division. Studies using 2-CdA in untreated newly diagnosed patients, and also using combinations of 2-CdA, mitoxanthrone and prednisone have been initiated [84]. A fluorinated derivative of 2-CdA (2-chloro-2-arabino-fluoro 2-deoxy adenosine) is currently being investigated for oral use [97].
2-CdA proved to be very effective also in Waldenström's macroglobulinaemia. A recent study showed that in 29 patients, 20 of whom had been previously treated, the response rate was 59% [98]. All untreated patients (9) achieved remission. It is remarkable that IgM reduction continued in responders even after discontinuation of treatment (Table 6) [98].
The toxicity of 2-CdA is mainly neutropenia with a nadir occurring between 7 and 14 days post therapy. Thrombocytopenia is also observed. Myelosuppression was found to be cumulative. Fever and opportunistic infections have been reported. Non-haematological side-effects included renal and CNS toxicity but only when the drug was administered at higher doses [96].
2-DcF: Studies regarding the efficacy of 2-DcF in LGNHL are not yet available.

Table 6. 2-Deoxychloroadenosine (2-CdA) in LGNHL

Author	No. of pts.	Schedule	Results	Duration of response
Kay 1992 [95]	40, pretreated 6 with histological transformation	0.1 mg/kg/d x 7 days i.v.	CR: 20% PR: 23% CR+PR: 33% in transformed LGNHL	Median duration of CR: 6 mo of PR: 3-6 mo
Dimopoulos 1992 [98]	29, Waldenström's macroglobulinaemia (9 untreated)	0.1 mg/kg/d x 7 days i.v.	Response: 59% (100% in untreated)	NG

CR: complete remission; PR: partial response; NG: not given

Attempts with Other, Novel Agents

In a phase II study by Rotarski et al. a new platinum analogue (oxaliplatin) was used in refractory or relapsed LGNHL at a dose of 65 mg/m^2 up to 130 mg/m^2 every 3 weeks [99]. The response rate was 42% with a CR of 17% [99]. In a study at Charing Cross Hospital 4-demethoxydaunorubicin (4-DMDNR-Idarubicin), a synthetic analogue of daunorubicin, was administered in a group of heavily pretreated refractory LGNHL patients [100]. Given the known antitumour effect of daunorubicin, the availability of the drug as an oral anthracycline analogue and its mild toxicity compared to daunorubicin, an attempt was made to test its efficacy in LGNHL [100]. The median number of prior treatments, incuding anthracycline regimens, was 4. Low doses of 15 mg/m^2 Idarubicin weekly for up to 6 months were used. The response rate was 26% (all partial) and the median duration of response was 10 weeks. The toxicity was very mild with no evidence of cumulative myelosuppression. Further studies with higher doses are needed to possibly achieve a higher response rate. Combination of Idarubicin with alkylating agents seems promising [100]. Alpha calcidol (1α-hydroxyvitamin D3) has proved to be active in LGNHL, although the mechanism of action is not clear [101]. It produced an overall response rate of 25% in a group of 34 patients, 19 of whom were pretreated. The median duration of response was 14 months [101].

Interleukin-2

Interference with the immune system and the induction of host effector mechanisms is the concept of the use of cytokines in the treatment of LGNHL [102].
Interleukin-2 (IL-2) is a cytokine produced by a subset of CD4+ T lymphocytes called TH1 [103]. There are 3 forms of IL-2 receptors: those with high, intermediate and low affinity [104-106]. T and B lymphocytes, NK cells and monocytes express IL-2 receptors, but only NK cells express the high-affinity IL-2 receptors in resting conditions, contrary to the other cell types, which must be activated [107-109].

Mechanism of Action

In cancer patients IL-2 may have a therapeutic impact by multiple mechanisms. IL-2 can generate cytotoxic effector cells, i.e., lymphokine-activated killer cells (LAK cells) that are capable of killing lymphoma cells [110,111]. It also induces the secretion of other immunomodulatory cytokines such as TNF and IFN-γ, which not only enhance the cytotoxic activity [112] but also lead to a direct antiproliferative effect on tumour cells [113]. Cancer patients showing an impaired immune response, although they are capable of tumour antigen recognition, may benefit from IL-2 treatment at low doses as IL-2 can boost the immune response against tumour antigens [114]. Improvement of impaired NK cell activity has been observed in patients with B-cell malignancies after IL-2 administration [115]. Several investigators have tested

Table 7. Interleukin-2 in LGNHL

Author	No. of pts.	Treatment - Schedule	Response	Duration of response
Rosenberg 1987 [124]	18 (histological type not given)	bolus i.v. 100,000 IU/kg q-8 ± LAK cells	CR: 6% PR: 17%	CR: 10 mo
West 1987 [125]	1	3.0×10^6 IU/m^2/day continuous i.v. infusion + LAK cells	PR: 100%	4+ mo
Alison 1989 [126]	7 (intermediate also included)	$1.5\text{-}3.0 \times 10^6$ IU/m^2/day bolus i.v.	PR: 43%	1-17 mo
Hesketh 1991 [118]	11 (5 cutaneous)	DAB_{486} IL-2 0.012-0.1 mg/kg/day for 5 days or 0.1 mg/kg/week for 5 weeks	CR: 9% PR: 18%	11+ - 12+ weeks
Tourani 1991 [121]	10	continuous i.v. infusion 2 induction cycles of 18×10^6 IU/m^2/day on days 1-5 and 12-16 4-monthly maintenance cycles 18×10^6 IU/m^2/d on days 1-5	CR: 10% PR: 40% MR: 20%	4 mo
Weber 1992 [120]	8	bolus i.v. 720,000 IU/kg q-8 ± LAK cells	CR: 12% PR: 38%	10-26 mo
LeMaistre 1992 [119]	9	DAB_{486} IL-2 0.0007 mg/kg/day - 11 doses 0.2 mg/kg/day - 10 doses	CR: 11%	18+ mo
Richards unpublished	3	3.0×10^6 IU/m^2/day continuous i.v. infusion + LAK cells	PR: 33%	9 mo

CR: complete remission; PR: partial response; MR: mixed response

the efficacy of DAB_{486} IL-2 [110], a recombinant fusion toxin in which the native receptor-binding domain of diphtheria toxin has been replaced by human IL-2 [117]. This molecule is extremely specific for the high-affinity IL-2 receptor [117]. After binding to this receptor, an intracellular mechanism of adenosine diphosphate ribosylation of the elongation factor 2 takes place, which leads to inhibition of protein synthesis resulting in cell death [117]. Administration of recombinant IL-2 (rIL-2) in combination with monoclonal antibodies directed against tumour markers leads to an enhancement of the MoAb-induced antibody-dependent cell cytotoxicity (ADCC), due to the natural killer cell expansion caused by IL-2 [103,117].

Efficacy of IL-2 (Table 7)

IL-2 may be used as induction therapy, but it is assumed to be more effective in minimal residual disease, where the proportion of tumour cells and cytokine effector cells is balanced [102]. DAB_{486} IL-2 has been used in phase I trials [110,118,119] in patients whose tumours expressed this form of receptor. Most of them had T-cell malignancies. Some, mostly partial, responses were observed [110,118, 119].

Furthermore, there are phase II studies demonstrating some therapeutic effect after administration of rIL-2 with or without LAK cells in high or moderate dose schedules to patients with B-cell lymphomas [110,120-124]. The responses observed were restricted mostly to LGNHL

[125,126]. Weber et al. used high doses of IL-2 given as a bolus i.v. with or without LAK cells and achieved an overall response rate of 50%, with one response lasting for 26 months [120]. Tourani et al. administered IL-2 in continuous i.v. infusion as induction and as maintenance treatment with an overall response rate of 70% [121]. The results of the above trials and of those listed in Table 7 are promising and give us a strong motive for further investigation of IL-2 efficacy in LGNHL.

Monoclonal Antibodies

In recent years a new, fascinating modality has emerged in the treatment of B cell non-Hodgkin's lymphomas: monoclonal antibodies (MoAbs). This treatment concept seems to be more specific than other modalities, as monoclonal antibodies target markers on malignant cells only, thus protecting normal cells from the cytotoxic effect of chemotherapy [123].

Different groups of MoAbs have been employed: 1) MoAbs against differentiation antigens restricted to lymphocyte subpopulations such as Campath 1-H [127,128]; 2) anti-idiotype antibodies that target the idiotypic determinants (on the variable region) of the surface immunoglobulin of the malignant cells [129-131]; 3) radionuclide-linked monoclonal antibodies, which not only bind the specific tumour markers, but also emit radioactivity to the tumour cells [132-134]; 4) combination of monoclonal antibodies with biological response modifiers such as IFN or IL-2, or with cytotoxic agents such as chlorambucil, in order to enhance the cytotoxicity through the independent synergistic antitumour effect of the above-mentioned agents [139,131]; 5) vaccination with the idiotypic immunoglobulin expressed on the malignant cells [135]; 6) cocktails of more than one antibody may be required to overcome the variability of the idiotypic determinants of surface immunoglobulin of the malignant cell clone [130,134,136]; 7) "chimaeric" or designer antibodies, which can be constructed by means of molecular engineering, is one of the future directions of MoAb therapy [123,137,138]. These sophisticated techniques allow us to select the valuable features of the immunoglobulin leading to reduction of the adverse effects of MoAb therapy.

Mechanism of Action

Monoclonal antibodies bind to specific antigens on the surface of the malignant cells and activate human effector mechanisms, such as ADCC [139] and complement fixation and cytolysis [140]. Some monoclonal antibodies, for example anti-CD20, can directly induce apoptosis [132]. As far as anti-idiotype antibodies are concerned, apart from the above-mentioned mechanisms they can directly alter the idiotype anti-idiotype network, which is important for the regulation of some malignant B-cell clones [130-141]. As regards radionuclide-linked MoAbs, additional mechanisms of action play an important role in the antitumour effect: the selective radiotherapy delivered to the targeted tumour cells by the monoclonal antibodies [132-134] and the non-specific whole body irradiation by the systemic administration of the radiolabeled MoAbs [132-134]. The radioactivity that is delivered to the tumour cells expressing the antigen to which the MoAb is bound, may also kill adjacent malignant cells which do not express this specific antigen [132-134].

The main obstacles in the treatment with monoclonal antibodies are the following: 1) the heterogeneity of tumour cells: not all cells express the particular antigen at different sites and within the same site [138]; 2) circulating antigens, usually idiotype proteins or antigens on the surface of normal cells, bind the injected MoAb and prevent the therapeutic effect on tumour cells [138]; 3) the vascularity of the tumour varies considerably and so does the penetration of the MoAb into the tumour [132, 138]; 4) the development of human antibodies against foreign (murine) immunoglobulins prevents the effective targeting of antibodies after repeated administration (HAMA response) [123,134,138]; 5) the simple binding of the MoAb to the surface antigen of the tumour cell, with the exception of MoAbs directed against growth factor receptors, does not predict tumour lysis because these mechanisms require complement components or host effector response which may not function optimally in patients with cancer [138]; 6) the emergence of idiotype-negative cells which may be selected after therapy with anti-idiotype antibodies, is responsible for recurrence of the disease after treatment [123,130,138,144,145].

Efficacy of MoAbs (Table 8)

In a preliminary trial by Hale et al. [128] Campath-1H, a monoclonal antibody against CDw52, was used in 2 patients with LGNHL at daily doses of 1-20 mg, resulting in disease reduction as established by clinical and laboratory criteria. Some severe adverse effects had been noted in these 2 patients. In a subsequent phase I trial by Clendennin dose regimens varying from 0.5 to 240 mg were given once, 3 or 5 times weekly [127]. The most promising schedule was the 3-weekly doses which led to disease reduction in 92% of patients with either LGNHL or CLL [127,127a]. Side-effects were acute, consisting of fever, rigours, rash, nausea, vomiting, headache, dyspnoea and hypotension, but they diminished with the continuation of treatment. Opportunistic infections were observed due to a dramatic fall in the lymphocyte count.

It must be kept in mind that the choice of the right antibody [128,132,133] and its isotype [128,132] are very important factors for the efficacy of treatment. CDw52 seems to be a good target, as it is widely distributed and does not show antigenic modulation [128].

As already mentioned, the variable region (idiotype) of the immunoglobulin molecule can serve as a specific tumour marker [130,135, 146,147]. The use of anti-idiotype antibodies as a therapeutic tool is extremely specific, as only the malignant cells are targeted, without affecting normal cells.

Levy et al. [129] administered unconjugated anti-idiotype antibodies to 14 heavily pretreated patients with B-cell lymphomas; a response was observed in 8 of these patients and one patient remained in CR for 6 years.

The existence of idiotype-negative cells among the tumour cell population - due to point mutations - is responsible for the recurrence of the disease after monoclonal antibody therapy [123,130,138,144,145]. This has triggered the hypothesis that this obstacle might be overcome by using biological agents [130,146,149] or cytotoxic drugs [131] with a different and independent antitumour activity in combination with MoAbs, thus targeting both idiotype-positive and idiotype-negative cells. Brown and colleagues [130] compared the efficacy of anti-idiotype antibodies alone and in combination with IFN-α in patients with LGNHL, including transformed lymphomas. In this study the addition of interferon did not prevent the emergence of idiotype-negative clones, but there was a trend towards higher remission rates (CR 6%, PR 44% with MoAbs alone vs CR 17%, PR 58% with combination of MoAbs and IFN).

Maloney et al. [131] have also tried to improve the therapeutic effect of MoAb therapy. They administered a pulse dose of chlorambucil after 2 courses of MoAbs at the site where idiotype-negative cells might proliferate, without any significant benefit.

The use of radiolabeled monoclonal antibodies seems very attractive due to the combination of the mechanisms of action of radiation [132,133,139,140] and MoAbs [132-134,142]. Radioactivity will be delivered to tumour sites only, and normal tissues will be protected from the catastrophic effects of radiotherapy [132, 133]. Kaminski et al. [132] used anti-B1 (anti-CD20) tracer labeled with ^{131}I, with a CR rate of 44% and a PR of 22%. When considering the LGNHL group only, the overall response rate was 100%. They performed pretreatment with unlabeled antibody in order to enhance the access of the radiolabeled antibody through competition between labeled and unlabeled antibody and saturation of non-specific binding sites of normal B cells, such as the spleen, by the unlabeled antibody. Splenomegaly and tumour sclerosis proved to be poor prognostic factors for the success of this form of therapy.

Press et al. [133] tested the efficacy of anti-CD20 and anti-CD37 labeled with ^{131}I in 43 patients with B-cell lymphoma. They used 10-fold higher doses of radioactivity and autologous bone marrow support. They performed biodistribution studies with tracer-labeled MoAbs before administering the therapeutic dose. Only patients with a favourable biodistribution were selected for the therapeutic infusions. The CR rate was very high (84%). They observed that patients without splenomegaly and a tumour burden less than 500 ml had a better biodistribution and would possibly respond. It was also demonstrated that anti-CD20 was superior to anti-CD37 [132,133] because of its lesser toxicity, more favourable biodistribution and slower internalization by the tumour cells [150].

In another trial by Czuczman et al. the MoAb OKB7 (anti-CD21) was administered to 18 patients, 10 of whom had LGNHL [134]. They observed responses in 80% of the LGNHL

Table 8. Monoclonal antibodies in LGNHL

Author	MoAb	No. of pts.	Dose	Response	Survival
Hale 1988 [128]	Campath 1-H	2	1-20 mg/d x 30-43 days	Both patients	Duration of response 100+ days
Clendennin 1993 [127]	Campath 1-H	160 (not only LGNHL)	0.5-240 mg i.v. 3x/weekly	CR+PR: 7% 25% disease reduction: 92%	NG
Brown 1989 [130]	anti-Id Ab ± IFN-α	a. 14 (11 LGNHL, 2 transformed) 2 pts treated twice	a. anti-Id Ab alone: 3xw for 3-4 w Total Ab dose: 500-15,500 mg	a. CR: 6%, PR: 44%, MR: 13%	a. duration of CR: 6 ys duration of PR: 1-25+ mo duration of MR:1-3 mo
		b. 11 (4 transf. LGNHL) 1 pt treated twice	b. + IFN: 12x10^{6} IU/m^{2} 3xw for 8 w 2h before Ab infusion Total Ab dose: 1680-8400 mg	b. CR: 17%, PR: 58%, MR: 17%	b. duration of CR: 21+ - 24+ mo duration of PR: 2-13 mo duration of MR: 5-6 mo
Levy 1990 [129]	unconjugated anti-Id Ab	14 2 pts treated twice	i.v. every 2-3 days for at least 2 weeks Total Ab dose: 500-15,000 mg	CR: 12.5% PR: 37.5%	FFP of CRs: 29 mo and 6 y FFP of PRs: 1-12 mo
Maloney 1992 [131]	Anti-idiotype antibody ± IFN-α	34 (B-cell lymphomas)	NG	CR: 18% PR: 50%	NG
"	Anti-idiotype antibody + pulse dose chlorambucil	13 (B-cell lymphomas)	NG	CR: 8% PR: 61% MR: 16%	median FFP: 7 mo
Kwak 1992 [135]	"vaccine with immunoglobulin idiotypic protein"	9 in CR or with minimal residual disease	0.5 mg + KLH s.c. at 0,2,6,10,14 w followed by booster injections at 24 and 28 weeks	immune responses in 77%	

Table 8. Monoclonal antibodies in LGNHL (continued)

Author	MoAb	No. of pts.	Dose	Response	Survival
Kaminski 1993 [132]	Anti-B1 (anti-CD20) labeled with ^{131}I	10 (9 treated) 5 with LGNHL	Pretreatment with unlabeled Ab: 135-685 mg Ab therapeutic dose: 15-700 mg Ab total dose: 30-1565 mg Whole body dose: 25-45 cGy 15 mg of Ab cont. 5mCi	CR: 44% (all pts) PR: 22% (all pts) CR+PR in LGNHL group: 100%	median PFS for all pts and for LGNHL: 8 mo
Press 1993 [133]	Anti-CD20) labeled Anti-CD37) with ^{131}I	24 (19 treated) intermediate and low grade	234-777mCi of ^{131}I 58-1168 mg of MoAb	CR: 84% PR: 10% MR: 5%	median duration CR: 10+ mo (3+ - 53+ mo) median duration PR: 4 mo median overall survival: 21+ mo
Czuczman 1993 [134]	OK-B7 (anti-CD21) labeled with ^{131}I	18 10 LGNHL	Ab dose: 25 mg individual doses of ^{131}I: 30-50mCi Total dose of ^{131}I: 90-160mCi	Response: 72% (all pts) PR: 10%, MR: 70% in LGNHL group	median duration of CR: 6 mo for all pts, 3.5 mo for LGNHL

CR: complete remission; PR: partial response; MR: mixed response; NG: not given; FFP: freedom from progression; PRS: progression-free survival group. They used a dose escalation schedule from 90 to 200 mCi. The antitumour activity was seen to depend on the total dose of ^{131}I-OKB7. A large tumour burden was found to be a limiting factor for MoAb uptake.

Kwak et al. [135] tried to determine whether there were specific immune responses after "vaccination" with the idiotypic determinants of the cell surface immunoglobulin of the malignant B cells. Seven of 9 patients had specific immune responses, humoural and/or cell mediated. This therapeutic approach, which should be further investigated, can be used either at the time of minimal residual disease, in order to prevent regrowth of tumour cells, or even as main therapy.

Therapy with monoclonal antibodies seems very attractive and promising. Future studies are expected using cytokines, local hyperthermia, vasoactive drugs in combination with MoAbs, or cocktails of different MoAbs, with the aim of improving their therapeutic efficacy and specificity [134].

Myeloablative Treatment and Bone Marrow Transplantation or Peripheral Stem Cell Support

This therapeutic modality is discussed in another chapter of this monograph.

Irradiation

Radiotherapy is one of the oldest approaches to the treatment of LGNHL and can be applied in the forms of involved field irradiation (IF) [151-153], whole body irradiation (WBI) [30, 151,154,155-158] or total lymphoid irradiation (TLI) [159,160]. In the rare situation of stage I or low tumour burden stage II at diagnosis, irradiation can lead to successful control of the disease [152,159]. The field size to be used is subject to controversy. With IF irradiation approximately 50% of the patients will be free of disease at 5 years [153]. Studies by Monfardini et al. and from the M.D. Anderson Cancer Center have shown the necessity of additional chemotherapy even in these early stages, because the conventional staging procedures might not detect the extent of the disease [161, 162]. In the first study LGNHL patients with PS I and II were treated with radiotherapy or radiotherapy and chemotherapy (CVP). A better 5-year survival in the group of patients treated with combined therapy was demonstrated [161]. In the second study the 5-year DFS for patients treated with combined chemotherapy and radiotherapy was better than for patients receiving radiotherapy alone (64% vs 37%) [162].

For the advanced stages (III-IV) several irradiation schedules have been used, for example WBI, WBI followed by IF or TLI. Hoppe et al. used fractionated WBI followed by low-dose IF. They randomized 51 patients to receive either radiotherapy or single-agent chemotherapy or the CVP combination [1]. The CR rates were similar (71%, 64% and 88%, respectively), while the time required for CR achievement was shorter for the irradiated group (3 months vs 5 months for CVP and 12 months for single agent). They did not observe any significant differences in overall survival and freedom from relapse. In a trial at the NCI combination chemotherapy (CVP or C-MOPP) was compared to radiotherapy (total body, total nodal or hemibody), and no significant differences were observed [154]. Identical results were obtained in another NCI trial comparing chemotherapy (CVP or C-MOPP) combined with WBI to chemotherapy alone [154].

In another study from the Gustave Roussy Institute, low-dose limited-field irradiation therapy (LDLRT) was given to LGNHL patients. Of the 27 evaluable patients 22 were at advanced clinical stages (III-IV) and 25 had received prior chemotherapy. The overall response rate after the first LDLRT course was 89% with 37% CR and the duration of response in the irradiated areas ranged from 4-30 months [163]. The authors concluded that in localized LGNHL there is no clear correlation between dose and response and that in advanced LGNHL low-dose fractionated WBI (1.5-2 Gy) can produce a long DFS.

Deferring Therapy

Although the majority of patients with LGNHL present with advanced disease, according to certain investigators a large proportion (up to 86%) do not require initial treatment (they are asymptomatic and have no organ compromise) and could be managed by the "watch-and-wait" policy [13,34]. Horning et al. compared 83 patients who were monitored without therapy and 73 patients who received treatment although it could have been omitted [164]. They concluded that actuarial survival at 5 years was the same for the two groups (84%). The incidence of transformation (44% vs 42%), the actuarial risk of transformation (19% vs 23%) and the median time to transformation (57 months vs 54 months) showed no significant differences. Of the group that did not receive treatment 23% presented spontaneous regression of the disease. Sixty-one percent of these patients required therapy at some time of their course and the median time for this was 3 years [164]. These results demonstrate that there is no need for immediate initiation of treatment in a large proportion of advanced LGNHL. In the study of Young et al. 89 patients were randomly assigned either to be watched without treatment or to receive aggressive chemotherapy (ProMACE/MOPP) followed by total nodal irradiation. Forty-four percent of the untreated patients required therapy at some time in their follow-up and the median time to cross over to ProMAC/MOPP was similar to that of the above-mentioned study (34 months) [34]. The overall survival was the same at 5 years (>78%), but DFS was significantly longer in the ProMACE/MOPP arm (51% vs 12%) [34].

Table 9. Treatment options available for LGNHL

"Traditional"

Stages I and II (Pathologically documented)

Involved field radiation
Total lymphoid radiation
Chemotherapy
Surgery

Stages II bulky, III and IV

Single-agent chemotherapy
Combination chemotherapy
Whole body irradiation
Chemotherapy/radiation therapy

"Newer Approaches"

Interferon-α
Fludarabine monophosphate
2-Chlorodeoxyadenosine
2-Deoxycoformycin
Idarubicin
Bone marrow transplantation
or peripheral stem cell support

"Investigational"

Newer drugs
Monoclonal antibodies
Interleukin-2
Antibiotics (MALT lymphomas)

Table 10. Features of aggressive disease in LGNHL

B Symptoms

Rapid increase in tumour burden

Leukaemic picture

Vital organ involvement (liver, lung, pleura, kidney)

Increased serum LDH levels

Elevated serum β_2M

Treatment Options and Therapeutic Strategies

The treatment options available for LGNHL may be divided into "traditional", "newer approaches" and "investigational" according to the experience gained so far (Table 9). Our therapeutic strategy for early stages (I and limited II) is an attempt to cure and this can be achieved by irradiation, chemotherapy plus irradiation or chemotherapy alone. In advanced stages single-agent chemotherapy, radiation therapy (total nodal or whole body) or combination chemotherapy (first generation) may be given. Deferring treatment in advanced stages may also be considered. When evidence of aggressive disease is present (Table 10) more intensive therapy is required and therefore combination chemotherapy (first or second generation) with or without Interferon-α is generally recommended. At the time of relapse the treatment of choice may be mitoxanthrone, crossover chemotherapy in relation to initial therapy, administration of newer drugs (mainly the purine analogues fludarabine monophosphate and 2-chlorodeoxyadenosine) or even more investigational approaches including monoclonal antibodies, interleukin-2 or megatherapy followed by autologous bone marrow transplantation or peripheral stem cell support. If a histological conversion is present, aggressive chemotherapy is needed (depending on previous therapy). Alternatively fludarabine monophosphate or 2-chlorodeoxyadenosine as monotherapy may be given [83,95]. In the case of histological conversion megatherapy with autologous bone marrow transplantation may also be considered. In cases of follicular mixed histology an effort should be made to achieve CR by using combination chemotherapy (CHOP-Bleo or C-MOPP) as first-line treatment. The rationale behind this approach is that NML is considered a curable disease on the basis of a plateau shown in the RFS curves of these patients.

Discussion

The low-grade non-Hodgkin's lymphomas are considered indolent lymphomas with a long natural history [1-3]. Little progress has been made towards a cure of these diseases, although many new cytotoxic drugs and combinations have been introduced. A multiple relapse pattern and development of refractoriness or histology evolution to intermediate-grade lymphomas is the rule after an excellent initial response [27].
Survival and DFS curves, whatever treatment is given, do not reach a plateau even at 10 years [2,25-27,36,165]. Not all patients have the same prognosis. Patients with a low tumour burden (defined by nodal size, number of extranodal sites involved and extent of bone marrow involvement) have a 10-year FFS of 32% and an overall survival of 73% [36,165]. The group with the best prognosis is females with a low tumour burden. Their 10-year survival curve has reached a plateau at 92% and their 10-year FFS at 50%. Stage I or small volume stage II disease can also be cured with local radiation plus chemotherapy. All other groups can be considered as incurable, males with a high tumour burden having a 10-year survival of practically 0% [36,165]. As far as the histological subtypes are concerned, only in the follicular mixed type progress has been made by using aggressive chemotherapy [37-39]. It seems that patients with nodular lymphomas respond better to treatment and survive longer than patients with diffuse lymphocytic well differentiated lymphomas, although only the nodular mixed type seems to be curable with currently available chemotherapy [44]. Earlier reports have shown that DLWD patients have a lower 1-year survival rate (75%) than NLPD (97%) and NM (90%) patients [44].
It is important to mention that in NLPD the quality of response does not affect survival, while patients with NML and DLWD who achieved a CR have a significantly longer survival than partial or non-responders [37-39,41,44]. Bearing in mind that NML can be cured, it is obvious that in this subtype the achievement of CR with first-line therapy is essential for survival. A proportion of patients with advanced disease can be followed up without treatment if their clinical situation allows it. They may not require therapy for 5-10 years [13,34,164]. Homing et al. found that the actuarial survival in initially untreated patients and in treated ones who could have avoided treatment, was the same [164]. They also confirmed that the incidence of transformation and median time to transformation were not influenced by the initiation of treatment [164]. As can be seen, the natural history of these diseases rarely changes and to the present day they can only be considered as incurable.
As regards the different regimens which can be used as first-line therapy, the results are controversial. The standard approach is a single alkylating agent such as cyclophosphamide or chlorambucil ± prednisone with high response rates (65-80%) [3,8-11]. Combination chemotherapy was introduced to obtain higher response rates and more durable results. Even more aggressive chemotherapy regimens were used by several groups without any convincing benefit and influence on the natural history. Survival did not prove to be better even with adriamycin containing regimens. No study has yet demonstrated a survival advantage with aggressive chemotherapy. Higher CR rates could be obtained with combined-modality treatments and a better DFS in some but not all studies, which does not reflect an overall survival improvement [14,28,30,31,34,37,38]. The median time for CR achievement is shorter with combination chemotherapy than with single agents [1]. Some studies have demonstrated

that CVP is a better induction regimen than single agent in nodular lymphomas, whereas single agent seems to produce better results in DWDL, so that single-agent chemotherapy should be the first approach in this subgroup [14,44].

The improvement achieved in all these years in comparing single-agent and combination chemotherapy concerned 4 parameters: a) in follicular mixed lymphoma the survival advantage with combined modality treatment, especially CHOP-Bleo, over single-agent chemotherapy has been confirmed. Considering the fact that CR achievement is a rather strong prognostic factor, it is of importance to produce a CR in these patients; therefore combined chemotherapy is the treatment of choice in this subgroup; b) combined modality seems to lead to a prolongation of the duration of response in patients with stage III disease; c) a longer duration of the initial treatment either with single-agent or combined modalities might be needed to obtain better results; d) the role of maintenance therapy seems to be essential. During the last years the role of maintenance treatment has been investigated. There is a suggestion that maintenance with IFN-α may prolong the duration of response, but further studies are needed for the determination of a survival advantage [72,73,75,76]. It also remains to be seen if it is better to use IFN-α simultaneously with initial treatment. LGNHLs are low growth fraction tumours, so they may become resistant to drugs or may be protected from their cytotoxic activity due to the fact that the malignant lymphocytes are not cycling. These residual cells may result in the relapses observed and this is the crucial point for the employment of biological agents such as IFN-α and other cytokines, when minimal residual disease is present and an immunomodulatory effect can be gained [52].

As already mentioned, the need for salvage treatment is the rule in these patients. After their initial indolent course the LGNHLs become refractory with a poor outcome. New agents such as purine analogues, mitoxanthrone and others may offer a solution [24,83-87,95]. Alternative approaches to eradicate the disease have to be further investigated, for example more aggressive regimens together with growth factors with ABMT or peripheral stem cell support.

Explanation of acronyms

CVP: Cyclophosphamide, vincristine, prednisone

ProMACE/MOPP: Cyclophosphamide, adriamycin, etoposide, nitrogen mustard, vincristine, procarbazine, methotrexate

CHOP-Bleo: Cyclophosphamide, adriamycin, vincristine, prednisone, bleomycin

COP-Bleo: CVP+bleomycin

CHOP-BCG: CHOP + bacillus Calmette - Guerin

COPP: Cyclophosphamide, vincristine, procarbazine, prednisone

BCVP: BCNU, cyclophosphamide, vincristine, prednisone

C-MOPP: Contains the same drugs as COPP

COPA: Contains the same drugs as CHOP

CHVP or CAP-VM26: Cyclophosphamide, adriamycin, prednisone, VM26

MEP: Mitoxanthrone, etoposide, prednisone

BP-VACOP: Bleomycin, cisplatin, etoposide, doxorubicin, cyclophosphamide, vincristine, prednisone

ESHAP: With VPIG-ara C, platinum

NOPP: Mitoxanthrone, vincristine, procarbazine, prednisone

CHOD-Bleo: Like CHOP-Bleo, but instead of prednisone, dexamethasone

REFERENCES

1 Hoppe RT, Kushlan P, Kaplan HS, Rosenberg SA, Brown BW: The treatment of advanced stage favorable histology non-Hodgkin's lymphoma: A preliminary report of a randomized trial comparing single agent chemotherapy, combination chemotherapy and whole body irradiation. Blood 1981 (58):592-598

2 Lister TA: The management of follicular lymphoma. Ann Oncol 1991 (2 suppl 2):131-135

3 Portlock CS: Management of the low grade non-Hodgkin's lymphoma. Semin Oncol 1990 (17):51-59

4 Jones SE, Fuks Z, Bull M, Kadin ME, Dorfman RF, Kaplan HS, Rosenberg SA, Kim H: Non-Hodgkin's lymphomas IV. Clinicopathologic correlation in 405 cases. Cancer 1973 (31):805-823

5 Cullen MH, Lister TA, Brearley RL, Shand WS, Stansfeld AG: Histological transformation of non-Hodgkin's lymphoma. A prospective study. Cancer 1979 (44):645-651

6 Risdall R, Hoppe RT, Warnke R: Non-Hodgkin's lymphoma: A study of the evolution of the disease based upon 92 autopsied cases. Cancer 1979 (44):529-542

7 Garvin AJ, Simon RM, Osborne CK, Merrill J, Young RC and Berard CW: An autopsy study of histological progression in non-Hodgkin's lymphoma: 192 cases from the National Cancer Institute. Cancer 1983 (52):393-398

8 Jones SE, Rosenberg SA, Kaplan HS, Kadin ME, Dorfman RF: Non-Hodgkin's Lymphomas. II. Single agent chemotherapy. Cancer 1972 (30):31-38

9 Bonadonna G, Lattuada A, Banfi A: Recent trends in the treatment of non-Hodgkin's lymphomas. Eur J Cancer 1976 (12):661-673

10 Bodey GP and Rodriguez V: Approaches to the treatment of acute leukemia and lymphoma in adults. Semin Hematol 1978 (15):221-261

11 Portlock CS: Management of the indolent non-Hodgkin's lymphomas. Semin Oncol 1980 (7):292-301

12 Pangalis GA, Tsekouras Ch, Boussiotis VA, Poziopoulos C, Angelopoulou MK, Gribabis DA, Kittas C: Treatment of low grade non-Hodgkin's lymphomas (LGNHL) with chlorambucil and α2b-Interferon (α2b-IFN). Fifth International Conference of Malignant Lymphoma, Lugano, June 1993, p 112 (abstract)

13 Mead GM: The low grade non-Hodgkin's lymphomas. Oncology Today 1992 (6):9-14

14 Kennedy BJ, Bloomfield CD, Kiang DT, Vosika G, Peterson BA, Theologides A: Combination versus successive single agent chemotherapy in lymphocytic lymphoma. Cancer 1978 (41):23-28

15 Pangalis GA, Roussou PA, Kokkinou S, Anagnostopoulos N, Hill RL, Meletis J, Fessas Ph: Treatment of non-Hodgkin's lymphomas with low grade malignancy. In: Sotto, Vrousos, Sotto and Vincent (eds) Non-Hodgkin's Lymphomas: New Techniques and Treatments. 4th Cancer Res Workshop, 1984, pp 210-214

16 Jones SE, Rosenberg SA, Kaplan HS, Kadin ME, Dorfman EF: Non-Hodgkin's Lymphomas. II. Single agent chemotherapy. Cancer 1972 (30):31-38

17 Ezdinli EZ, Costello WG, Silverstein MN, Berard C, Hartsock RJ, Sokal JE: Moderate versus intensive chemotherapy of prognostically favorable non-Hodgkin's lymphoma. Cancer 1980 (46):29-33

18 Morisson VA and Peterson BA: Combination chemotherapy in the treatment of follicular low grade lymphoma. Leukemia and Lymphoma 1993 (10 suppl):29-33

19 Montserrat E, Lopez-Guillermo A, Rozman C: B-cell low grade malignant lymphomas. In: Proceedings of the Educational Programme of the XIIth Meeting of the International Society of Haematology. Vienna 1993, pp 56-79

20 Durr FE, Wallace RF, Citarella RV: Molecular and biochemical pharmacology of mitoxanthrone. Cancer Treat Rev 1983 (10 suppl B):3-11

21 Alberts DS, Peng YM, Leigh S, Davis TP, Woodward DL: Disposition of mitoxanthrone in patients. Cancer Treat Rev 1983 (10 suppl B):23-27

22 Gams RA, Keller JW, Golomb HM, Steinberg J, Dukart G: Mitoxanthrone in malignant lymphomas. Cancer Treat Rev 1983 (10 Suppl B):69-72

22a Coltman CA, McDaniel TM, Balcerzak SP, Morrison FS, VanHoff DD: Mitoxanthrone hydrochloride in lymphoma. Cancer Treat Rev 1983 (10 suppl B):73-76

23 Nissen NI and Hansen SW: High activity of daily schedule mitoxanthrone in newly diagnosed low-grade non-Hodgkin's lymphomas: A 5 year follow up. Semin Oncol 1990 (17 suppl 10):10-13

24 Angelopoulou MK, Lafioniatis SN, Pangalis GA: Low grade non-Hodgkin's lymphomas: Disease control with mitoxanthrone monotherapy in patients refractory to conventional therapy. Leukemia and Lymphoma 1994 (12):253-258

25 Brittinger G, Bartels H, Common H et al (Kiel Lymphoma Study Group): Clinical and prognostic relevance of the Kiel classification of non-Hodgkin's lymphomas: results of a prospective multicenter study by the Kiehl Lymphoma Study Group. Haematol Oncol 1984 (2):269-306

26 Gallagher CJ and Lister TA: Follicular non-Hodgkin's lymphomas. Bailliere's Clinical Haematology 1987 (1):1-19

27 Erbsoll J, Schultz HB, Pedersen-Bjergaard J, Nissen N: Follicular low grade non-Hodgkin's lymphoma: Long term outcome with or without tumor progression. Eur J Haematol 1989 (42):155

28 Luce JK, Gamble JF, Wilson HE et al: Combined cyclophosphamide, vincristine and prednisone therapy of malignant lymphoma. Cancer 1971 (28): 306-317

29 Hoogstraten B, Owens AH, Lenhard RE et al: Combination chemotherapy in lymphosarcoma and reticulum cell sarcoma. Blood 1969 (33):370-378

30 Portlock CS, Rosenberg SA, Glatstein E, Kaplan HS: Treatment of advanced non-Hodgkin's lymphomas with favorable histologies: Preliminary results of a prospective trial. Blood 1976 (47):747-756

31 Portlock CS and Rosenberg SA: Chemotherapy of the non-Hodgkin's lymphomas: The Stanford experience. Cancer Treat Rep 1978 (61):1049-1055
32 Schein PS, Chabner BA, Canellos GP, Young RC, Berard C, DeVita VT: Potential for prolonged disease free survival following combination chemotherapy of non-Hodgkin's lymphoma. Blood 1974 (43):181-189
33 Anderson T, Bender RA, Fischer RI et al: Combination chemotherapy in non-Hodgkin's lymphoma: Results of a long term follow up. Cancer Treat Rep 1977 (61):1057-1066
34 Young RC, Longo DL, Glatsein E, Ihde DC, Jaffe ES, DeVita VT: The treatment of indolent lymphomas: Watchful waiting vs aggressive combined modality treatment. Semin Hematol 1988 (25 suppl 2):11-16
35 McLaughlin P, Cabanillas F, Hagemeister F et al: CHOP-Bleo plus interferon (IFN) in stage IV low grade lymphoma (LGL). Proc Am Soc Clin Oncol 1992 (11):326 (abstract)
36 Romaguera JE, McLaughlin P, North L et al: Multivariate analysis of prognostic factors in stage IV follicular low-grade lymphomas. A risk model. J Clin Oncol 1991 (9):762-769
37 Peterson BA, Frizzera G, Anderson JR et al: Response of low grade lymphomas to cyclophosphamide (CTX) or cyclophosphamide, adriamycin, vincristine, prednisone and bleomycin (CAVPB). Proc Am Soc Clin Oncol 1985 (4):211 (abstract)
38 Peterson BA, Anderson JR, Frizzera G, Bloomfield CD, Gottlieb AJ and Holland JF: Nodular mixed lymphoma (NML): A comparative trial of cyclophosphamide (CTX) and cyclophosphamide, adriamycin, vincristine, prednisone and bleomycin (CAVPB). Blood 1985 (66 suppl 1):216 (abstract)
39 Peterson BA, Andrson JR, Frizzera G, Bloomfield CD, Propert KJ and Gottlieb AJ: Combination chemotherapy prolongs survival in follicular mixed lymphoma (FML). Proc Am Soc Clin Oncol 1990 (9):259 (abstract)
40 Jones SE, Grozea PN, Metz EN et al: Superiority of adriamycin containing combination chemotherapy in the treatment of diffuse lymphoma. Cancer 1979 (43):417-425
41 Longo DL, Young RC, Hubbard SM et al: Prolonged initial remission in patients with nodular mixed lymphoma. Ann Inter Med 1984 (100):651-656
42 Smalley RV, Andersen JW, Hawkins MJ et al: Interferon alfa combined with cytotoxic chemotherapy for patients with non-Hodgkin's lymphoma. N Engl J Med 1992 (327):1336-1341
43 Solal-Celigny Ph, Lepage E, Brousse N et al: Recombinant interferon alfa-2b combined with a regimen containing doxorubicin in patients with advanced follicular lymphoma. N Engl J Med 1993 (329):1608-1614
44 Ezdinli E, Pocock S, Berard CW et al: Comparison of intensive vs moderate chemotherapy of lymphocytic lymphomas. Cancer 1976 (38):1060-1068
45 Klasa RJ, Hoskins PJ, O'Reilly SE et al: BP-VACOP and extensive lymph node irradiation (RT) for advanced stage low grade lymphoma. Proc Am Soc Clin Oncol 1992 (11):328 (abstract)
46 Caplan SN, Shustik C, Joyce LJ: Mitoxanthrone, etoposide and prednisone (MEP) in relapsed low and intermediate grade non-Hodgkin's lymphoma (NHL). Proc Am Soc Clin Oncol 1992 (11):335 (abstract)
47 Simon S, Mucenski J, Zidar B, Viverette F, Pugh R: Effective palliative chemotherapy with bleomycin, vincristine and methyloprednisolone for patients with refractory non-Hodgkin's lymphoma. Proc Am Soc Clin Oncol 1992 (11):320 (abstract)
48 George P and Coleman M: The C3 regimen for resistant lymphoma: Daily oral etoposide, chlorambucil, procarbazine and prednisone. Proc Am Soc Clin Oncol 1993 (12):379 (abstract)
49 McLaughlin P, Hagemeister FB, Swan F et al: A new intensive regimen for stage IV low grade lymphoma: High remission rate with stringent molecular monitoring. Proc Am Soc Clin Oncol 1993 (12):377 (abstract)
50 Einat M, Resmitzky D and Kimchi A: Close link between reduction of c-myc expression by interferon and Go-G1 arrest. Nature 1985 (31) :597-600
51 Schlom J: Monoclonal antibodies: They are more and less than you think. In: Broder S (ed) Molecular Foundation of Oncology. William and Wilkins, Baltimore 1990 pp 95-134
52 McLaughlin P: The role of interferon in the therapy of low-grade lymphoma. Leukemia and Lymphoma 1993 (10 suppl):17-20
53 Merigan TC, Sikora K, Breeden JH, Levy R, Rosenberg SA: Preliminary observations on the effet of human leukocyte interferon in non-Hodgkin's lymphoma. N Engl J Med 1978 (299): 1449-1453
54 Gutterman JU, Blumenschein GR, Alexanian R et al: Leukocyte interferon induced tumor regression in human metastatic breast cancer, multiple myeloma and malignant lymphoma. Ann Intern Med 1980 (93):399-406
55 Louie AC, Gallagher JC, Sikora K, Levy R, Rosenberg SA, Merigan TC: Follow up observations on the effect of human leukocyte interferon in non-Hodgkin's lymphoma. Blood 1981 (58):712-718
56 Horning SJ, Levine JF, Miller RA, Rosenberg SA, Merigan TC: Clinical and immunologic effects of recombinant leukocyte A interferon in 8 patients with advanced cancer. JAMA 1982 (247):1718-1722
57 Foon KA, Roth MS, Bunn PA Jr: Interferon therapy of non-Hodgkin's lymphoma. Cancer 1987 (59 suppl 1):601-604
58 Gams R, Gordon D, Guaspari A, Tuttle R: Phase II trial of human polyclonal lymphoblastoid interferon (Welferon) in the management of malignant lymphomas. Proc Am Assoc Clin Oncol 1984 C-253 (abstract)
59 Quesada JR, Hawkins M, Horning S et al: Collaborative phase I-II study of recombinant DNA produced leukocyte interferon (Clone A) in meta-

static breast cancer, malignant lymphoma and multiple myeloma. Am J Med 1984 (77):427-432
60 Horning S, Merigan TC, Krown SE et al: Human interferon alpha in malignant lymphoma and Hodgkin's disease. Cancer 1985 (56):1305-1310
61 Bunn PA, Ihde DC, Foon KA: The role of recombinant interferon alpha-2a in the therapy of cutaneous T cell lymphomas. Cancer 1986 (57): 1689-1695
62 Wagstaff J, Loynds P, Growther D: A phase II study of human rDNA alpha-2 interferon in patients with low grade non-Hodgkin's lymphoma. Cancer Chemother Pharmacol 1986 (18):54-58
63 O'Connell MJ, Colgan JP, Oken MM, Ritts RE, Kay NE, Itri LM: Clinical trial of recombinant leukocyte A interferon as initial therapy for favorable histology non-Hodgkin's lymphomas and chronic lymphocytic leukemia. An Eastern Cooperative Oncology Group Pilot Study. J Clin Oncol 1986 (4):128-136
64 Foon KA, Sherwin SA, Abrams PG et al: Treatment of advanced non-Hodgkin's lymphoma with recombinant leukocyte A interferon. New Engl J Med 1984 (311):1148-1152
65 Leavitt RD, Ratanatharathorn V, Ozer U, Ultmann JE, Portlock C, Meyers JW: Alpha-2b interferon in the treatment of Hodgkin's disease and non-Hodgkin's lymphoma. Semin Oncol 1987 (14 suppl 2):18-23
66 Mantovani L, Guglielmi C, Martelli M et al: Recombinant alpha interferon in the treatment of low-grade non-Hodgkin's lymphoma: Results of a cooperative phase II trial in 31 patients. Haematologica 1989 (74):571-575
67 Karanes C, Ratanathanathorn V, Jones S et al: Sequential chlorambucil and recombinant DNA alpha-2b IFN (Intron-A) in the treatment of low-grade lymphomas. A SWOG phase II study. Blood 1986 (68 suppl 1):239a (abstract)
68 Ozer H, Anderson JR, Peterson BA et al: Combination trial of subcutaneous interferon alpha-2b and oral cyclophosphamide in favorable histology, non-Hodgkin's lymphoma. Invest New Drugs 1987 (5 suppl):27-33
69 Rohatimer AZS, Richards MA, Barnett MJ, Stansfeld AJ, Lister TA: Chlorambucil and interferon for low grade non-Hodgkin's lymphoma. Br J Cancer 1987 (55):225-226
70 Chisesi T, Capnist G, Vespignani M, Dini E: The role of interferon alpha-2b and chlorambucil in the treatment of non-Hodgkin's lymphoma. Cancer Treat Rev 1988 (15 suppl A):27-33
71 Clark RH, Dimitrov NV, Axelson JA, Charamella LJ, Stott PB: A phase II trial of intermittent leukocyte interferon and high dose chlorambucil in the treatment of non-Hodgkin's lymphoma resistant to conventional therapy. Am J Clin Oncol 1989 (12):75-77
72 Chisesi T (Non-Hodgkin's Lymphoma Cooperative Study Group): Randomized study of chlorambucil (CB) compared to interferon (alpha-2b) combined with CB in low grade non-Hodgkin's lymphoma: an interim report of a randomized study. Eur J Cancer 1991 (27 suppl 4):31-33
73 Price CGA, Rohatimer AZS, Steward W et al: Interferon alpha-2b in addition to chlorambucil in the treatment of follicular lymphoma: preliminary results of a randomized trial in progress. Eur J Cancer 1991 (27 suppl 4):S34-S36
74 Peterson BA, Petroni G, Oken MM, Ozer H for CALBG and ECOG: Cyclophosphamide versus cyclophosphamide plus interferon alfa-2b in follicular low grade lymphomas: A preliminary report of an intergroup trial. Proc Am Soc Clin Oncol 1993 (12):366 (abstract)
75 McLaughlin P, Hagemeister F, Romaguera J et al: CHOP-Bleo plus α-interferon for stage IV low grade lymphoma. Blood 1988 (72 suppl 1):165a (asbtract)
76 Hiddemann W, Unterhalt M, Koch P, Nahler M, Hermann R, Van de Loo J: Alpha interferon maintenance therapy in patients with low grade non-Hodgkin's lymphomas after cytoreductive chemotherapy with prednimustine and mitoxanthrone. Eur J Cancer 1991 (27 suppl 4):37-39
77 Hagenbeek A, Carde P, Somers R et al: Maintenance of remission with human recombinant alpha-2 interferon (Roferon-A) in patients with stages III and IV low grade malignant non-Hodgkin's lymphoma. Results from a prospective, randomized phase III clinical trial in 331 patients. Blood 1992 (80 suppl 1):74a (abstract)
78 Montgomery JA and Hewson K: Synthesis of potential anticancer agents. Part XX 2 - Fluoropurines. J Am Chem Soc 1960 (82):463-468
79 Hang P, Chubb S, Plunkett W: Termination of DNA synthesis by 9-ß-D-arabinosyl-2-fluoroadenine. A mechanism for cytotoxicity. J Biol Chem 1990 (265):16617-16625
80 Spriggs D, Robbins G, Mitchell T, Kufe D: Incorporation of 9-ß-D-arabinofuranosyl-2 fluoroadenine into HL60 cellular RNA and DNA. Biochem Pharmacol 1986 (35):247-252
81 Keating MJ, Kantarjian H, Talpaz M, Redman J, Koller C: Fludarabine: A new agent with major activity against chronic lymphocytic leukemia. Blood 1989 (74):19-25
82 Ross SR, McTavish D, Faulds D: Fludarabine: A review of its pharmacological properties and therapeutic potential in malignancy. Drugs 1993 (45):737-759
83 Hochster HS, Kim K, Green MD et al: Activity of fludarabine in previously treated non-Hodgkin's low grade lymphoma. Results of an Eastern Cooperative Oncology Group Study. J Clin Oncol 1992 (10):28-32
84 Leiby JM, Snider KM, Kraut EH, Metz EN, Malpeis L: Phase II trial of 9-ß-D-arabinosyl-2-fluoroadenine 5-monophosphatase in non-Hodgkin's lymphoma: prospective comparison of response with deoxycytidine kinase activity. Cancer Res 1987 (47):2719-2722
85 Redman JR, Cabanillas F, Velasquez WS, McLaughlin P, Hagemeister FB: Phase II trial of fludarabine phosphate in lymphoma: an effective new agent in low grade lymphoma. J Clin Oncol 1992 (10):970-974

86 Whelan JS, Davis CL, Rule S et al: Fludarabine phosphate for the treatment of low grade lymphoid malignancy. Br J Cancer 1991 (64):120-123

87 Pangalis GA, Angelopoulou MK, Poziopoulos Ch: Fludarabine monophosphate in leukemias and lymphomas. In: Pavlidis N (ed) New Drugs in Cancer Therapy. European School of Oncology Seminar, Corfu, Greece 1993 pp 191-210

88 Hochster H and Cassileth P: Fludarabine phosphate therapy of non-Hodgkin's lymphoma. Semin Oncol 1990 (17 suppl 8):63-65

89 Whelan JS, Ganjoo R, Johnson PWM, Rohatimer AZSS, Lister TA: Treatment of low grade non-Hodgkin's lymphomas with fludarabine. Leukemia and Lymphoma 1993 (10 suppl):35-37

90 Kantarjian HM, Alexanian R, Koller CA, Kurzrock R, Keating MJ: Fludarabine therapy in macroglobulinemic lymphoma. Blood 1990 (75):1928-1931

91 Carson DA, Kaye J, Seegmiller JE: Lymphospecific toxicity in adenosine deaminase deficiency and purine nucleoside phosphorylase deficiency: possible role of nucleoside kinase(s). Proc Natl Acad Sci USA 1977 (74):5677-5681

92 Carson DA, Wasson DB, Teatle R and Yu A: Specific toxicity of 2-chloroadenosine toward resting and proliferating human lymphocytes. Blood 1983 (62):737-743

93 Beutler E: Cladribine (2-chlorodeoxyadenosine). The Lancet 1992 (340):952-956

94 O'Dwyer PJ, Wagner B, Leyland-Jones B, Wittes RE, Cheson BD, Hoth DF: 2-Deoxycoformycin (Pentostatin) for lymphoid malignancies. Ann Intern Med 1988 (108):733-743

95 Kay AC, Saven A, Carrera CJ, Carson DA, Thurston D, Beutler E, Piro LD: 2-Chlorodeoxyadenosine treatment of low grade lymphomas. J Clin Oncol 1992 (10):371-377

96 Saven A and Piro LD: 2-chlorodeoxyadenosine: A new nucleoside agent effective in the treatment of lymphoid malignancies. Leukemia and Lymphoma 1993 (10 suppl):43-49

97 Carson DA, Wasson DB, Esparza LM, Carrera CJ, Kipps TJ, Cottam HB: Oral antilymphocytic activity and induction of apoptosis by 2-chloro-2-ARA-2-deoxyadenosine (CAFdA) Proc Natl Acad Sci USA 1992 (89):2970-2974

98 Dimopoulos MA, Kantarjian H, Estey E et al: Treatment of Waldenström macroglobulinemia with 2-chlorodeoxyadenosine. Ann Inter Med 1993 (118):195-198

99 Rotarski M, Brienza S, Gastiaburu J et al: A new platinum analogue: Active in refractory relapsed intermediate and low grade non-Hodgkin lymphoma (NHL). A phase II study. Proc Am Soc Clin Oncol 1993 (12):375 (abstract)

100 Steward WP, Smith DB, Crowther D: Weekly oral 4-demethoxydaunorubicin in patients with relapsed low grade non-Hodgkin's lymphoma. Ann Oncol 1991 (2):605

101 Raina V, Cunningham D, Gilchrist N, Soukop M: Alfacalcidol is a non toxic effective treatment of follicular small-cleaved cell lymphoma. Br J Cancer 1991 (63):463-465

102 Brenner MK: Interleukin 2 and the treatment of leukemia and lymphoma. Leuk Lymph Rev 1992 (1):339-346

103 Caligiuri MA: Low-dose recombinant interleukin-2 therapy: Rationale and potential clinical applications. Semin Oncol 1993 (20 suppl 9):3-10

104 Minami Y, Kono T, Yamada K, Taniguchi T: The interleukin-2 receptors: insights into a complex signalling mechanism. Biochem Biophys Acta 1992 (1114):163-177

105 Wang HM and Smith KA: The interleukin-2 receptor: Functional consequences of its biomolecular structure. J Exp Med 1987 (166):1055-1069

106 Taniguchi T and Yasuhiro M: The IL-2/IL-2 receptor system. A current overview. Gill 1993 (73):5-8

107 Smith KA: Interleukin-2: Inception, impact and implications. Science 1988 (240):1169-1176

108 Cantrell DA and Smith KA: The interleukin-2 T-cell system: A new cell growth model. Science 1984 (224):1312-1316

109 Caligiuri MA, Zmuidzinas A, Manley TJ, Levine H, Smith KA and Ritz J: Functional consequences of interleukin-2 receptor expression on resting human lymphocytes: Identification of a novel natural killer cell subset with high affinity receptors. J Exp Med 1990 (171):1509-1526

110 Dutcher JP and Wiernik PH: The role of recombinant interleukin-2 in therapy for hematologic malignancies. Semin Oncol 1993 (20 suppl 9):33-40

111 Van der Marst D, Brand A, Van Luxemburg-Heys SAP, Kooy-Winkelaar EMC, Vanrood JJ: Lymphokine activated killer cells functions in patients with leukemic B-lymphoproliferative diseases. Blood 1989 (74):2464-2470

112 Gottlieb DJ, Prendice HG, Heslop HE et al: Effects of recombinant interleukin-2 administration on cytotoxic function following high dose chemotherapy for haematologic malignancy. Blood 1989 (74):2335-2342

113 Broxmeyer HE, Williams DE, Lu L et al: The suppressive influences of human tumor necrosis factor on bone marrow hematopoietic progenitor cells from normal donors and patients with leukemia: Synergism of tumor necrosis factor and interferon-gamma. J Immunol 1986 (136):4487-4495

114 Fearon ER, Pardoll DM, Itaya T et al: Interleukin-2 production by tumor cells bypasses T helper function in the generation of an antitumor response. Cell 1990 (60):397-403

115 Kay N and Zarling J: Restoration of impaired natural killer cell activity of B-chronic lymphocytic leukemia patients by recombinant interleukin-2. Am J Hematol 1987 (24):161-167

116 Williams DP, Snider SE, Strom TB, Murphy JR: Structure function analysis of interleukin-2 toxin (DAB_{486} IL-2). Fragment B sequences required for the delivery of fragment A to the cytosol of target cells. J Biol Chem 1990 (265):11885-11889

117 Caligiuri MA, Murray C, Robertson MJ et al: Selective immune modulation of NK cells following prolonged infusions of low dose recombinant IL-2. J Clin Invest 1993 (91):123-132

118 Hesketh P, Caguioa P, Bulger K et al: Complete response of a cutaneous T-cell lymphoma to an IL-2 diphtheria hybrid toxin (DAB_{486} IL-2). Proc Am Soc Clin Oncol 1991 (19):285 (abstract)
119 Le Maistre CF, Meneghetti C, Rosenblum M et al: Phase I trial of an interleukin-2 (IL-2) fusion toxin (DAB_{486} IL-2) in hematologic malignancies expressing the IL-2 receptor. Blood 1992 (79):2547-2554
120 Weber JS, Yang JC, Topalian SL, Schwartzentruber DJ, White DE, Rosenberg SA: The use of interleukin-2 and lymphokine activated killer cells for the treatment of patients with non-Hodgkin's lymphoma. J Clin Oncol 1992 (10):33-40
121 Tourani JM, Levy V, Briere J, Levy R, Franks C, Andrieu JM: Interleukin-2 therapy for refractory and relapsing lymphomas. Eur J Cancer 1991 (27): 1676-1680
122 Gisselbrecht C, Maraninchi D, Pico JL et al: Interleukin-2 in lymphoma: A phase II multicentric study. Proc Am Assoc Cancer Res 1992 (33): A1360 (abstract)
123 Ellis ED, Williams SF, Golomb HM: Current advances and guidelines in therapy of non-Hodgkin's lymphomas: In: Pangalis GA and Polliack A (eds) Benign and Malignant Lymphadenopathies. Clinical and Laboratory Diagnosis. 1993 pp 319-332
124 Rosenberg SA, Lotze MT, Muul LM et al: A progress report on the treatment of 157 patients with advanced cancer using lymphokine activated killer cells and interleukin-2 or high dose interleukin-2 alone. N Engl J Med 1987 (316):889-897
125 West WH, Taner KW, Yannelli JR et al: Constant infusion recombinant interleukin-2 in adoptive immunotherapy of advanced cancer. N Engl J Med 1987 (316):898-905
126 Allison MAK, Jones SE, McGuffey P: Phase II trial of outpatient interleukin-2 in malignant lymphoma, chronic lymphocytic leukemia and selected solid tumors. J Clin Oncol 1989 (7):75-80
127 Clendeninn NJ, Nethersell ABW, Scott JE, Offenhansen KO, Collier MA: Early safety and efficacy results using Campath-1H (CP-1H), a humanized anti-lymphocyte monoclonal antibody (MAB), in non-Hodgkin's lymphoma (NHL) and chronic lymphocytic leukemia (CLL). Proc Am Soc Clin Oncol 1993 (12):378 (abstract)
127a Tsekouras Ch, Angelopoulou MK, Pangalis GA: Treatment of B-chronic lymphocytic leukaemia (B-CLL) with the monoclonal antibody Campath-1H. Br J Haematol 1994 (87 suppl 1):237
128 Hale G, Clark MR, Marcus R et al: Remission induction in non-Hodgkin lymphoma with reshaped human monoclonal antibody Campath-1H. Lancet 1988 (ii):1394-1399
129 Levy R and Miller RA: Therapy of lymphoma directed at idiotypes. NCI Monographs 1990 (10): 61-68
130 Brown SL, Miller RA, Horning SJ et al: Treatment of B-cell lymphomas with anti-idiotype antibodies alone and in combination with alpha interferon. Blood 1989 (73):651-661
131 Maloney DG, Brown S, Czerwinski DK et al: Long term remissions following monoclonal anti-idiotype antibody therapy of B cell lymphoma. Proc Am Soc Clin Oncol 1992 (11):321 (abstract)
132 Kaminski MS, Zasadny KR, Francis IR et al: Radioimmunotherapy of B-cell lymphoma with [^{131}I] anti-B1 (anti-VD20) antibody. N Engl J Med 1993 (329):495-465
133 Press OW, Eary JF, Appelbaum FR et al: Radiolabeled antibody therapy of B-cell lymphoma with autologous bone marrow support. N Engl J Med 1993 (329):1219-1224
134 Czuczman MS, Straus DJ, Divgi CR et al: Phase I dose escalation trial of iodine labeled monoclonal antibody OKB7 in patients with non-Hodgkin's lymphoma. J Clin Oncol 1993 (11):2021-2029
135 Kwak LW, Campell MJ, Czerwinski DK, Hart S, Miller RA, Levy R: Induction of immune responses in patients with B-cell lymphoma against the surface immunoglobulin idiotype expressed by their tumors. N Engl J Med 1992 (327):1209-1215
136 Sugita K, Majdic O, Stockinger H et al: Use of cocktail of monoclonal antibodies and human complement in selective killing of acute lymphocytic leukemia cells. Int J Cancer 1986 (37):351-357
137 Hamblin TJ, Cattan AR, Glennie MJ et al: Initial experience in treating human lymphoma with a chimeric univalent derivative of monoclonal anti-idiotype antibody. Blood 1987 (69):790-797
138 Bast RC: Progress in radioimmunotherapy. N Engl J Med 1993 (329):1266-1268
139 Buchsbaum DJ, Wahl RL, Normolle DP, Kaminski MS: Therapy with unlabeled and ^{131}I labeled pan-B-cell monoclonal antibodies in nude mice bearing Raji Burkitt's lymphoma xenografts. Cancer Res 1992 (52):6476-6481
140 Bast RC Jr, Ritz J, Lipton JM et al: Elimination of leukemic cells from human bone marrow using monoclonal antibody and complement. Cancer Res 1983 (43):1389-1394
141 Geha RS: Regulation of the immune response by idiotype anti-idiotype interactions. N Engl J Med 1981 (305):25-28
142 Macklis RM, Lin JY, Beresford B, Atcher RW, Hines JJ, Humm JL: Cellular kinetics, dosimetry and radiobiology of alpha-particle radioimmunotherapy: induction and apoptosis. Radiat Res 1992 (130):220-226
143 Nourigat C, Badger CC, Bernstein ID: Treatment of lymphoma with radiolabeled antibody: elimination of tumor cells lacking target antigen. JNCI 1990 (82):47-50
144 Meeker T, Lowder J, Cleary ML, Stewart S, Warnkke R, Sklar J, Levy R: Emergence of idiotype variants during treatment of B-cell lymphomas with anti-idiotype antibodies. N Engl J Med 1985 (312):1658-1665
145 Starnes CO, Carroll WL, Campbell MJ, Houston LL, Apell G, Levy R: Heterogeneity of a murine B cell lymphoma. Isolation and characterization of idiotypic variants. J Immunol 1988 (141):333-339
146 Stevenson GT, Elliott EV, Stevenson FK: Idiotypic determinants on the surface immunoglobulin of neoplastic lymphocytes: a therapeutic target. Fed Proc 1977 (36):2268-2271
147 Levy R, Warnke R, Dorfman RF, Haimovich J: The monoclonality of human B cell lymphoma. J Exp J Med 1977 (145):1014-1028

148 Berinstein N and Levy R: Treatment of a murine B cell lymphoma with monoclonal antibodies and IL-2. J Immunol 1987 (139):971-976
149 Basham TY, Kaminski MS, Kitamura K, Levy R, Merigan TC: Synergistic antitumor effect of interferon and anti-idiotype monoclonal antibody in murine lymphoma. J Immunol 1986 (137):3019-3024
150 Press OW, Farr AG, Borroz KI, Anderson SK, Martin PJ: Endocytosis and degradation of monoclonal antibodies targeting human B-cell malignancies. Cancer Res 1989 (49):4906-4912
151 Thar TL, Million RR, Noyes WD: Total body irradiation in non-Hodgkin's lymphoma. Int J Radiat Biol 1979 (5):171-176
152 Jones SE, Fuks Z, Kaplan HS, Rosenberg SA: Non-Hodgkin's lymphomas: V. Results of radiotherapy. Cancer 1973 (32):682-691
153 Mead GN: Clinical aspects of early stage NHL. Br J Cancer 1991 (61):7-8
154 Young RC, Johnson RE, Canellos GP, Chabner BA, Brereton HD, Berard CW, DeVita VT: Advanced lymphocytic lymphoma: Randomized comparisons of chemotherapy and radiotherapy alone or in combination. Cancer Treat Rep 1977 (61): 1153-1159
155 Chaffey JT, Hellman S, Rosenthal DS, Moloney WC: Total body irradiation in the treatment of lymphocytic lymphoma. Cancer Treat Rep 1977 (61): 1149-1152
156 Johnson RE: Evaluation of fractionated total body irradiation in patients with leukemia and disseminated lymphomas. Radiology 1966 (86): 1085-1089
157 Carabell SC, Chaffey JT, Rosenthal DS, Maloney WC, Hellman S: Results of total body irradiation in the treatment of advanced non-Hodgkin's lymphomas. Cancer 1979 (43):994-1000
158 Choi NC, Timothy AR, Kaufman SD, Carey RW, Aisenberg AC: Low dose fractionated whole body irradiation in the treatment of advanced non-Hodgkin's lymphoma. Cancer 1979 (43):1636-1642
159 Rosenberg SA: Is intensive treatment of favorable non-Hodgkin's lymphoma necessary? In: Wiernik PH (ed) Contraversies in Oncology. John Wiley and Sons, New York 1982 pp 45-60
160 Glatstein E, Fuks Z, Goffiner DR, Kaplan HS: Non-Hodgkin's lymphomas of stage II extent: Is total lymphoid irradiation appropriate treatment? Cancer 1976 (37):2806-2812
161 Monfardini S, Banfi A, Bonadonna G et al: Improved 5-year survival after combined chemotherapy-radiotherapy for stage I-II non-Hodgkin's lymphoma. Int J Radiat Oncol Biol Phys 1980 (6): 125-134
162 McLaughlin P, Fuller L, Velasquez WS, Sullivan-Halley JA, Butler JJ, Cabanillas F: Stage I-II follicular lymphoma: Treatment results for 76 patients. Cancer 1986 (58):1596-1602
163 Ganem G, Lambin Ph, Socie G, Girinsky T, Bosq J, Pico JL, Solal-Celigny Ph, Cosset JM: Low dose limited field radiation therapy (2x2 grays) in the management of low grade non-Hodgkin's lymphomas. Proc Am Soc Clin Oncol 1992 (11): 336 (abstract)
164 Horning SJ and Rosenberg SA: The natural history of initially untreated low-grade non-Hodgkin's lymphomas. New Engl J Med 1984 (311):1471-1475
165 Romaguera JE: Can we identify patients with low grade lymphoma for frontline ABMT? Leukemia and Lymphoma 1993 (10 suppl):9-15

Prognostic Factors in Aggressive Non-Hodgkin's Lymphoma

Bertrand Coiffier

Service d'Hématologie, Hospices Civils de Lyon, Centre Hospitalier Lyon-Sud, 69495 Pierre-Bénite Cedex, France

What is the Main Interest of Prognostic Factors?

Every disease, and particularly non-Hodgkin's lymphomas (NHL), is heterogeneous. In NHL, the major causes of this heterogeneity derive from the numerous different histological subtypes, the lymphoma's origin from either nodal or extranodal sites, and its capacity to remain localized or disseminate in the whole body. This heterogeneity is further complicated by the patient's age and possible associated diseases. In order to propose the best therapeutic options to a patient, a physician should take into account all prognostic implications of this heterogeneity. Because of the diverse manifestations of the lymphoma and the different histological subtypes, it is impossible to predict accurately the outcome for each patient. Large studies on the description of subgroups have been based on series of patients having the same profile and manifestations.

The first step towards the definition of such subgroups was the application to NHL patients of the Ann Arbor staging system [1], originally designed for Hodgkin's disease. This staging system was applied to lymphoma patients for more than 20 years; however, its limitations became apparent with the improvement of therapeutic results, an improvement that was associated with more intensive chemotherapy regimens. During the years 1980-1990 new prognostic parameters were described, some of which with a better capability to distinguish patient subgroups than the Ann Arbor staging system [2]. The definition of these new prognostic indicators has led to the description of prognostic indexes that include the more useful prognostic parameters. Finally, the major centres involved in NHL management have decided to unite their efforts and an International Prognostic Index has recently been formulated [3].

The new area opened up by the study of prognostic factors will allow us to clarify the heterogeneity of lymphoma, to understand why some patients do not respond to therapy as well as expected, to stratify patients before treatment so that comparable subgroups of patients can be described, and to compare results from different trials around the world; moreover, it constitutes a great improvement in the decision making related to the treatment of lymphoma patients.

Description of Major Prognostic Parameters

A variety of clinical features have been identified as being of influence on response to treatment and on survival. The features that have most frequently been associated with the ability to achieve a complete remission after treatment and with a long overall survival are listed in Table 1.

Histological Subtypes

A substantial tissue specimen of the tumour should be obtained in order to establish the diagnosis of lymphoma and its subtype. Additional studies may be useful to obtain or confirm the diagnosis and to establish biological and molecular prognostic factors.

Numerous lymphoma subtypes have been described [4,5]. The disease course associated

Table 1. Prognostic factors associated with achievement of complete remission, long time to treatment failure, and long-term survival in univariate analyses in all lymphoma subtypes

Age (<60 years versus ≥60 years)
Performance status (ECOG scale 0 or 1 versus ≥2)
B symptoms (absence versus presence)
Stage (local [I or II] versus disseminated [III or IV])
Tumour size (<10 cm versus ≥10 cm)
Number of extranodal sites of disease (0 or 1 versus ≥2)
Bone marrow involvement (absence versus presence)
Serum LDH level (normal versus increased)
Serum ß2-microglobulin level (<3 mg/l versus ≥3 mg/l)
Serum albumin level (<35 g/l versus ≥35 g/l)

with each of these subtypes varies from indolent to very aggressive. The histological classifications used in Europe and North America attempt to reflect these different outcomes and categorize histological subtypes into subgroups with a low, intermediate or high risk of progression. However, clinical outcome changes with time as therapeutic strategies improve and some histological subtypes now have a better prognosis than several years ago. On the other hand, in some subtypes no therapeutic improvement may have been achieved and the relative prognosis may thus change from low to high risk. Mantle cell lymphoma represents an example of the latter [6,7].

Diffuse large cell lymphomas (B-cell or T-cell subtypes)

Diffuse large cell lymphomas comprise diffuse mixed lymphomas (F subtype), large cell lymphomas (G subtype), and immunoblastic lymphomas (H subtype) in the Working Formulation for Clinical Usage [4] and may have a B-cell or a T-cell phenotype. In the Kiel classification, they are described as centroblastic or immunoblastic subtypes. No difference was observed between these subtypes in several studies [3,8].

Since the definition of the Working Formulation and the Kiel classification new subtypes of large cell lymphomas have been described [9,10]: anaplastic large cell lymphomas [11,12] and mediastinal clear cell lymphoma [13-15]. Anaplastic large cell lymphomas were initially characterized by their positivity for the CD30 or Ki-1 antigen [16-18]; however, CD30-positive lymphomas can be observed with different morphological aspects [16,19-24] and with various phenotypes [25,26]. No prognostic value has been associated with these different lymphoma subtypes. Cutaneous anaplastic large cell lymphoma patients have been reported to have a longer survival than systemic CD30+ lymphoma patients [27-31], but this better outcome must be compared with the good prognosis of all cutaneous large cell lymphoma patients, either CD30-positive or not [32]. In our experience [33] as well as that of others [34], patients with CD30+ lymphoma from T-cell, B-cell or undetermined lineage have a prognosis similar to that of patients with CD30- large cell lymphomas and the same clinico-biological adverse parameters.

Mediastinal B-cell lymphoma with sclerosis was originally associated with a poor outcome [35-37] but studies involving larger patient series showed that cure can be achieved in mediastinal B-cell lymphoma with the same frequency as in other large cell lymphomas of the mediastinum [13,15,38,39]. Prognostic indicators in these patients are not different from those found in other patients with large cell lymphomas: presence of tumour outside the thorax, number of extranodal sites, and LDH level (see below). In fact, there is nothing in favour of a therapeutic individualization of these patients [40,41].

Patients with immunoblastic lymphomas seemed to have a worse prognosis a few years ago and thus were classified as high grade in the Working Formulation for Clinical Usage. However, more recent studies did not find a worse outcome for these patients when compared to centroblastic lymphoma or other large cell subtype patients [8,42,43]. There was also no significant difference in prognosis between diffuse large cell cases additionally subclassified as large cleaved cell and those with large non-cleaved cells [42].

Burkitt's lymphoma

Burkitt's lymphoma represents 50% of childhood lymphomas and 3% to 5% of adult lymphomas. In children, efficient treatments have been described and these patients have a long survival, except for those with bone marrow or central nervous system involvement [44].

In adult patients, Burkitt's lymphoma is usually associated with a highly proliferative picture, disseminated disease, and very high LDH levels. These patients are at risk for acute tumour lysis syndrome [45] but they respond to therapy, and with high-dose regimens their survival is not different from that of other patients with similar adverse prognostic factors [46].
Small non-cleaved cell lymphomas also represent 50% of the lymphomas seen in HIV-positive patients or in immunocompromised patients after transplantation [47-50]. In such conditions these lymphomas are associated with a poor prognosis.

Lymphoblastic lymphoma

Lymphoblastic lymphoma represents 30% of childhood lymphomas and 1% or 2% of adult lymphomas. However, in the Kiel classification the term lymphoblastic lymphoma is used for undifferentiated lymphomas [5] and pathologists using this classification may find a larger number of lymphoblastic lymphomas. True immature T-cell lymphoblastic lymphoma patients usually have a large mediastinal tumour mass, 50% of them have bone marrow involvement, and 20% meningeal involvement. Thus, the clinical picture of these patients resembles that of adult lymphoblastic leukaemia patients. In these patients, short survival was associated with failure to reach a complete remission, older age, B symptoms, high LDH level, and haemoglobin <10 g/dl [51].

Non-cutaneous T-cell lymphomas

Although the prognostic significance of the lymphoma cell phenotype will be described below, we will briefly mention here the difference between the T-cell lymphoma subtypes. T-cell lymphomas are characterized by their diversity and there exists no good classification to list them. These neoplasms are classified as small lymphocytic, mixed small and large cell, large cell, lymphoepithelioid cell, angiocentric, and adult T-cell leukaemia/lymphoma type [52]. Some cases are associated with angioimmunoblastic or Hodgkin-like features. Patients with small cell disease (small lymphocytic, lymphoepithelioid) have a better outcome than those with larger cell types (large cell, angiocentric). However, these differences in response to treatment and in survival were not found in all studies [53,54]. Among these entities, patients whose lymphoma expresses the CD30 antigen or who have an anaplastic T-cell lymphoma seem to have a longer survival [55].

Immunological Parameters Associated with Prognosis

Lymphoma cells may exhibit a B-cell or a T-cell phenotype or may not be immunologically characterized because of the lack of B or T-cell specific markers or because of the expression of markers from both lineages. If some histological subtypes are always of B-cell lineage (Burkitt's lymphoma) or T-cell lineage (CTCL), large cell lymphomas may have a B or T-cell phenotype. Moreover, a large proportion of diffuse mixed lymphoma in the Working Formulation have a T-cell phenotype and are described as T-cell lymphomas in the Kiel classification. Do large T-cell lymphoma patients have a different outcome from those with large B-cell lymphomas? Do "diffuse mixed" T-cell lymphoma patients have a similar outcome to large cell lymphoma patients and should they be treated with the same regimens or do they need a specific approach? Most T-cell lymphomas are not low grade lymphomas as described in the Kiel classification because the median survival of these patients is usually shorter than that of large cell lymphoma patients [56-61].
Preliminary reports considering small numbers of patients with T-cell lymphomas described an aggressive course with a poor outcome in most cases [62-65]. However, studies on larger patient series including T-cell and B-cell lymphomas treated in the same way reported heterogeneous outcomes without an adverse prognosis for T-cell lymphoma patients in some studies [58,61] but with a shorter disease-free survival or a shorter survival in others [57,59, 60,66,67].
T-cell lymphoma patients more often have a poor performance status, disseminated stage with B symptoms, extranodal sites of disease, and high LDH levels. It is unknown if the poor outcome associated with T-cell phenotype is related to the immunological phenotype of lymphoma cells or to the frequent concomitant adverse parameters seen in these patients.

True histiocytic lymphomas have been described [68-70] but the patient numbers are too small to provide any real prognostic indicators.

Karyotypic Abnormalities Associated with Prognosis

Certain karyotypic translocations have been closely associated with some histological subtypes. It is currently unknown if the presence or absence of these characteristic translocations have a prognostic value within specific histological subgroups. It is also unclear if the presence of such karyotypic abnormalities in other histological subtypes carries a particular prognostic value.

The t(8;14) (q24;q32) and variant translocations [t(2;8) and t(8;22)], which rearrange the proto-oncogene c-*myc* on 8q24 with the immunoglobulin genes, result in a deregulation of the expression of c-*myc* messenger RNA and protein. These abnormalities were first identified in small non-cleaved cell (SNCC) Burkitt's lymphomas and were thought to be associated with the poorer prognosis of this particular histological subtype. The presence of the t(8;14) (q24;q32) translocation has also been reported in large cell lymphomas and follicular lymphomas [71].

Abnormalities of either the long (1q21-23) or short (1p32-36) arms of chromosome 1 have been associated with adverse outcome for intermediate and low-grade lymphoma [71,72]. Multiple chromosomal abnormalities involving chromosome 6 have been reported in up to one third of lymphomas and may be associated with an adverse outcome in large cell lymphomas [71-73]. Recent molecular analyses indicate, however, that several distinct breakpoints in 6q21-27 may be implicated in different histological subtypes, and further analysis is needed to assess if these abnormalities are really of prognostic significance [74,75]. Structural abnormalities or monosomy of chromosomes 7 and 17 have also been reported as having an adverse prognostic value [71,72,76, 77], as well as trisomy 7 [71]. A small multiparametric analysis showed that trisomy 5, 6, or 8, chromosome 5 abnormalities, and 14q11-12 aberrations were significantly associated with adverse prognosis [78]. A larger multivariate analysis performed on a cohort of 205 large cell lymphoma patients demonstrated that breaks at 1q21-23 or the presence of 4 marker chromosomes were significantly and independently associated with shortened survival [71]. It will be of interest to determine if the rearrangement of the *bcl*-6 gene located on 3q27 and recently identified in 15% to 35% of diffuse large cell lymphomas [79,80] carries a particular prognosis [81].

As outlined, recurrent karyotypic abnormalities result in direct changes in gene structure or expression that dramatically influence the biology of lymphoma cells. Therefore, the molecular lesions encountered in NHL may profoundly influence the clinical behaviour of the disease and patient outcome. Given the complexity of karyotypic changes, the identification of genes involved in these changes is slow, although many of them have been characterized over the past 10 years. This - and the difficulty of routine molecular investigations - explain the scarcity of clinical data correlating patients' prognosis to molecular abnormalities. As a result, only 3 genes have been more extensively studied: c-*myc*, *bcl*-2 and *p53*.

C-*myc* rearrangement is more frequent in primary extranodal lymphomas than in primary nodal lymphomas [82]. Acquired abnormalities of c-*myc* have been well documented in some cases of histological progression in follicular lymphomas [83,84], but these cases seem to be infrequent [85].

Expression of the *bcl*-2 protein has no influence on the outcome in follicular lymphoma patients [86]. In large cell lymphomas, expression of the *bcl*-2 protein may be associated with a poor outcome [87].

Recent data suggest that mutations of the *p53* gene, a tumour suppressor gene localized on chromosome 17, may occur in a certain subset of NHL with an adverse prognosis. Mutations of *p53* in NHL were first detected in Burkitt's lymphoma, in a substantial (38%) number of cases [88]. *p53* mutations were also reported to be more often found in patients with advanced disease [89]. Other reports suggest that the occurrence of *p53* mutations is frequently associated with histological transformation of follicular lymphomas, and in some cases may even precede the clinical occurrence of transformation [90,91]. If these findings are confirmed in larger series, it may turn out that *p53* mutation can affect the outcome of some subsets of lymphoma patients.

Parameters Related to the Patient

Age

The effect of age on treatment results has been analysed in various ways in a number of published studies. In a Southwest Oncology Group (SWOG) study, older patients had a worse outcome because they responded less well to treatment and relapsed more often. This poorer outcome was related to a decrease in chemotherapy dose intensity because aged patients should receive only 50% of the drug dosage [92]. In another study, aged patients were observed to die more often during the first courses of treatment but those who responded to this treatment did well after response was achieved [93,94]. It was then concluded that aged patients are more likely to present complications after chemotherapy because of their age and possible disabilities. Whatever the reason, age was isolated as an adverse prognostic factor in all studies [3,8,95-101].

The cutoff between young and old patients is between 60 and 65 years for patients with large cell lymphomas [3]. As an example, Figure 1 shows the survival of patients treated for an aggressive lymphoma in the Groupe d'Etude des Lymphomes de l'Adulte (GELA) in 3 subgroups: patients younger than 55 with the best outcome, those aged between 55 and 65 with an intermediate outcome, and those older than 65 with the worst outcome.

When prognostic parameters were analysed separately for patients younger or older than 60, few differences could be found between the groups [95,97,102]. Older patients often have a poorer performance status or stage IV disease but these differences are rarely statistically significant. Finally, the predictive capacity of chronological age and the tolerability of therapy are related to poor performance status (PS), the presence of concomitant diseases, the dose intensity of chemotherapy, and the patients' physiological resources. In an elderly patient with a good PS and few or no debilitating concomitant diseases, there is no reason to withhold curative treatment.

Infection by the Human Immunodeficiency Virus (HIV)

The development of non-Hodgkin's lymphomas is frequently observed in HIV-seropositive individuals. It has been suggested that survival prolongation of HIV-infected individu-

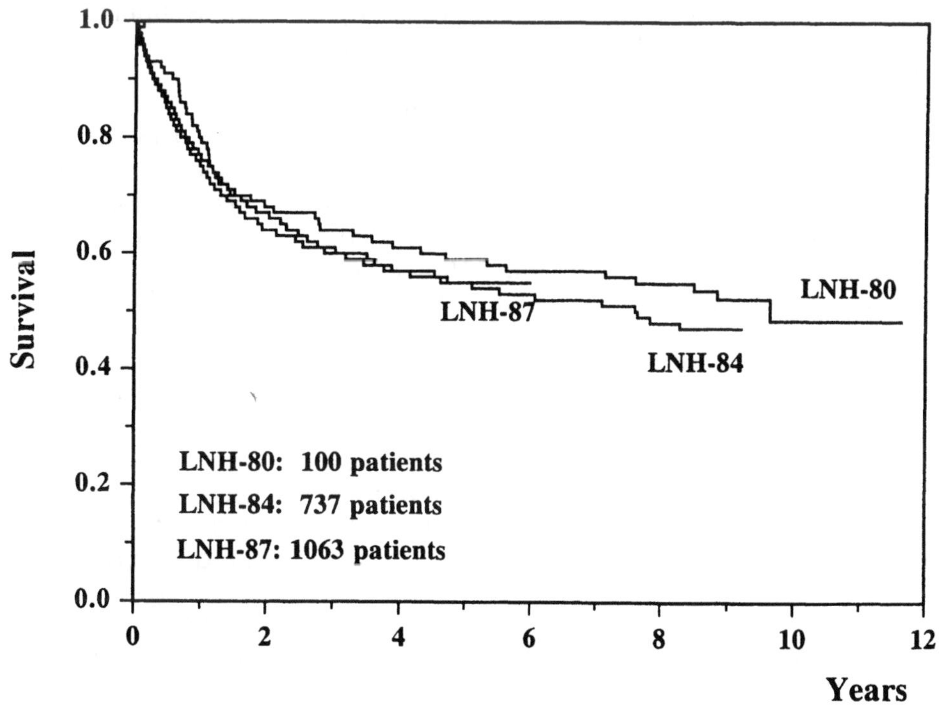

Fig. 1. Overall survival of aggressive lymphoma patients included in the LNH-80, LNH-84 and LNH-87 trials [43,46]

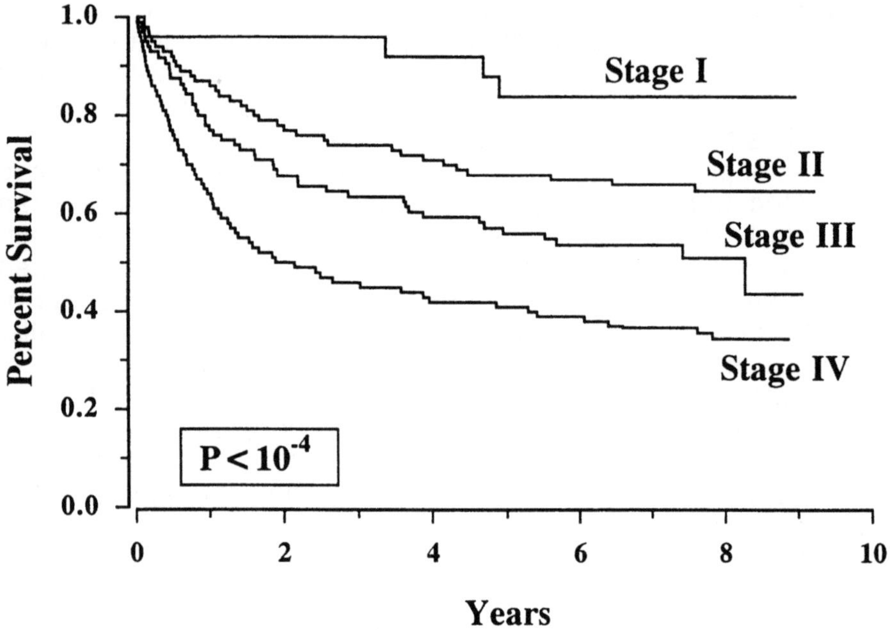

Fig. 2. Advanced stage patients have a poorer outcome than patients with localized disease. Overall survival of patients included in the LNH-84 regimen [43] according to disease stage ($p < 0.10^{-4}$)

als secondary to the use of specific anti-viral therapy and improved treatment of opportunistic infections will result in an increased frequency of NHLs in such patients [103]. Patient status and history regarding HIV infection allow us to distinguish histologically aggressive and disseminated NHLs occurring early in the disease, which may even be the first AIDS manifestation, from primary CNS lymphomas that appear later in the evolution of AIDS and bear an extremely poor prognosis [47]. Several studies have identified prognostic factors for AIDS-related lymphoma patients [104-106]. In 141 patients prospectively treated with an intensive chemotherapy regimen, multivariate analysis identified 4 major prognostic factors predicting outcome: 1) CD4+ lymphocyte count below 100×10^6/l; 2) performance status greater than 1; 3) immunoblastic histological subtype; 4) manifestation of AIDS prior to the onset of the lymphoma [106]. Therefore, HIV-induced severe immunosuppression seems to be the main adverse factor affecting outcome, although a substantial proportion of patients without adverse prognostic factors can benefit from durable lymphoma remission.

Prognostic Parameters Related to Tumour Mass

A large tumour mass has long been recognized as an important adverse parameter. However, the estimation of tumour mass differs widely from one study to another. Parameters associated with a large tumour mass and with prognosis are: number of nodal sites, number of extranodal sites, specific sites, largest diameter of the tumour, stage, LDH level, and ß2-microglobulin level. We will describe each of these factors and discuss their relative power to distinguish poor-outcome patients.

Stage

The Ann Arbor staging system was originally devised for Hodgkin's disease [1] but it has always been applied to non-Hodgkin's lymphoma patients as well. However, since it was devised for an essentially nodal disease, it is rather difficult to use it for NHLs because of 1) their diffusion to bone marrow; 2) the extranodal primary localizations in up to 40% of large cell subtype patients; 3) the weak correlation between extranodal diffusion and outcome in some lymphoma subtypes.

Stage is somehow related to outcome and in most studies stage I patients typically have a longer survival than stage IV patients [8,98, 100,107-110]. The results observed for patients included in the LNH-84 study [43] are shown in Figure 2; they illustrate the poorer outcome of advanced stages.

Number of nodal sites

The spreading of the lymphoma may reflect its tumour mass and this point has been taken into account in the Ann Arbor staging system. Patients with truly localized disease (stage I) have a better outcome than patients with locally disseminated disease (stage II) or patients with enlarged lymph nodes in the whole body (stage III). However, the number of nodal areas involved by the lymphoma has never been studied, probably because this can only be done after biopsies of all lymph node areas and because an elaborate estimation of lymphoma cell dissemination is not really useful for prognosis or choice of treatment.

The number of lymph node areas with nodes larger than 2 cm has been described as a strong prognostic parameter [99,111-113]. It is, however, related to other important prognostic parameters and disappears in multivariate analysis.

Nowadays the number of involved nodal sites is no longer considered as a prominent prognostic indicator. Estimation of disease stage, either localized or disseminated, is more powerful and easier to obtain.

Number of extranodal sites

The number of lymphoma localizations to be found depends on the number and the extent of specialized examinations (e.g. CT scan, endoscopy, fluid examinations, biological tests). Patients with extranodal sites of disease may either have a localized lymphoma with involvement of only one site with or without regional dissemination, or disseminated disease. The number of extranodal localizations is probably a reflection of the disease's propensity to disseminate through the whole body. More than one extranodal site has been associated with a poor prognosis [8,98,99,110,112-117]. The number of extranodal sites of disease is one of the most relevant prognostic factors in aggressive (large cell) lymphomas and it keeps its prognostic value in multivariate analyses (Table 2) [3,8].

Table 2. Frequency of extranodal sites of disease among patients included in the LNH-84 regimen, aggressive lymphoma patients with primary and secondary involvement [101], and patients recorded in the Danish NHL registry; all histological types but only primary involvement [201]

Extranodal sites of disease	**LNH-84 regimen patients**		**Danish NHL registry patients**	
	N (%)	Prognostic value	N (%)	Prognostic value
Bone marrow	173 (23)	0.001	89 (19)	0.031
Spleen	158 (21)	0.01		
GI tract	124 (17)			
- Stomach			87 (19)	
- Intestine			52 (11)	
Liver	117 (16)	0.01	27 (6)	0.001
Pleura	98 (13)	0.01		
Head and neck	85 (12)			
Bone	68 (9)		41 (9)	
Lung	64 (9)		24 (5)	
Skin	46 (6)		56 (12)	
CNS	37 (5)		33 (7)	
Salivary glands			17 (4)	
Thyroid			25 (5)	
Testes			15 (3)	0.015

Largest diameter of the tumour

Another means for expressing the aggressiveness of a lymphoma is by measuring the largest diameter of the largest (nodal) tumour on CT scans. Poor outcome has been associated with the largest tumours but the cutoff may vary from 5 cm to 10 cm [8,99,112,114-116, 118]. Large tumours are thought to be associated with an increased risk of development of more aggressive clones of the lymphoma cells but this adverse prognosis does not persist in some multiparametric analyses [3] because it is closely associated with other adverse parameters.

Specific extranodal localizations

Lymphoma cells may originate in every organ or lymph node of the body and thus the extranodal sites may be as diverse as the number of body parts. Some of these extranodal sites may be associated with poorer outcome in retrospective studies. However, all multiparametric analyses have shown that a poorer outcome was observed in patients with a large number of extranodal sites [3,8,112-115,117] and not in patients with specific localizations.

Patients with bone marrow involvement have disseminated disease and thus have a poorer outcome than those with normal marrow. Burkitt's and lymphoblastic lymphoma patients with bone marrow involvement have a considerably worse prognosis than those without marrow involvement and are generally treated as leukaemia patients [51,119-123]. Only 20% to 25% of large cell lymphoma patients in various studies had bone marrow involvement at the time of diagnosis but these patients showed a poorer response to therapy and a shorter survival [98,110,118,124,125]. This poorer outcome, however, was not observed in all studies and its prognostic significance was rarely conserved in multiparametric analysis [3,8,114,126]. Recently, bone marrow infiltration was subdivided into infiltration by large cells similar to those seen in the lymph node and infiltration by small cells [127-129]. Patients with large cell lymphoma and bone marrow involvement by small cell lymphoma have a higher risk of relapse but a longer survival than patients with involvement by large cells [127-129].

Gastrointestinal localization is the most frequent extranodal site in lymphomas but its prognostic value as well as its therapy have been discussed for more than 30 years [130]. Gastrointestinal involvement is sometimes confounded with MALT lymphoma but large cell lymphoma is more frequent than MALT subtypes and has a poorer outcome. The idea of a more favourable outcome associated with gastrointestinal tract lymphomas may be related to the fact that 80% are gastric lymphomas, that 30% to 40% of gastric lymphomas have a MALT subtype, and that half of the large cell lymphomas from gastric or intestine sites are localized. However, compared to another population with localized nodal or extranodal but non-gastrointestinal sites, patients with histologically localized gastrointestinal lymphomas did not have a statistically different outcome [131].

Central nervous system (CNS) lymphomas have always been considered as a special localization requiring specific treatments. In fact CNS lymphomas comprise 4 different subgroups of patients: those with meningeal localization; those with an extradural spinal space lymphoma with spinal cord compression; those with primary large cell lymphoma of hemispheric or non-hemispheric localization; and immunocompromised patients with lymphoma as a secondary manifestation, particularly HIV-positive patients. Meningeal involvement may be seen in small cell lymphomas or large cell lymphomas but is more frequent in lymphoblastic or Burkitt's subtypes [132,133]. This involvement reflects disseminated disease and is always associated with a poor outcome. However, patients with CNS disease do not seem to have a worse prognosis than patients without CNS involvement but with similar degrees of LDH elevation or with bone marrow involvement, suggesting that extensive disease rather than CNS involvement is responsible for the poor prognosis [44]. CNS localizations at the time of relapse are always an indicator of poor prognosis [134]. Lymphoma of the extradural spinal space associated with spinal cord compression has been associated with a poor outcome but this localization has never been studied in large series or in multiparametric analysis [135]. Primary CNS lymphomas are usually large cell lymphomas and are rarely associated with nodal or other extranodal sites of lymphoma [136-138]. Adverse prognostic factors associated with these lymphomas are identical to those isolated in non-CNS lymphoma patients: high LDH level, poor PS, age older than 60. Specific adverse prognostic parameters have been isolated in large series of patients: high CSF protein at diagnosis, impaired neurological function, particularly memory dysfunction, non-hemispheric tumour site [138,139]. High-dose methotrexate in the treatment has resulted in longer survival [138, 140]. Intraocular lymphoma is associated with primary CNS lymphomas [141-143].

Primary cutaneous lymphomas are polymorphic in appearance, clinical manifestation, histological subtype, and outcome. Apart from the cutaneous T-cell lymphoma of the *mycosis fungoides* subtype with its characteristic epidermoid infiltration, all other subtypes may occur as a primary cutaneous lymphoma but the most frequent subtypes are large B-cell lymphoma and CD30-positive lymphomas [144, 145]. Large B-cell lymphomas are often localized, indolent in their evolution, and have a good prognosis [32,146]. They may, however, disseminate to non-cutaneous sites after months or years. Because of this favourable outcome they have been compared to MALT lymphoma of the skin [147]. The most common cutaneous lymphoma is a large cell lymphoma, CD30-positive, with a T-cell phenotype or a null phenotype [24]. These patients often have several cutaneous localizations that may appear or disappear with time before becoming larger. This lymphoma has a favourable outcome [28]. The better survival of cutaneous CD30-positive cell patients could not be ascribed to differences in age, stage, or initial mode of treatment [148].

Lactic dehydrogenase (LDH) level

LDH is a cytoplasmic enzyme whose level increases in blood when cells are lysed by any mechanism (viral hepatitis, infarction, spontaneous death). In neoplastic disease the LDH blood level is a marker of increased cell turnover and a substitute for tumoural mass [149, 150]. Increased LDH level has been Isolated as a prognostic factor in lymphoma patients since the first prognostic factor studies [151-153] and in nearly all published prognostic analyses [2,8,98,99,101,107,110,112,154]. A general finding is that the higher the LDH level, the poorer is the outcome [2,8].

Recent multivariate analyses have established that an above normal LDH level is one of the most important prognostic factors [2,3,8].

ß2-microglobulin level

The adverse prognosis associated with a high level of ß2-microglobulin was recognized in lymphoma patients as well as myeloma patients years ago [155-157], but this parameter has not been widely used since. This explains why too few patients had a result for ß2-microglobulin level in the International Prognostic Index study and why this parameter did not appear to be of interest for prognosis in large cell lymphoma patients.

A high ß2-microglobulin level has been defined as greater than 3 mg/l, i.e., between 1.25 and 1.4 times the normal value (2.1 to 2.4 mg/ml). The putative importance of ß2-microglobulin level was recognized and applied in some centres [158-160]. In the M.D. Anderson Cancer Center, Houston, LDH level and ß2-microglobulin level are the two most important parameters to predict outcome of large cell lymphoma [159]. Like LDH level, ß2-microglobulin level seems to be one of the parameters that may predict the risk of relapse for complete remission patients [161].

Prognostic Parameters Related to Patient-Tumour Relationship

Under this heading we have assembled parameters not directly related to tumour measurement such as largest diameter of the tumoural mass or LDH level. These parameters are B symptoms, performance status, albumin and haemoglobin levels. They are clearly interrelated and one prognostic study may only isolate one of them as being prominently statistically important. They probably reflect the same phenomenon, i.e., cytokine secretion by either tumour cells or, more likely, the patient's immune cells responding to the tumour. Whereas older studies favour B symptoms, more recent ones, such as the International Prognostic Index, prefer performance status, while statisticians will select serum albumin or haemoglobin levels because they are more easily measurable.

Table 3. Equivalence of performance status as defined originally by the Eastern Cooperative Oncology Group and the Karnovsky index

	ECOG scale		Karnofsky index
0	No symptoms	90-100%	Normal activity
1	Symptoms but continued ability to ambulate	80%	Decreased ability to work
2	Bedridden status less than 50% of the day	70%	Home work possible but efforts impossible
3	Bedridden status greater than 50% of the day	50-60%	Limited home work with need for help
4	Chronic bedridden status and requirement of daily maintenance	10-40%	Chronic bedridden status and requirement of daily maintenance

B symptoms

B symptoms have been originally described for Hodgkin's disease patients [1]. They are defined as either weight loss greater than 10%, fever higher than 38°C for more than one week, or abundant night sweats, requiring a change of nightclothes 2 or 3 times a night. Fever or night sweats are indirect manifestations which are difficult to define; they are related to interleukin secretion but not to tumour burden. Therefore, the B symptom parameter was primarily used in older studies [118,124,162] and has been supplanted by its main component, important weight loss, or by performance status. We propose to abandon these two symptoms. Weight loss may be related to interleukin secretion too but may be secondary to other manifestations of the lymphoma such as GI tract localization, age of the patient, poor PS. It has some prognostic importance in itself [8,43].

Performance status

The ability to lead a normal life may be measured by the performance status (PS) according to the scales described by the Eastern Clinical Oncology Group (ECOG) or D.A. Karnovsky [163,164] (Table 3). This type of functional status assessment has been widely used in oncology to measure loss of normal functions, as well as physiological and psychological effects. The ECOG scale is simpler and more generally used, but both scales have been validated in a large number of patients. Even if this type of measurement is somewhat subjective, the reliability of these indexes has been validated in prospective studies where the measurementes were carried out independently by two physicians and by the patient [165]. Patients with a PS equal to or greater than 2 are non-ambulatory and not able to carry out everyday tasks by themselves. Lymphoma patients with B symptoms, older age, weight loss or large tumour burden frequently have a PS of 2.

Poor PS was associated with an adverse prognosis in nearly all analyses which considered it as a potential prognostic parameter [2,3, 100,110,114,115]. PS allows the physician to globally appreciate if a patient tolerates the lymphoma or if the tumour is poorly tolerated.

Serum albumin level

Four recent analyses of prognostic factors [8,107,166,167] showed that the serum albumin level is a strong prognostic indicator in large cell lymphomas. Patients with serum albumin lower than 35 g/l have a high death rate during treatment (Fig. 3). This was associated with a higher toxicity of treatment courses, particularly haematological, and a higher failure rate. In our personal analyses, serum albumin level is closely correlated with B symptoms, weight loss, and poor PS. This parameter was not taken into account in the International Prognostic Index study because too few patients had this measurement done.

Haemoglobin level

The haemoglobin level at diagnosis, like the serum albumin level, has been related to death rate during treatment and response to treatment [101,166]. Anaemia is usually defined as a haemoglobin level of less than 12 g/dl. The shorter survival for anaemic patients is independent of bone marrow infiltration by lymphoma cells [168].

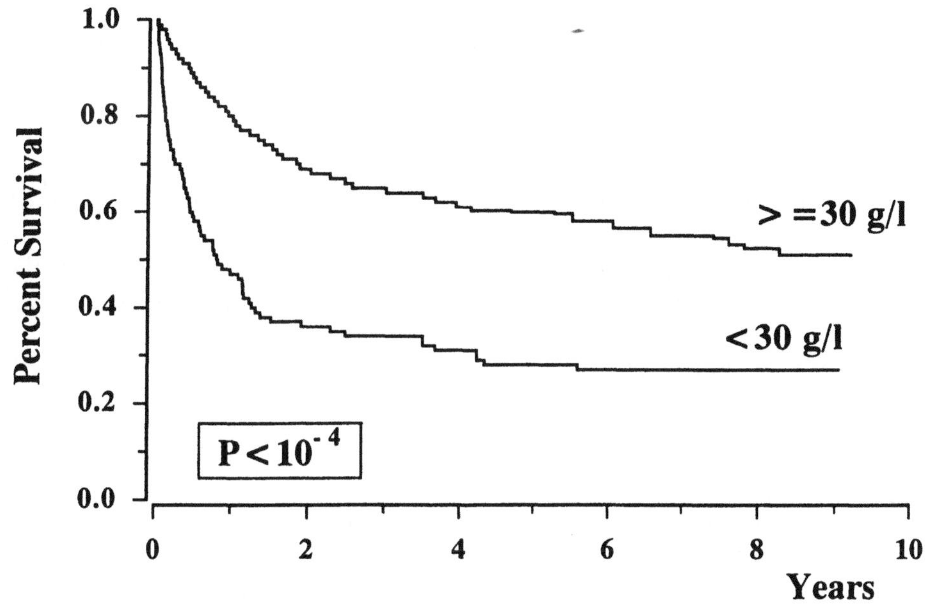

Fig. 3. Survival of the patients treated with the LNH-84 regimen [43] according to serum albumin level

Prognostic Parameters Related to the Physician

Although it has not been proved unequivocally and is still under discussion, the outcome of lymphoma patients is also influenced by the physician who treats the patient. Non-Hodgkin's lymphoma is a complicated disease and physicians must have a wide experience in this field to correctly treat a patient. To be aware of the different clinical aspects, treatment-related complications, and therapeutic interventions, a physician should see at least 40 patients a year. Contacts with a large cooperative lymphoma group are recommended. In addition, increasing experience with any treatment regimen seems to be associated with improved treatment results, particularly with a decrease in treatment-related mortality [169].

Choice of treatment

As pointed out above, physicians must have good experience with the treatment regimen they prefer, in order to decrease the occurrence of treatment-related complications and treatment-related deaths [94]. Moreover, the treatment must be adapted to the patient and the aggressiveness of the lymphoma and, therefore, the physician has to take into account all the most important prognostic parameters described in this chapter.
The first aim of treatment must be to achieve complete remission as quickly as possible. Irrespective of the lymphoma subtype and the treatment, PR patients have a poorer outcome than complete remission patients [107,110, 170]. Moreover, the speed at which they reach this complete remission may be important [171].
Involvement of the CNS was frequent in relapsed patients with large cell lymphomas or other aggressive subtypes treated with CVP or CHOP regimens before the introduction of regimens containing high-dose i.v. methotrexate: 5% of 1039 patients in a SWOG study [172], 16% of 174 patients in the M.D. Anderson Cancer Center [173], 9% of 592 patients from Boston [133]. As high-dose i.v. methotrexate is very effective in treating CNS localizations [174], the use of high-dose methotrexate (greater than 200 mg/m^2) in front-line chemotherapy regimens has dramatically decreased this recurrence and has probably increased the cure rate. For example, less than 1% of the patients included in the LNH-84 regimen without initial CNS localization recurred in the CNS (meningeal or hemispheric sites) [43].

Dose-intensity importance

The dose intensity (DI) of a regimen can be modified by increasing individual drug doses or adding new drugs [175]. Several regimens containing 4 to 5 drugs have been reported on, with CR and survival rates comparable to regimens using smaller numbers of drugs [176, 177]. The identical results obtained with Pro-

MACE-MOPP and ProMACE-MOPP "flexitherapy" (in which MOPP sequences were delivered later) also suggest that the number of non-crossresistant drugs administered over a short induction period is not a determinant factor for outcome [178]. Attempts to increase CHOP or MACOP-B dose intensity with the addition of bleomycin or etoposide also did not improve CR rates or survival [179,180]. In most cases, the addition of new drugs to a regimen results in decreased doses of the drugs already administered in this regimen to avoid unacceptable toxicity. The resulting decreased DI of drugs such as doxorubicin and cyclophosphamide may affect the final outcome.

Although it has been suggested that increased DI may improve the survival of aggressive lymphoma patients [175,181], no randomized study has investigated whether the same combination regimen used at an increased DI is associated with improved survival. However, many studies have shown that patients receiving low doses of therapy due to old age or other adverse factors (e.g. bone marrow involvement) have a very poor outcome [92, 182]. Several retrospective analyses conducted in patients who received CHOP, CHOP-like, or high-dose CHOP regimens suggested that the delivered DI could influence survival [183-185]. The largest study analyzed the outcome of 311 patients included in the prospective LNH-87 trial according to the received relative DI of doxorubicin and cyclophosphamide [185]. Significantly decreased response (65% versus 79%) and survival rates (61% versus 72%) were observed in patients receiving a DI below 70% of the planned dose, and this difference remained significant in multiparametric analysis (p=0.004) [185]. However, in several phase II SWOG studies, the relative DI after 12 weeks was associated with CR and survival but was not found to be an independent prognostic variable. The retrospective character of all these studies is an important limitation since the physician's choice to administer drugs at high DI is heavily influenced by pretreatment prognostic factors such as age, performance status, or B symptoms [181].

Taken together, these data suggest that the number of drugs administered is less important than the DI of "standard" drugs such as cyclophosphamide and doxorubicin. These data and others [178] further suggest that increased DI may improve the outcome of aggressive lymphoma patients. Regimens with a high DI (especially of cyclophosphamide) have been utilized for selected patients with a predicted poor outcome with interesting preliminary results [186-189]. However, the definition of "high-risk" patients in these studies is quite heterogeneous. A consensus definition of poor-prognosis patients [3] will facilitate the identification of these patients and the interpretation of such studies.

Therapeutic innovations based on small alterations of existing regimens are unlikely to result in significant differences in outcome and may actually compromise the original results of the regimen.

Prognostic Indexes

A number of investigators have utilized the subset of clinical features that retained independent significance in multivariate analysis of their patients to develop prognostic factor models predictive of an individual patient's risk of shortened survival. Although the specific clinical features utilized in the prognostic factor models differed, each model incorporated features that reflected the volume of disease and the extent of tumour involvement at diagnosis [2].

Previous Indexes

The Dana-Farber Cancer Institute (Boston, MA) developed a prognostic factor model in aggressive lymphoma patients treated with M-BACOD or m-BACOD regimens based on pretreatment performance status, tumour mass, and number of extranodal sites [114,115]. Investigators at M.D. Anderson Cancer Center (Houston) developed several prognostic factor models [99,112,158,159,190], including one based on pretreatment serum LDH levels and assessment of tumour burden (number of extranodal and extensive nodal sites of involvement). Memorial Sloan-Kettering Cancer Center (New York) investigators defined a prognostic factor model based on pretreatment serum LDH levels and assessment of the location and size of nodal and extranodal sites of disease (level of site involvement) [117].

Recently the GELA (Groupe d'Etude des Lymphomes de l'Adulte, France) compared the predictive value of these prognostic factor models and found that they were equally predictive of survival in the 737 aggressive lymphoma patients treated with the LNH-84 regimen [2]. The GELA also developed its own prognostic factor model which included an assessment of pretreatment serum LDH level, Ann Arbor stage, the number of extranodal sites of disease, and tumour bulk [8]. This model identified 3 groups of large cell lymphoma patients with rates of complete remission and 3-year survival of 93% and 88%, 83% and 71%, and 62% and 41%, respectively.

In addition to identifying clinical prognostic features that predict the likelihood of large cell lymphoma patients achieving a complete remission and surviving for 5 years, investigators have identified clinical characteristics associated with the risk of relapse. This parameter is important because patients at high risk of relapse may benefit from more intensive consolidation chemotherapy. In several independent studies, increased pretreatment serum LDH level and disseminated disease (Ann Arbor stage III or IV) have been associated with the likelihood of relapse [8,191].

International Non-Hodgkin's Lymphoma Prognostic Index (IPI)

In 1990 there was a consensus that an international classification system based on clinically relevant prognostic factors in large cell lymphoma should be developed and utilized [192]. Consequently, 16 single institutions and cooperative groups in the United States, Europe and Canada participated in the International Non-Hodgkin's Lymphoma Prognostic Factor Project [3]. In 2031 patients of all ages the model, based on age, tumour stage, serum lactate dehydrogenase concentration, performance status and number of extranodal disease sites, identified 4 risk groups with predicted 5-year survival rates of 73%, 51%, 43% and 26% (Table 4). In 1274 patients of 60 years or younger, an age-adjusted model based on tumour stage, lactate dehydrogenase level and performance status identified 4 risk groups with predicted 5-year survival rates of 83%, 69%, 46% and 32%. In both models, an increased mortality risk was due to both a lower complete response rate and a higher relapse rate.

These two indexes, the IPI and the age-adjusted international index, were significantly

Table 4. The International Non-Hodgkin's Lymphoma Prognostic Factor Index (adapted from Shipp MA and coll. [3])

Model		**Age-adjusted model**	
Age			
Ann Arbor stage		Ann Arbor stage	
Performance status		Performance status	
Serum LDH		Serum LDH	
Number of extranodal sites of disease			
Survival according to risk groups			
Number of factors and percentage of patients	Complete remission rate	5-year DFS	5-year survival
0 or 1 (35)	87	70	73
2 (27)	67	50	51
3 (22)	55	49	43
4 or 5 (16)	44	40	26
Age-adjusted index in patients below 60			
Number of factors and percentage of patients	Complete remission rate	5-year DFS	5-year survival
0 (22)	92	86	83
1 (32)	78	66	69
2 (32)	57	53	46
3 (14)	46	58	32

more accurate than the Ann Arbor classification in predicting long-term survival. The expectation is that the international index and the age-adjusted international index will be used in the design of future therapeutic trials in patients with aggressive non-Hodgkin's lymphoma and in the selection of appropriate therapeutic approaches for individual patients.

LDH plus ß2-Microglobulin-Based Index

Because very few centres determined ß2-microglobulin levels 10 years ago, the IPI could not incorporate this important prognostic indicator into multivariate analyses. However, the M.D. Anderson Cancer Center team has developed multivariate studies including ß2-microglobulin level and other important parameters [158,193]. An index based on LDH and ß2-microglobulin level was proposed and was shown to be effective in discriminating patients with good or poor risk whatever the lymphoma subtype.

Parameters Influencing the Relapse Rate in CR Patients

Parameters Associated with Relapse in CR Patients

Depending on the histological subtype, 30% to 100% of complete remission patients will eventually relapse. If patients with a high risk of relapse could be recognized, treatment might be adapted in an attempt to decrease this risk. Very few of the previously described prognostic indicators are also associated with a high relapse rate.

Cabanillas and coworkers [194] studied relapses arising after 30 months in 503 CR patients. The overall risk was 6.8% and a greater risk was associated with divergent histology (large cells in nodes and small cells in bone marrow), sclerosing large cell lymphoma, or a diagnosis based on extranodal site. When none of these features were present, the risk of relapse was only 3%. When any one of these features was present, the risk was 14%. Patients with divergent histology had a risk of 43% of late relapse. Five of the 8 B-cell lymphoma patients with late relapse had a low S-phase, suggesting a chemotherapy selection of a cell clone with a low proliferative potential that could have given rise to the late relapse. Immunophenotypic analysis of 3 cases at diagnosis and after relapse failed to support the hypothesis of a second primary lymphoma and were consistent with a true recurrence of the original tumour. However, a second lymphoma may be seen in very late relapses [195].

In our prognostic factor analysis for patients treated with the LNH-84 regimen [8], the only initial parameters that were associated with a higher relapse rate were high LDH level, advanced stage, non-large cell subtype, and T-cell phenotype. However, these parameters were only associated with relapse during the first 2 or 3 years after treatment and we were not able to find specific indicators of late relapses [189]. For CR patients at the end of their treatment, no indicator of early relapse may be found (see below).

Residual disease

Scanographic masses

With modern radiological examinations, nearly all patients with initial bulky tumour have persistent radiological abnormalities at the end of their treatment. These patients may be in true CR with persisting fibronecrotic masses or may have persisting lymphoma cells. The problem is really important for patients having persistent masses larger than 3 cm. In larger tumours, cytological or histological examination of persisting tissue must be performed, particularly in young patients, because an intensive therapy may be proposed in these true PR patients to reach CR and to achieve cure [169].

Among the patients treated with the LNH-84 regimen [43], 518 of the 553 CR patients were evaluated for persisting radiological masses and 150 patients were found to have a so-called persisting fibronecrotic mass. Thirty-seven percent of the patients with a persisting tumour mass relapsed, compared to 35% without persisting radiological abnormalities. Disease-free survival was not different for the 2 subgroups (Fig. 4). This observation was confirmed in studies from the Dana-Farber Cancer Institute (Boston, MA) and the National Cancer Institute [191,196]. Patients with persisting radiological abnormalities might relapse but

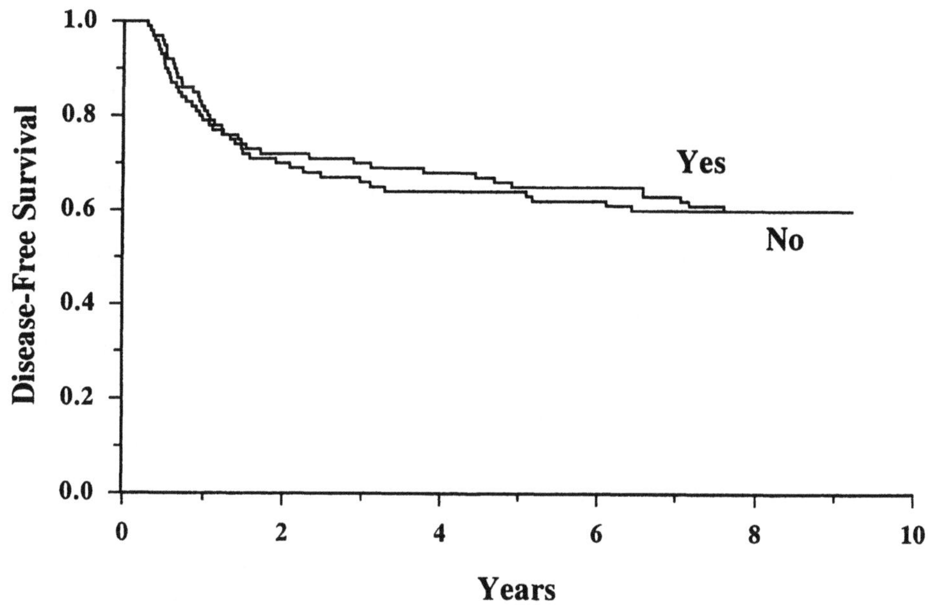

Fig. 4. Risk of relapse in aggressive lymphoma patients treated with the LNH-84 regimen according to the presence or not of a persisting tumour mass after completion of chemotherapy

they did not relapse more frequently than patients without these abnormalities and the site of relapse did not often involve the persisting abnormal mass.

Gallium-67 imaging

Gallium-67 imaging has been proposed to distinguish patients with a persisting fibronecrotic mass from patients with a persisting lymphoma mass [197,198]. Persisting lymphoma cells show gallium-67 uptake and therefore patients with a persisting mass and an image on gallium scan are thought to have a higher relapse risk than those without any gallium uptake. However, very few prospective studies exist to demonstrate that gallium imaging is useful in all patients and some cases of abnormal mediastinal gallium-67 uptake without secondary relapse have been described [199].

Conclusions

As already outlined, the first prognostic variable essential for selecting adequate therapy is the exact histological subtype of lymphoma. This information is indispensable at diagnosis and useful at subsequent relapse if a potentially curative treatment is still available. When a patient is referred to a specialized centre, tissue specimens should be available for review. If slide review is not possible or if the slides are not informative, the physician should repeat the biopsy as histology remains the most valuable prognostic indicator. Before the revision of the Working Classification for Clinical Usage, the use of this histological classification, although imprecise for some lymphoma subtypes, allows a good understanding by most physicians. Other classifications can be used, but a clear histological description of the tumour should be provided to enable the physician to establish a histology-based prognosis.

The prognostic factors described by the International Non-Hodgkin's Lymphoma Prognostic Factor Index are then assembled so that the patient can be included in a comparable group of patients with a similar outcome (Table 4).

In addition to detailed clinical examination, CT scans and bone marrow examination should be performed to assess the clinical stage and the number of extranodal sites of disease. Measurement of performance status should be done according to the objective criteria described for this index to avoid physician subjectivity. Serum LDH should be assessed after correct sampling and sample management to avoid haemolysis which could lead to overestimated results.

Measurement of tumour mass is not required for prognostic estimation but constitutes an essential reference for further follow-up. Careful extranodal examination is recommended in particular circumstances to complete the assessment of disease extent: CSF examination in aggressive lymphomas (large cells, T-cell lymphomas, small non-cleaved and lymphoblastic cells); GI tract exploration in case of clinical symptoms or oropharyngeal involvement.

Although ß2-microglobulin is not a prognostic factor included in the IPI, its measurement provides useful information and can be used in addition to the IPI.

Most of the other prognostic factors are provided by further analysis of the lymphoma specimen. Their routine evaluation cannot be recommended and they have not proved to be superior to histology and the International Index in predicting outcome. However, large studies analyzing the predictive value of these new parameters should be performed and may provide new insights into the influence of biological parameters on clinical outcome. Immunological phenotyping usually helps the histological diagnosis (B or T-cell discriminatory markers, additional markers [CD5, CD10, CD23, and SIg]) and is useful to further classify the histological subtypes. It also permits to evaluate the expression of other markers such as adhesion molecules. Karyotypic analysis also provides important information but is only available in highly specialized centres. The preservation of tumour specimens in liquid nitrogen is strongly recommended to perform further immunohistological and molecular tests, to assess the presence of PCR amplifiable markers useful for monitoring minimal residual disease, and to carry out other biological studies.

Preservation of frozen plasma or serum samples is also advisable for the future evaluation of new serological markers.

We have reviewed in this chapter the main prognostic parameters that have led to the definition of the International Non-Hodgkin's Lymphoma Prognostic Index and we have mentioned new directions of study and research. The international prognostic index will help physicians to design new treatment strategies but it should only be considered as an interim analysis of the history of prognostic factors and will have to be redefined in a few years.

The definition of prognostic factors and prognostic indexes has allowed us to propose treatment strategies adapted to the status of individual patients and thus to increase the number of patients who tolerate their treatment, who respond to their treatment, and who are cured by it [200]. Even if this may not be considered as an improvement in the efficacy of treatments, it is certainly an improvement in patient care.

REFERENCES

1 Carbone PP, Kaplan HS, Musshoff K et al: Report of the Committee on Hodgkin's disease staging classification. Cancer Res 1971 (31):1860-1861

2 Coiffier B and Lepage E: Prognosis of aggressive lymphoma: a study of five prognostic models with patients included in the LNH-84 regimen. Blood 1989 (74):558-564

3 The International Non-Hodgkin's Lymphoma Prognostic Factors Project: A predictive model for aggressive non-Hodgkin's lymphoma. N Engl J Med 1993 (329):987-994

4 The Non-Hodgkin's Lymphoma Pathologic Classification Project: National Cancer Institute sponsored study of classifications of non-Hodgkin's lymphomas. Summary and description of a Working Formulation for Clinical Usage. Cancer 1982 (49): 2112-2135

5 Lennert K, Mohri N, Sein H, Kaiserling E: The histopathology of malignant lymphoma. Br J Haematol 1975 (31):193-203

6 Berger F, Felman P, Sonet A et al: Nonfollicular small B-cell lymphomas: A heterogeneous group of patients with distinct clinical features and outcome. Blood 1994 (83):2829-2835

7 Banks PM, Chan J, Cleary ML et al: Mantle cell lymphoma. A proposal for unification of morphologic, immunologic, and molecular data. Am J Surg Pathol 1992 (16):637-640

8 Coiffier B, Gisselbrecht C, Vose JM et al: Prognostic factors in aggressive malignant lymphomas. Description and validation of a prognostic index that could identify patients requiring a more intensive therapy. J Clin Oncol 1991 (9):211-219

9 Banks PM: Newly recognized variant forms of non-Hodgkin's lymphomas. Hematol/Oncol Clin NA 1991 (5):935-952

10 Burke JS: The histopathologic classification of non-Hodgkin's lymphomas. Ambiguities in the Working Formulation and two newly reported categories. Sem Oncol 1990 (17):3-10

11 Penny RJ, Blaustein JC, Longtine JA, Pinkus GS: Ki-1-positive large cell lymphomas, a heterogenous group of neoplasms. Morphologic, immunophenotypic, genotypic, and clinical features of 24 cases. Cancer 1991 (68):362-373

12 Kadin ME: Ki-1 positive anaplastic large-cell lymphoma: A clinicopathologic entity. J Clin Oncol 1991 (9):533-536

13 Jacobson JO, Aisenberg AC, Lamarre L et al: Mediastinal large cell lymphoma. An uncommon subset of adult lymphoma curable with combined modality therapy. Cancer 1988 (62):1893-1898

14 Moller P, Lammler B, Eberlein-Gonska M et al: Primary mediastinal clear cell lymphoma of B-cell type. Virchows Arch Pathol Anat 1986 (409):79-92

15 Perrone T, Frizzera G, Rosai J: Mediastinal diffuse large-cell lymphoma with sclerosis. A clinicopathologic study of 60 cases. Amer J Surg Pathol 1986 (10):176-191

16 Bitter MA, Franklin WA, Larson RA et al: Morphology in Ki-1 (CD30)-positive non-Hodgkin's lymphoma is correlated with clinical features and the presence of a unique chromosomal abnormality, t(2;5)(p23;q35). Amer J Surg Pathol 1990 (14):305-316

17 Mason DY, Bastard C, Rimokh R: CD30-positive large cell lymphomas (Ki-1 lymphoma) are associated with a chromosomal translocation involving 5q35. Br J Haematol 1990 (74):161-168

18 Perkins PL, Ross CW, Schnitzer B: CD30-positive, anaplastic large-cell lymphomas that express CD15 but lack CD45. A possible diagnostic pitfall. Arch Pathol Lab Med 1992 (116):1192-1196

19 Bellas C, Molina A, Montalban C, Mampaso F: Signet-ring cell lymphoma of T-cell type with CD30 expression. Histopathology 1993 (22):188-189

20 Feller AC and Sterry W: Large cell anaplastic lymphoma of the skin. Br J Dermatol 1989 (121): 593-602

21 Kinney MC, Collins RD, Greer JP et al: A small-cell-predominant variant of primary Ki-1 (CD-30)+ T-cell lymphoma. Am J Surg Pathol 1993 (17):859-868

22 Leoncini L, Del Vecchio MT, Kraft R: Hodgkin's disease and CD30-positive anaplastic large cell lymphomas: A continuous spectrum of malignant disorders. A quantitative morphometric and immunohistologic study. Am J Pathol 1990 (137):1047-1057

23 Pileri S, Falini B, Delsol G et al: Lymphohistiocytic T-cell lymphoma (anaplastic large cell lymphoma CD30+/Ki-1+ with a high content of reactive histiocytes). Histopathology 1990 (16):383-391

24 Willemze R and Beljaards RC: Spectrum of primary cutaneous CD30 (Ki-1)-positive lymphoproliferative disorders. A proposal for classification and guidelines for management and treatment. J Am Acad Dermatol 1993 (28):973-980

25 Carbone A, Gloghini A, Volpe R: Immunohistochemistry of Hodgkin and non-Hodgkin lymphomas with emphasis on the diagnostic significance of the BNH9 antibody reactivity with anaplastic large cell (CD30 positive) lymphomas. Cancer 1992 (70): 2691-2698

26 Piris M, Brown DC, Gatter KC, Mason DY: CD30 expression in non-Hodgkin's lymphoma. Histopathology 1990 (17):211-218

27 Banerjee SS, Heald J, Harris M: Twelve cases of Ki-1 positive anaplastic large cell lymphoma of skin. J Clin Pathol 1991 (44):119-125

28 Beljaards RC, Kaudewitz P, Berti E et al: Primary cutaneous CD30-positive large cell lymphoma: Definition of a new type of cutaneous lymphoma with a favorable prognosis. A European multicenter study of 47 patients. Cancer 1993 (71):2097-2104

29 Kadin ME: The spectrum of Ki-1+ cutaneous lymphomas. Curr Prob Dermatol 1990 (19):132-143

30 Willemze R, Meijer CJLM, Sentis HJ et al: Primary cutaneous large cell lymphomas of follicular center cell origin. A clinical follow-up study of nineteen patients. J Am Acad Dermatol 1987 (16):518-526

31 Offit K, Ladanyi M, Gangi MD et al: Ki-1 antigen expression defines a favorable clinical subset of non-B cell non-Hodgkin's lymphoma. Leukemia 1990 (4):625-630

32 Santucci M, Pimpinelli N, Arganini L: Primary cutaneous B-cell lymphoma: A unique type of low-

grade lymphoma. Clinicopathologic and immunologic study of 83 cases. Cancer 1991 (67):2311-2326
33 d'Agay MF, Brière J, Lepage E et al: Primary anaplastic large cell non Hodgkin's lymphoma in adults: a clinicopathological study of 122 cases compared to a cohort of 1173 non anaplastic large cell lymphoma. A GELA study. Thity-fifth meeting of the American Society of Hematology, St. Louis, MO, 1993 (82):135a (abstract # 525)
34 Shulman LN, Frisard B, Antin JH et al: Primary Ki-1 anaplastic large-cell lymphoma in adults: Clinical characteristics and therapeutic outcome. J Clin Oncol 1993 (11):937-942
35 Miller JB, Variakojis D, Bitran JD et al: Diffuse histiocytic lymphoma with sclerosis: a clinicopathologic entity frequently causing superior venacaval obstruction. Cancer 1981 (47):748-756
36 Levitt LJ, Aisenberg AC, Harris NL et al: Primary non-Hodgkin's lymphoma of the mediastinum. Cancer 1982 (50):2486-2492
37 Trump DL and Mann RB: Diffuse large cell and undifferentiated lymphomas with prominent mediastinal involvement. A poor prognostic subset of patients with non-Hodgkin's lymphoma. Cancer 1982 (50):277-282
38 Todeschini G, Ambrosetti A, Meneghini V et al: Mediastinal large-B-cell lymphoma with sclerosis. A clinical study of 21 patients. J Clin Oncol 1990 (8): 804-808
39 Kirn D, Mauch P, Shaffer K et al: Large-cell and immunoblastic lymphoma of the mediastinum: Prognostic features and treatment outcome in 57 patients. J Clin Oncol 1993 (11):1336-1343
40 Lister TA: Sclerosing B-cell lymphoma of the mediastinum: entity or non-entity? Ann Oncol 1991 (2):707-708
41 Aisenberg AC: Primary large-cell lymphoma of the mediastinum. J Clin Oncol 1993 (11):2291-2294
42 Kwak LW, Wilson M, Weiss LM et al: Clinical significance of morphologic subdivision in diffuse large cell lymphoma. Cancer 1991 (68):1988-1993
43 Coiffier B, Gisselbrecht C, Herbrecht R et al: LNH-84: a multicenter study of intensive chemotherapy in 737 patients with aggressive malignant lymphoma. J Clin Oncol 1989 (7):1018-1026
44 Haddy TB, Adde MA, Magrath IT: CNS involvement in small noncleaved-cell lymphoma: Is CNS disease per se a poor prognostic sign? J Clin Oncol 1991 (9):1973-1982
45 Cohen LF, Balow JE, Macgrath IT et al: Acute tumor lysis syndrome. A review of 37 patients with Burkitt's lymphoma. Am J Med 1980 (68):486-491
46 Coiffier B, Bryon PA, Berger F et al: Intensive and sequential combination chemotherapy for aggressive malignant lymphomas (Protocol LNH-80). J Clin Oncol 1986 (4):147-153
47 Levine AM: Acquired immunodeficiency syndrome-related lymphoma. Blood 1992 (80):8-20
48 Raphael M, Gentilhomme O, Tulliez M et al: Histopathologic features of high-grade non-Hodgkin's lymphomas in acquired immunodeficiency syndrome. Arch Pathol Lab Med 1991 (115):15-20
49 Nalesnik MA, Jaffe R, Starzl TE et al: The pathology of posttransplant lymphoproliferative disorders occurring in the setting of cyclosporine A - prednisone immunosuppression. Amer J Pathol 1988 (133):173-192
50 Penn I: Lymphomas complicating organ transplantations. Transplant Proc 1983 (15):2790-2797
51 Morel P, Lepage E, Brice P et al: Prognosis and treatment of lymphoblastic lymphoma in adults: A report on 80 patients. J Clin Oncol 1992 (10):1078-1085
52 Pinkus GS, O'Hara CJ, Said JW: Peripheral post-thymic T-cell lymphomas: A spectrum of disease. Clinical, pathologic, and immunologic features of 78 cases. Cancer 1990 (65):971-998
53 Liang R, Loke SL, Chan ACL: The prognostic factors for peripheral T-cell lymphomas. Hematol Oncol 1992 (10):135-140
54 De Bruin PC, Noorduyn AL, Van der Valk P et al: Noncutaneous T-cell lymphomas. Recognition of a lymphoma type (large cell anaplastic) with a relatively favorable prognosis. Cancer 1993 (71):2604-2612
55 Nakamura S, Koshikawa T, Koike K et al: Phenotypic analysis of peripheral T cell lymphoma among the Japanese. Acta Pathol Jpn 1993 (43):396-412
56 Coiffier B, Berger F, Bryon PA, Magaud JP: T-cell lymphomas: immunologic, histologic, clinical, and therapeutic analysis of 63 cases. J Clin Oncol 1988 (6):1584-1589
57 Coiffier B, Brousse N, Peuchmaur M et al: Peripheral T-cell lymphomas have a worse prognosis than B-cell lymphomas: a prospective study of 361 immunophenotyped patients treated with the LNH-84 regimen. Ann Oncol 1990 (1):45-50
58 Horning SJ, Doggett RS, Warnke RA et al: Clinical relevance of immunologic phenotype in diffuse large cell lymphoma. Blood 1984 (63):1209-1215
59 Shimizu K, Hamajima N, Ohnishi K et al: T-cell phenotype is associated with decreased survival in non-Hodgkin's lymphoma. Jpn J Cancer Res 1989 (80):720-726
60 Lippman SM, Miller TP, Spier CM et al: The prognostic significance of the immunotype in diffuse large-cell lymphoma: a comparative study of the T-cell and B-cell phenotype. Blood 1988 (72):436-441
61 Kwak LW, Wilson M, Weiss LM et al: Similar outcome of treatment of B-cell and T-cell diffuse large-cell lymphomas: The Stanford experience. J Clin Oncol 1991 (9):1426-1431
62 Watanabe S, Sato Y, Shimoyama M et al: Immunoblastic lymphadenopathy, angioimmunoblastic lymphadenopathy, and IBL-like T-cell lymphoma. A spectrum of T-cell neoplasia. Cancer 1986 (58):2224-2232
63 Greer JP, York JC, Cousar JB et al: Peripheral T-cell lymphoma: a clinicopathologic study of 42 cases. J Clin Oncol 1984 (2):788-798
64 Grogan TM, Fielder K, Rangel C et al: Peripheral T-cell lymphoma: aggressive disease with heterogeneous immunotypes. Am J Clin Pathol 1985 (83): 279-288
65 Chan JK, Ng CS, Ngan KC et al: Angiocentric T-cell lymphoma of the skin. An aggressive lymphoma distinct from mycosis fungoides. Amer J Surg Pathol 1988 (12):861-876

66 Armitage JO, Vose JM, Linder J et al: Clinical significance of immunophenotype in diffuse aggressive non-Hodgkin's lymphoma. J Clin Oncol 1989 (7): 1783-1790
67 Schuurman HJ, Huppes W, Verdonck LF et al: Immunophenotyping of non-Hodgkin's lymphoma. Correlation with relapse-free survival. Am J Pathol 1988 (131):102-111
68 Van der Valk P, Van Oostveen JW, Stel HV et al: Phenotypic and genotypic analysis of large-cell lymphomas, formerly classified as true histiocytic lymphoma. Identification of an unusual group of tumors. Leuk Res 1990 (14):337-346
69 Levine EG, Hanson CA, Jaszcz W, Peterson BA: True histiocytic lymphoma. Sem Oncol 1991 (18): 39-49
70 Hsu SM, Ho YS, Hsu PL: Lymphomas of true histiocytic origin: Expression of different phenotypes in so-called true histiocytic lymphoma and malignant histiocytosis. Am J Pathol 1991 (138):1389-1404
71 Offit K, Wong G, Filippa DA et al: Cytogenetic analysis of 434 consecutively ascertained specimens of non-Hodgkin's lymphoma. Clinical correlations. Blood 1991 (77):1508-1515
72 Levine EG, Arthur DC, Frizzera G et al: Cytogenetic abnormalities predict clinical outcome in non-Hodgkin lymphoma. Ann Inter Med 1988 (108): 14-20
73 Schouten HC, Sanger WG, Weisenburger DD, Armitage JO: Abnormalities involving chromosome 6 in newly diagnosed patients with non-Hodgkin's lymphoma. Cancer Genet Cytogenet 1990 (47):73-82
74 Offit K, Parsa NZ, Gaidano G et al: 6q deletions define distinct clinico-pathologic subsets of non-Hodgkin's lymphoma. Blood 1993 (82):2157-2162
75 Romaguera JE, Pugh W, Luthra R et al: The clinical relevance of t(14;18)/BCL-2 rearrangement and DEL 6q in diffuse large cell lymphoma and immunoblastic lymphoma. Ann Oncol 1993 (4):51-54
76 Cabanillas F, Pathak S, Grant G et al: Refractoriness to chemotherapy and poor survival related to abnormalities of chromosome 17 and 7 in lymphoma. Am J Med 1989 (87):167-172
77 Rodriguez MA, Ford RJ, Goodacre A et al: Chromosome 17p and p53 changes in lymphoma. Br J Haematol 1991 (79):575-582
78 Schouten HC, Sanger WG, Weisenburger DD et al: Chromosomal abnormalities in untreated patients with non-Hodgkin's lymphoma: Associations with histology, clinical characteristics, and treatment outcome. Blood 1990 (75):1841-1847
79 Ye BH, Lista F, Lococo F et al: Alterations of a zinc finger encoding gene, Bcl-6, in diffuse large-cell lymphoma. Science 1993 (262):747-750
80 Kerckaert JP, Deweindt C, Tilly H et al: LAZ3, a novel zinc-finger encoding gene, is disrupted by recurring chromosome 3q27 translocations in human lymphomas. Nature Genetics 1993 (5):66-70
81 Offit K, LoCoco F, Louie D et al: Bcl-6 rearrangements defines a clinical and prognostic subset of diffuse large cell lymphoma. Thirty-fifth meeting of the American Society of Hematology, St. Louis, MO, 1993 (82 suppl 1):133a (abstract # 517)
82 Raghoebier S, Kramer MHH, Vankrieken JHJM et al: Essential differences in oncogene involvement between primary nodal and extranodal large cell lymphoma. Blood 1991 (78):2680-2685
83 Lee JT, Innes DJ, Williams ME: Sequential bcl-2 and c-myc oncogene rearrangements associated with the clinical transformation of non-Hodgkin's lymphoma. J Clin Invest 1989 (84):1454-1459
84 de Jong D, Voetdijk BMH, Beverstock GC et al: Activation of the c-myc oncogene in a precursor-B-cell blast crisis of follicular lymphoma, presenting as composite lymphoma. N Engl J Med 1988 (318):1373-1377
85 Yano T, Jaffe ES, Longo DL, Raffeld M: MYC rearrangements in histologically progressed follicular lymphomas. Blood 1992 (80):758-767
86 Pezzella F, Jones M, Ralfkiaer E et al: Evaluation of bcl-2 protein expression and 14-18 translocation as prognostic markers in follicular lymphoma. Br J Cancer 1992 (65):87-89
87 Hermine O, Haioun C, Lepage E et al: Bcl-2 protein expression in aggressive non-Hodgkin's lymphoma. A new adverse prognostic factor? A GELA Study. Fifth International Conference on Malignant Lymphoma, Lugano 1993 (abstract # 16)
88 Gaidano G, Ballerini P, Gong JZ et al: P53 mutations in human lymphoid malignancies. Association with Burkitt lymphoma and chronic lymphocytic leukemia. Proc Natl Acad Sci USA 1991 (88):5413-5417
89 Ichikawa A, Hotta T, Takagi N et al: Mutations of p53 gene and their relation to disease progression in B-cell lymphoma. Blood 1992 (79):2701-2707
90 Sander CA, Yano T, Clark HM et al: P53 mutation is associated with progression in follicular lymphomas. Blood 1993 (82):1994-2004
91 Lo Coco F, Gaidano G, Louie DC et al: P53 mutations are associated with histologic transformation of follicular lymphoma. Blood 1993 (82):2289-2295
92 Dixon DO, Neilan B, Jones SE et al: Effect of age on therapeutic outcome in advanced diffuse histiocytic lymphoma: the Southwest Oncology Group experience. J Clin Oncol 1986 (4):295-305
93 Armitage JO and Potter JF: Aggressive chemotherapy for diffuse histiocytic lymphoma in the elderly: increased complications with advancing age. J Am Geriat Soc 1984 (32):269-273
94 Vose JM, Armitage JO, Weisenburger DD et al: The importance of age in survival of patients treated with chemotherapy for aggressive non-Hodgkin's lymphoma. J Clin Oncol 1988 (6):1838-1844
95 Dumontet C, Anderson JR, Sebban C et al: Elderly non-Hodgkin lymphoma patients have comparable prognostic factors but a poorer outcome than younger patients. 11th American Society of Clinical Oncology Meeting, San Diego, CA, 1992 (11):328 (abstract # 1118)
96 Solal-Celigny P, Chastang C, Herrera A et al: Age as the main prognostic factor in adult aggressive non-Hodgkin's lymphoma. Am J Med 1987 (83): 1075-1080
97 Ansell SM, Falkson G, van der Merwe R, Uys A: Chronological age is a multifactorial prognostic variable in patients with non-Hodgkin's lymphoma. Ann Oncol 1992 (3):45-50

98 Stein RS, Greer JP, Flexner JM et al: Large-cell lymphomas. Clinical and prognostic features. J Clin Oncol 1990 (8):1370-1379

99 Velasquez WS, Jagannath S, Tucker SL et al: Risk classification as the basis for clinical staging of diffuse large-cell lymphoma derived from 10-year survival data. Blood 1989 (74):551-557

100 Hayward RL, Leonard RCF, Prescott RJ: A critical analysis of prognostic factors for survival in intermediate and high grade non-Hodgkin's lymphoma. Br J Cancer 1991 (63):945-952

101 Coiffier B, Bryon PA, Ffrench M et al: Intensive chemotherapy in aggressive lymphomas: updated results of LNH-80 protocol and prognostic factors affecting response and survival. Blood 1987 (70): 1394-1399

102 Carbone A, Volpe R, Gloghini A et al: Non-Hodgkin's lymphoma in the elderly. 1. Pathologic features at presentation. Cancer 1990 (66):1991-1994

103 Gail MH, Pluda JM, Rabkin CS: Projections of the incidence of non-Hodgkin's lymphoma related to acquired immunodeficiency syndrome. JNCI 1991 (83):695-701

104 Kaplan LD, Abrams DI, Feigal E et al: AIDS-associated non-Hodgkin's lymphoma in San Francisco. JAMA 1989 (261):719-724

105 Levine AM, Sullivan-Halley J, Pike MC et al: Human immunodeficiency virus-related lymphoma. Prognostic factors predictive of survival. Cancer 1991 (68):2466-2472

106 Gisselbrecht C, Oksenhendler E, Tirelli U et al: Human immunodeficiency virus-related lymphoma: treatment with intensive combination chemotherapy. Am J Med 1993 (95):188-196

107 Cowan RA, Jones M, Harris M et al: Prognostic factors in high and intermediate grade non-Hodgkin's lymphoma. Br J Cancer 1989 (59):276-282

108 Jones SE, Miller TP, Connors JM: Long-term follow-up and analysis for prognostic factors for patients with limited-stage diffuse large-cell lymphoma treated with initial chemotherapy with or without adjuvant radiotherapy. J Clin Oncol 1989 (7:)1186-1191

109 Nakamine H, Bagin RG, Vose JM et al: Prognostic significance of clinical and pathologic features in diffuse large B-cell lymphoma. Cancer 1993 (71): 3130-3137

110 Lopez-Guillermo A, Montserrat E, Reverter JC et al: Large-cell lymphoma: a study of prognostic factors and assessment of five recently proposed predictive systems. Leukemia and Lymphoma 1993 (10):101-109

111 Cabanillas F, Burke JS, Smith TL et al: Factors predicting for response and survival in adults with advanced non-Hodgkin's lymphoma. Arch Int Med 1978 (138):413-418

112 Jagannath S, Velasquez WS, Tucker SL et al: Tumor burden assessment and its implication for a prognostic model in advanced diffuse large-cell lymphoma. J Clin Oncol 1986 (4):859-865

113 Hoskins PJ, Ng V, Spinelli JJ et al: Prognostic variables in patients with diffuse large-cell lymphoma treated with MACOP-B. J Clin Oncol 1991 (9):220-226

114 Shipp MA, Harrington DP, Klatt MM et al: Identification of major prognostic subgroups of patients with large-cell lymphoma treated with m-BACOD or M-BACOD. Ann Inter Med 1986 (104):757-765

115 Shipp MA, Yeap BY, Harrington DP et al: The m-BACOD combination chemotherapy regimen in large-cell lymphoma: Analysis of the completed trial and comparison with the M-BACOD regimen. J Clin Oncol 1990 (8):84-93

116 Kaminski MS, Coleman CN, Colby TV et al: Factors predicting survival in adults with stage I and II large-cell lymphoma treated with primary radiation therapy. Ann Int Med 1986 (104):747-756

117 Danieu L, Wong G, Koziner B, Clarkson B: Predictive model for prognosis in advanced diffuse histiocytic lymphoma. Cancer Res 1986 (46):5372-5379

118 Fisher RI, Hubbard SM, DeVita VT et al: Factors predicting long-term survival in diffuse mixed, histiocytic, or undifferentiated lymphoma. Blood 1981 (58):45-51

119 Bernasconi C, Brusamolino E, Lazzarino M et al: Lymphoblastic lymphoma in adult patients: clinicopathological features and response to intensive multiagent chemotherapy analogous to that used in acute lymphoblastic leukemia. Ann Oncol 1990 (1): 141-146

120 Sweetenham JW, Mead GM, Whitehouse JMA: Adult lymphoblastic lymphoma: high incidence of central nervous system relapse in patients treated with the Stanford University protocol. Ann Oncol 1992 (3):839-841

121 Pees HW, Radtke H, Schwamborn J, Graf N: The BFM-protocol for HIV-negative Burkitt's lymphomas and L3 ALL in adult patients. A high chance for cure. Ann Hematol 1992 (65):201-205

122 Hagemeister FB: Results of treatment of small non-cleaved cell lymphoma in patients without positive HIV serology. Leukemia and Lymphoma 1993 (10):21-27

123 McMaster ML, Greer JP, Greco FA et al: Effective treatment of small-noncleaved-cell lymphoma with high-intensity, brief-duration chemotherapy. J Clin Oncol 1991 (9):941-946

124 Todd MB, Portlock CS, Farber LR et al: Prognostic indicators in diffuse large-cell (histiocytic) lymphoma. Int J Radiat Oncol Biol Phys 1986 (12):593-601

125 Vitolo U, Bertini M, Brusamolino E: MACOP-B treatment in diffuse large-cell lymphoma: Identification of prognostic groups in an Italian multicenter study. J Clin Oncol 1992 (10):219-227

126 Bennett JM, Cain KC, Glick JH et al: The significance of bone marrow involvement in non-Hodgkin's lymphoma: the Eastern Cooperative Oncology Group experience. J Clin Oncol 1986 (4):1462-1469

127 Conlan MG, Bast M, Armitage JO, Weisenburger DD: Bone marrow involvement by non-Hodgkin's lymphoma: The clinical significance of morphologic discordance between the lymph node and bone marrow. J Clin Oncol 1990 (8):1163-1172

128 Fisher DE, Jacobson JO, Ault KA, Harris NL: Diffuse large cell lymphoma with discordant bone marrow histology. Clinical features and biological implications. Cancer 1989 (64):1879-1887

129 Robertson LE, Redman JR, Butler JJ et al: Discordant bone marrow involvement in diffuse large-cell lymphoma: A distinct clinical-pathologic entity associated with a continuous risk of relapse. J Clin Oncol 1991 (9):236-242
130 Rossi A, Rohatiner AZS, Lister TA: Primary gastrointestinal non-Hodgkin lymphoma: still an unresolved question? Ann Hematol 1993 (4):802-803
131 Salles G, Herbrecht R, Tilly H et al: Aggressive primary gastrointestinal lymphomas. Review of 91 patients treated with the LNH-84 regimen. A study of the Groupe d'Etude des Lymphomes Agressifs. Am J Med 1991 (90):77-84
132 Mackintosh FR, Colby TV, Podolsky WJ et al: Central nervous system involvement in non-Hodgkin's lymphoma: an analysis of 105 cases. Cancer 1982 (49):586-595
133 Levitt LJ, Dawson DM, Rosenthal DS, Moloney WC: CNS involvement in the non-Hodgkin's lymphomas. Cancer 1980 (45):545-552
134 Recht L, Straus DJ, Cirrincione C et al: Central nervous system metastases from non-Hodgkin's lymphoma: Treatment and prophylaxis. Am J Med 1988 (84):425-435
135 Perry JR, Deodhare SS, Bilbao JM et al: The significance of spinal cord compression as the initial manifestation of lymphoma. Neurosurgery 1993 (32):157-162
136 O'Sullivan MG, Whittle IR, Gregor A, Ironside JW: Increasing incidence of CNS primary lymphoma in South-East Scotland. Lancet 1991 (338):895-896
137 Jellinger KA and Paulus W: Primary central nervous system lymphomas. An update. J Cancer Res Clin Oncol 1992 (119):7-27
138 Blay JY, Lasset C, Carrie C et al: Multivariate analysis of prognostic factors in patients with non HIV-related primary cerebral lymphoma. A proposal for a prognostic scoring. Br J Cancer 1993 (67): 1136-1141
139 Michalski JM, Garcia DM, Kase E et al: Primary central nervous system lymphoma. Analysis of prognostic variables and patterns of treatment failure. Radiology 1990 (176):855-860
140 Skarin AT, Zuckerman KS, Pitman SW et al: High-dose methotrexate with folinic acid in the treatment of advanced non-Hodgkin lymphoma including CNS involvement. Blood 1977 (50):1039-1047
141 Fredrick DR, Char DH, Ljung BM, Brinton DA: Solitary intraocular lymphoma as an initial presentation of widespread disease. Arch Ophthalmol 1989 (107):395-397
142 Peterson K, Gordon KB, Heinemann MH, Deangelis LM: The clinical spectrum of ocular lymphoma. Cancer 1993 (72):843-849
143 Whitcup SM, Desmet MD, Rubin BI et al: Intraocular lymphoma. Clinical and histopathologic diagnosis. Ophthalmology 1993 (100):1399-1406
144 Joly P, Charlotte F, Leibowitch M: Cutaneous lymphomas other than mycosis fungoides. Follow-up study of 52 patients. J Clin Oncol 1991 (9): 1994-2001
145 Mukai K, Sato Y, Wanatabe S et al: Non-Hodgkin's lymphoma of the skin excluding mycosis fungoides and cutaneous involvement of adult T-cell leukemia/lymphoma. J Cutan Pathol 1988 (15):193-200
146 Willemze R, Meijer CJLM, Scheffer E et al: Diffuse large cell lymphomas of follicular center cell origin presenting in the skin. A clinicopathologic and immunologic study of 16 patients. Am J Pathol 1987 (126):325-333
147 Giannotti B and Santucci M: Skin-associated lymphoid tissue (SALT)-related B-cell lymphoma (primary cutaneous B-cell lymphoma). A concept and a clinicopathologic entity. Arch Dermatol 1993 (129):353-355
148 De Bruin PC, Beljaards RC, Van Heerde P et al: Differences in clinical behaviour and immunophenotype between primary cutaneous and primary nodal anaplastic large cell lymphoma of T-cell or null cell phenotype. Histopathology 1993 (23):127-135
149 Pan L, Beverley PCL, Isaacson PG: Lactate dehydrogenase (LDH) isoenzymes and proliferative activity of lymphoid cells. An immunocytochemical study. Clin Exp Immunol 1991 (86):240-245
150 Vose JM and Armitage JO: Diffuse "histiocytic" lymphoma. Sem Oncol 1991 (18):50-60
151 Ferraris AM, Giuntini P, Gaetani GF: Serum lactic dehydrogenase as a prognostic tool for non-Hodgkin lymphomas. Blood 1979 (54):928-932
152 Csako G, Magrath IT, Elin RJ: Serum total and isoenzyme lactate dehydrogenase activity in American Burkitt's lymphoma patients. Am J Clin Pathol 1982 (78):712-717
153 Koziner B, Little C, Passe S et al: Treatment of advanced diffuse histiocytic lymphoma. An analysis of prognostic variables. Cancer 1982 (49): 1571-1579
154 Shimamoto Y, Suga K, Nishimura J et al: Major prognostic factors of Japanese patients with lymphoma-type adult T-cell leukemia. Am J Hematol 1990 (35):232-237
155 Cassuto JP, Krebs BP, Viot G et al: ß2-microglobulin, a tumour marker of lymphoproliferative disorders. Lancet 1978 (ii):108-109
156 Child JA, Spati B, Illingworth S et al: Serum beta-2 microglobulin and C-reactive protein in the monitoring of lymphomas. Finding in a multicentre study and experience in selected patients. Cancer 1980 (45):318-323
157 Hagberg H, Killander A, Simonsson B: Serum ß2-microglobulin in malignant lymphoma. Cancer 1983 (51):2220-2225
158 Swan F, Velasquez WS, Tucker S et al: A new serologic staging system for large-cell lymphomas based on initial ß2-microglobulin and lactate dehydrogenase levels. J Clin Oncol 1989 (7):1518-1527
159 Litam P, Swan F, Cabanillas F: Prognostic value of serum ß2-microglobulin in low-grade lymphoma. Ann Intern Med 1991 (114):855-860
160 Johnson PWM, Whelan J, Longhurst S et al: ß2-microglobulin: A prognostic factor in diffuse aggressive non-Hodgkin's lymphomas. Br J Cancer 1993 (67):792-797
161 Aviles A, Narvaez BR, Diaz-Maqueo JC et al: Value of serum beta 2 microglobulin as an indicator of early relapse in diffuse large cell lymphoma. Leukemia and Lymphoma 1993 (9):377-380
162 Anderson T, DeVita VT, Simon RM et al: Malignant lymphoma. II. Prognostic factors and response to

treatment of 473 patients at the National Cancer Institute. Cancer 1982 (50):2708-2721
163 Karnovsky DA, Abelmann WH, Craver LF, Buchenal JH: The use of nitrogen mustards in the palliative treatment of cancer. Cancer 1948 (1): 634-656
164 Zubrod CG, Schneiderman M, Frei E et al: Appraisal of methods for the study of chemotherapy of cancer in man: Comparative therapeutic trial of nitrogen mustard and triethylene thiophosphoramide. J Chron Dis 1960 (11):7-33
165 Conill C, Verger E, Salamero M: Performance status assessment in cancer patients. Cancer 1990 (65):1864-1866
166 Dhaliwal HS, Rohatiner AZS, Gregory W et al: Combination chemotherapy for intermediate and high grade non-Hodgkin's lymphoma. Br J Cancer 1993 (68):767-774
167 Mackintosh JF, Cowan RA, Jones M et al: Prognostic factors in stage I and II high and intermediate grade non-Hodgkin's lymphoma. Eur J Cancer Clin Oncol 1988 (24):1617-1622
168 Conlan MG, Armitage JO, Bast M, Weisenburger DD: Clinical significance of hematologic parameters in non-Hodgkin's lymphoma at diagnosis. Cancer 1991 (67):1389-1395
169 Armitage JO: Treatment of non-Hodgkin's lymphoma. N Engl J Med 1993 (328):1023-1030
170 Bosly A, Coiffier B, Gisselbrecht C et al: Bone marrow transplantation prolongs survival after relapse in aggressive lymphoma patients treated with the LNH-84 regimen. J Clin Oncol 1992 (10): 1615-1623
171 Armitage JO, Weisenburger DD, Hutchins M et al: Chemotherapy for diffuse large-cell lymphoma. Rapidly responding patients have more durable remissions. J Clin Oncol 1986 (4):160-164
172 Herman TS, Hammond N, Jones SE et al: Involvement of the central nervous system by non-Hodgkin's lymphoma. The Southwest Oncology Group experience. Cancer 1979 (43):390-397
173 Litam JP, Cabanillas F, Smith TL et al: Central nervous system relapse in malignant lymphomas: risk factors and implications for prophylaxis. Blood 1979 (54):1249-1257
174 Ervin T and Canellos GP: Successful treatment of recurrent primary central nervous system lymphoma with high-dose methotrexate. Cancer 1980 (45): 1556-1557
175 DeVita VT, Hubbard SM, Longo DL: The chemotherapy of lymphomas: Looking back, moving forward. The Richard and Linda Rosenthal Foundation Award lecture. Cancer Res 1987 (47): 5810-5824
176 Zuckerman KS, LoBuglio AF, Reeves JA: Chemotherapy of intermediate grade and high grade non-Hodgkin's lymphomas with a high-dose doxorubicin-containing regimen. J Clin Oncol 1990 (8): 248-256
177 Lee R, Cabanillas F, Bodey GP, Freireich EJ: A 10-year update of CHOP-Bleo in the treatment of diffuse large-cell lymphoma. J Clin Oncol 1986 (4): 1455-1461
178 Longo DL, Duffey PL, Devita VT et al: The calculation of actual or received dose intensity: A comparison of published methods. J Clin Oncol 1991 (9):2042-2051
179 Sweetenham JW, Mead GM, Whitehouse JMA: Intensive weekly combination chemotherapy for patients with intermediate-grade and high-grade non-Hodgkin's lymphoma. J Clin Oncol 1991 (9): 2202-2209
180 Gottlieb AJ, Anderson JR, Ginsberg SJ: A randomized comparison of methotrexate dose and the addition of bleomycin to CHOP therapy for diffuse large cell lymphoma and other non-Hodgkin's lymphomas. Cancer and Leukemia Group B Study 7851. Cancer 1990 (66):1888-1896
181 Meyer RM, Hryniuk WM, Goodyear MDE: The role of dose intensity in determining outcome in intermediate-grade non-Hodgkin's lymphoma. J Clin Oncol 1991 (9):339-347
182 Dana BW, Dahlberg S, Miller TP et al: m-BACOD treatment for intermediate-grade and high-grade malignant lymphomas: A Southwest Oncology Group phase II trial. J Clin Oncol 1990 (8):1155-1162
183 Epelbaum R, Faraggi D, Ben-Arie Y et al: Survival of diffuse large cell lymphoma. A multivariate analysis including dose intensity variables. Cancer 1990 (66):1124-1129
184 Kwak LW, Halpern J, Olshen RA, Horning SJ: Prognostic significance of actual dose intensity in diffuse large cell lymphoma: Results of a tree structured survival analysis. J Clin Oncol 1990 (8): 963-977
185 Lepage E, Gisselbrecht C, Haioun C et al: Prognostic significance of received relative dose intensity in non-Hodgkin's lymphoma patients: Application to LNH-87 protocol. Ann Oncol 1993 (4):651-656
186 Gulati SC, Shank B, Black P et al: Autologous bone marrow transplantation for patients with poor-prognosis lymphoma. J Clin Oncol 1988 (6):1303-1313
187 McMaster ML, Greer JP, Wolff SN et al: Results of treatment with high intensity, brief duration chemotherapy in poor prognosis non-Hodgkin's lymphoma. Cancer 1991 (68):233-241
188 Philip T, Hartmann O, Biron P et al: High-dose therapy and autologous bone marrow transplantation in partial remission after first-line induction therapy for diffuse non-Hodgkin's lymphoma. J Clin Oncol 1988 (6):1118-1124
189 Coiffier B, Tilly H, Bosly A et al: Long term follow-up of the 737 aggressive lymphoma patients treated in the LNH-84 protocol: Very few late relapses after 5 years. Thity-fifth meeting of the American Society of Hematology, St. Louis, MO, 1993 (82):444a (abstract # 1760)
190 Romaguera JE, Mclaughlin P, North L et al: Multivariate analysis of prognostic factors in stage-IV follicular low-grade lymphoma: A risk model. J Clin Oncol 1991 (9):762-769
191 Shipp MA, Klatt MM, Yeap B et al: Patterns of relapse in large-cell lymphoma patients with bulk disease: implications for use of adjuvant radiation therapy. J Clin Oncol 1989 (7):613-518
192 Coiffier B, Shipp MA, Cabanillas F et al: Report of the first workshop on prognostic factors in large-cell lymphomas. Ann Oncol 1991 (2):213-217
193 Rodriguez J, Cabanillas F, McLaughlin P et al: A proposal for a simple staging system for intermediate grade lymphoma and immunoblastic lym-

phoma based on the 'tumor score". Ann Oncol 1992 (3):711-717
194 Cabanillas F, Velasquez WS, Hagemeister FB et al: Clinical, biological, and histologic features of late relapses in diffuse large cell lymphoma. Blood 1992 (79):1024-1028
195 Dumontet C, Bastion Y, Felman P et al: Long-term outcome and sequelae in aggressive lymphoma patients treated with the LNH-80 regimen. Ann Oncol 1992 (3):639-644
196 Surbone A, Longo DL, DeVita VT et al: Residual abdominal masses in aggressive non-Hodgkin's lymphoma after combination chemotherapy: significance and management. J Clin Oncol 1988 (6): 1832-1837
197 Anderson KC, Leonard RCF, Canellos GP et al: High-dose gallium imaging in lymphoma. Am J Med 1983 (75):327-331
198 Kaplan WD, Jochelson MS, Herman TS et al: Gallium-67 imaging: A predictor of residual tumor viability and clinical outcome in patients with diffuse large-cell lymphoma. J Clin Oncol 1990 (8): 1966-1970
199 Peylan-Ramu N, Haddy TB, Jones E et al: High frequency of benign mediastinal uptake of Gallium-67 after completion of chemotherapy in children with high-grade non-Hodgkin's lymphoma. J Clin Oncol 1989 (7):1800-1806
200 Salles G, Shipp MA, Coiffier B: Chemotherapy of non-Hodgkin's aggressive lymphomas. Sem Hematol 1994 (31):46-69
201 d'Amore F, Christensen BE, Brincker H et al: Clinicopathological features and prognostic factors in extranodal non-Hodgkin lymphomas. Eur J Cancer 1991 (27):1201-1208

Treatment of Non-Hodgkin's Diffuse Large Cell Lymphomas

Gilles Salles and Bertrand Coiffier

Service d'Hématologie, Hospices Civils de Lyon, Centre Hospitalier Lyon-Sud, 69495 Pierre-Bénite Cedex, France

In the past 20 years, the advent of intensive combination chemotherapy has transformed non-Hodgkin's diffuse large cell lymphoma (DLCL) from a disease that was very often fatal to one that is often curable [1]. In the last decade, multi-agent regimens have been developed in an attempt to increase both the complete response rate and long-term survival [2-5]. This improvement in complete response and survival rates has been associated with an increase in the treatment toxicity and it is not yet formally established that these new regimens are truly improving overall long-term survival. More recently, intensified therapy in the form of high-dose chemotherapy with bone marrow transplantation (BMT) has been utilized in patients who either failed initial or salvage treatment or have a high risk of relapse [6-8]. The definition of the optimal strategy for a specific patient is complicated by the multiplicity of potentially active combination regimens and the diversity of strategic approaches. Clinical and biological parameters have also been identified that stratify patients into subgroups with markedly different prognoses, facilitating the individualization of therapy for patients in different risk groups and the comparison of therapeutic approaches in similar groups of patients [9]. However, randomized trials are still needed to resolve many questions regarding the ideal treatment for several subgroups of aggressive malignant lymphomas. Although in this review we will address the treatment of diffuse large cell lymphomas (groups F, G and H), the therapeutic approaches are similar in all aggressive histological subtypes [10,11].

Clinical Trials: Endpoints

In order to compare the therapeutic results obtained in DLCL trials, it is important to clearly define clinical endpoints. Despite improvements in staging procedures, it is difficult to specifically define a complete response (CR). Firstly, the complete remission rate can be assessed at different time points depending on the therapeutic regimen used: after 3 courses of chemotherapy, at the end of "induction therapy", or at the end of "consolidation therapy". Secondly, residual masses observed at the end of induction therapy, particularly in patients with bulky tumours, can be variably considered as partial response (PR) or as CR [12]. Thirdly, the heterogeneity in bone marrow infiltration by malignant cells represents an important difficulty in the assessment of CR. Although the percentage of patients achieving CR may be a useful parameter in a single-institution trial, this percentage does not constitute a reliable endpoint to compare therapeutic results between trials and institutions. For these reasons, variables such as overall survival (OS), or time to treatment failure (TTF) (which excludes unrelated causes of death) should be considered as primary reproducible endpoints. If one wishes to consider only the results of first-line therapy, freedom-from-progression (FFP) survival should be preferred to disease-free survival (DFS).

Patients' deaths during therapy may result from treatment toxicity or progressive disease (treatment failure). It is sometimes difficult to formally

Table 1. Principles for systemic therapy of diffuse large cell lymphoma

1.	A high rate of complete remissions must be obtained by a regimen to be curative
2.	Cure must be accomplished with front-line therapy
3.	Drugs must be delivered at curative doses
4.	Rapidity of achieving a CR might be related to the chance of cure
5.	Prolonged treatment for aggressive malignant lymphomas is unnecessary
6.	Aggressive chemotherapy for aggressive lymphomas is toxic

Reproduced from Armitage and Cheson [14]

distinguish between these two causes of death, especially in elderly patients or in those with altered performance status. Hence, the percentage of deaths during therapy should be considered as an important endpoint to evaluate the toxicity and the efficacy of different regimens.

Chemotherapy of DLCL

Principles for Combination Chemotherapy in DLCL

The combination chemotherapy regimens developed and utilized in DLCL are based on various concepts: 1) association of multiple synergistic drugs; 2) increased dosage of drugs for which a dose-response relationship has been experimentally or clinically demonstrated and for which relatively few non-haematological toxicities are found; 3) administration of multiple drugs over a short period of time, in order to take advantage of tumour growth and repopulation characteristics; 4) utilization of multiple drugs without cross-resistance at the onset of treatment in an attempt to overcome the appearance of drug-resistant cells, according to the Goldie and Coldman hypothesis; 5) utilization of chemotherapeutic agents with different patterns of haematological and non-haematological toxicity (myelotoxicity, mucosal toxicity, etc.).

The combination of these distinct but complementary approaches has led to the definition of the dose intensity (DI) concept [13]. The delivered DI for a given drug represents the dose administered over a defined period of time in comparison with the theoretical dose which would be administered over the theoretical period defined in the protocol. Adequate measurement of relative (delivered/projected) DI should reflect both treatment delays and modifications in drug dosages for each individual patient [4,13].

Clinical experience with multiple chemotherapy regimens has resulted in the enunciation of some important principles for the treatment of patients with DLCL [14] (Table 1).

Maturity of Modern Chemotherapy Regimens

Numerous combination chemotherapy regimens have been described as treatment for advanced DLCL in the last two decades. Table 2 summarizes selected anthracycline containing regimens and trials which fulfil 3 criteria: evaluation of a minimum of 50 previously untreated patients with the same regimen, median follow-up at least 2 years, and full publication of the trial (excluding preliminary results presented at meetings and in abstracts). These regimens were classified as follows: 1) CHOP (cyclophosphamide, doxorubicin, vincristine and prednisone administered every 3 or 4 weeks [15]) with CHOP-Bleo (CHOP plus bleomycin) and CHOP-like regimens; 2) regimens using the CHOP drug combination and scheduled as a framework with the addition of one or several drugs (methotrexate, bleomycin, etc.) during chemotherapy administration; 3) alternating cycling regimens where two different drug combinations are administered at regular intervals (for example ProMACE-MOPP); 4) sequential regimens where the first part of treatment includes one type of combination chemotherapy regimen and the second part another (for example LNH-80). At least 3 criteria are useful to evaluate the feasibility and the efficacy of a given regimen: reproducibility at other institutions and in multicentre trials, randomized comparison to other regimens, and publication of long-term results.

As outlined in Table 2, only 6 regimens have been reproduced out of their original institution by other centres or multicentre groups: CHOP and CHOP-Bleo, CAP-BOP, M/m-BACOD,

Table 2. Experience and reproducibility of modern chemotherapy regimens

Regimen	Ref.	No. pts.*	CR rate	Early death rate	Follow-up (y)	2/3-year survival rate	5-year survival rate
CHOP, CHOP-B and CHOP-like regimens							
CHOP	[24]	153/M	44	15	4		35-40
CHOP ± B	[17]	418/M	53	NA	5		30-40
CHOP-B	[78]	105/S	70	NA	6		50
COPA	[108]	70/M	46	0	5		34
COPA-B	[108]	133/M	46	2	5		45
CHOP	[109]	116/S	47	NA	5		35
CHOP ± B	[31]	177/M	47	5	5		38
CHVmP	[26]	70/M	49	2	5		29
CHOP	[21]	225/M	44	1	3	41	
CHOP-frame reinforced regimens							
CAP-BOP	[108]	129/M	43	2	5		45
CAP-BOP	[65]	157/M	65	7	3		42
Continuous CHOP	[110]	108/S	78	6	3		53
CHVmP-VB	[26]	71/M	79	4	5		53
COPBLAM III	[111]	51/S	84	10	2	65	
F-MACHOP	[80]	113/S	78	3	5.7		72
m/M-BACOD	[5,18]	215/S	65	2	4.5	63	57
m-BACOD	[37]	78/M	65	6	3.5	61	
m-BACOD	[112]	92/S	71	5	2.5	56	
m-BACOD	[21]	223/M	48	5	3	46	
MACOP-B	[3]	126/S	84	5	6	69	62
MACOP-B	[113]	70/S	54	7	2	56	
MACOP-B	[114]	109/M	50	5	4	51	
MACOP-BE	[34]	61/S	57	8	2.8	47	
MACOP-B	[115]	180/M	71	5	2	60	
MACOP-B	[21]	218/M	51	6	3	41	
Alternating chemotherapy regimens							
ProMACE-MOPP	[30]	99/S	7	2	5		53
ProMACE-CytaBOM	[30]	94/S	86	6	5		69
ProMACE-CytaBOM	[116]	78/M	65	6	3	57	
ProMACE-CytaBOM	[21]	233/M	56	3	3	46	
CHOP/VIM-B	[117]	81/M	73	1	2.5	6	
Sequential regimens							
ProMACE-MOPP Flexi	[118]	74/S	74	10	5	65	53
LNH-80	[20,119]	100/S	84	5	9.2	65	61
LNH-84	[10]	737/M	75	8	3	59	53

* S = single institution, M = multicentre; NA = not available

MACOP-B, ProMACE-CytaBOM and LNH-80. The differences in the therapeutic results obtained by investigators at different institutions can in part be explained by the heterogeneity in the treated patient populations, with variable numbers of patients older than 60 years, and with patients having adverse prognostic factors or particular histological subtypes (small cleaved cell lymphoma, small noncleaved cell lymphoma, immunoblastic lymphoma). In addition, some regimens are associated with substantial toxicity and are therefore difficult to deliver in unfamiliar settings [2,3, 5,16].

Significant differences in CR rate, death during induction rate, and survival are often observed when cooperative groups attempt to reproduce the results obtained by the original institution. In addition to the factors previously described, some centres participating in such studies and treating small numbers of patients may not have sufficient experience with a given regimen. Delivery of chemotherapy may then be altered (delayed administration of some courses, lower doses of myelotoxic drugs) and toxicity management may be suboptimal. These confounding factors can partly be assessed by 1) comparison of early death rates between single-institution and multicentre trials; 2) analysis of the average dose intensity administered in single-institution and multicentre trials. This does not mean that intensive combination chemotherapy regimens can only be administered at highly specialized centres but it does underscore the necessity of experience for the administration of these regimens. Choices between regimens with similar reported efficacy should be based on familiarity and ease of administration of particular regimens in a particular cancer centre.

Long-term results in patients treated with CHOP indicated that approximately 30% of these patients were cured with 10 years of follow-up [17]. Long-term survivors from the pilot studies for M-BACOD [18], MACOP-B [19] and LNH-80 [20] represent 50% (median follow-up 8 years), 62% (median follow-up over 6 years) and 52% (median follow-up over 9 years) of the treated patient populations, respectively.

Randomized Trials Comparing Modern Chemotherapy Regimens

In order to compare these different chemotherapy regimens, randomized trials have been undertaken by several collaborative groups (SWOG, Eastern Cooperative Oncology Group [ECOG], GELA, European Organization for Research and Treatment of Cancer [EORTC], Cancer and Leukaemia Group B [CALGB], and others). The SWOG-8516 phase III trial comparing CHOP vs m-BACOD vs MACOP-B vs ProMACE-CytaBOM [21] included 1138 total patients and 899 eligible patients (79%) with intermediate and high-grade lymphoma. The median age was 57 years, which was higher than in most of the previously reported large series. With a median follow-up of 35 months, the expected overall survival is not statistically different between the 4 regimens with 50 to 55% of the patients expected to survive at 3 years [21].

Although randomized trials are the best way to compare the results of different regimens, several important considerations must be kept in mind when current and future trials are analysed. The first consideration is the statistical power of the trial. It is unlikely that any modern regimen can improve survival by an order of magnitude of 20%. Detection of smaller although clinically and statistically significant differences will require a very large number of patients. For instance, a trial will have to include more than 500 patients per arm to detect a 10% difference in survival if the 5-year survival is 50% [22]. Moreover, clinical trials tend to include a large number of patients with various risk profiles. In such a heterogeneous population, some patient subgroups are more likely to benefit from an intensive regimen than others. Only an initial stratification allows valid statistical comparison of these subgroups [22] and, again, a large number of patients in each prognosis subset have to be analysed in order to obtain valuable conclusions. Finally, one should keep in mind that regimens more intensive than the classical CHOP are also more toxic. Therefore, if a regimen reduces the relapse rate at 2 or 3 years but is more toxic, a resulting improvement in survival may not be apparent in early reported results. In conclusion, current results suggest that the more intensive combination chemotherapy regimens are not clearly superior to CHOP in unselected populations of patients with DLCL. More trials addressing chemotherapy intensification in specific subgroups of patients are needed.

Long-Term Follow-up of Patients Treated with Modern Chemotherapy Regimens

Actuarial results projected with a median follow-up of less than 5 years are insufficient to assess the true number of DLCL patients who are potentially "cured" of their disease. As recently outlined in several studies [18,20,23], late relapses can be observed beyond 10 years after the achievement of CR. Long-term follow-up of patients treated with the CHOP regimen indicated that 30% to 40% of the patients were long-term survivors and that relapses could occur for at least 7 years following the completion of therapy [17]. In patients treated with m/M-BACOD, the risk of relapse was 13% per year during the first 2 years after treatment, approximately 8% per year until the fifth year, and one or two percent per year thereafter [18,20].

May New Regimens or Approaches Improve the Outcome of DLCL Patients?

A considerable amount of time and effort has been devoted to determining whether more intensive combination chemotherapy is associated with an improved outcome. In unselected patients, there appears to be no significant improvement in outcome associated with regimens developed in the last decade. However, several trends are apparent in these studies.

The Role of Dose Intensity

Despite the necessary reservations about the use of CR as a valid endpoint and the difficulties in comparing non-randomized trials, most intensive regimens developed after CHOP were associated with higher CR rates (65% to 85%) than those reported with CHOP (45% to 75%) (Table 2). So far, no randomized trial has shown a significant increase in CR rate with new regimens. Although CR rates are not synonymous with long-term survival rates, it is likely that any improvements achieved in long-term survival are associated with improvements in the number of complete responders [24,25]. For instance, recent results of the EORTC randomized study [26] of CHVmP (CHOP with VM26 instead of vincristine) versus CHVmP plus vincristine and bleomycin demonstrated statistical differences in CR rates (50% versus 80%) resulting in an improvement in 5-year overall survival (29% versus 53%, $p = 0.002$).

The dose intensity of a regimen can be modified by increasing individual drug doses or adding new drugs [27]. Several regimens containing 4 to 5 drugs have been reported with CR and survival rates comparable to regimens using smaller numbers of drugs [28,29] (see also Table 2). The identical results obtained with ProMACE-MOPP and ProMACE-MOPP "flexitherapy" (in which the MOPP sequences were delivered later) also suggest that the number of non-cross-resistant drugs administered over a short induction period is not a determinant factor for outcome [30]. Attempts to increase CHOP or MACOP-B "dose intensity" with the addition of bleomycin or etoposide also did not improve CR rates or survival [31-34]. In most cases, the addition of new drugs to a regimen results in decreased doses of the drugs already contained in this regimen to avoid unacceptable toxicity. The resulting decreased DI of drugs such as doxorubicin and cyclophosphamide may affect the final outcome.

Although it has been suggested that increased DI may improve the survival of patients with aggressive lymphoma [27,35], no randomized study has specifically investigated whether the same combination regimen used at an increased DI was associated with improved survival [36]. However, many studies have shown that patients receiving low doses of therapy because of old age or other adverse factors (such as bone marrow involvement) had a very poor outcome [37,38]. Two retrospective analyses conducted in patients who received CHOP or CHOP-like regimens suggested that the delivered DI could influence survival [39,40]. The actual relative DI of doxorubicin was identified as the single most important predictor for survival using multivariate recursive partitioning analysis in a small series of DLCL patients [40]. In another study, multivariate analysis also identified average relative DIs of doxorubicin and cyclophosphamide as predictive for survival of complete responders [39]. However, in several phase II SWOG studies, relative DI after 12 weeks was associated with CR and survival but was not found to be an independent prognostic variable [41]. The retrospective nature of all these studies is an important limitation since DI is also heavily influenced by pre-treatment prognostic factors such as age, performance status, or B symptoms. In the recent prospective NCI randomized trial comparing ProMACE-MOPP with ProMACE-CytaBOM, the delivered DI was substantially higher for cyclophosphamide (+43%) and doxorubicin (+42%) in the ProMACE-CytaBOM arm [30]. The 5-year survival was also found to be higher in the ProMACE-Cyta-

BOM arm, with a borderline significance (69% versus 53%, $p = 0.082$) [30]. This improvement was related to the increased DI because replacement of mechlorethamine and procarbazine (in MOPP) by cytarabine and bleomycin (in CytaBOM) is unlikely to account for all the improvement.

Taken together, these data suggest that the number of drugs administered is less important than the DI of "standard" drugs such as cyclophosphamide and doxorubicin. These data further indicate that increased DI may improve the outcome of DLCL patients. Regimens with a high DI (especially regarding cyclophosphamide) have been utilized in selected patients with a predictable poor outcome, with interesting preliminary results [42-45]. However, the definition of the "high-risk" patients in these studies is quite heterogeneous. It is now time to specifically and prospectively address the problem of the DI in aggressive lymphomas and to see if an increase in the administered dose of selected drugs can modify the outcome for patients with aggressive lymphomas. The availability of haematopoietic growth factors will allow delivery of higher drug doses without unacceptable toxicity [46,47] and such randomized trials are a priority for the future.

Recent Progress in Bone Marrow Transplantation

Bone marrow transplantation (BMT) has been initially developed for relapsing or refractory patients to support the use of high-dose therapy [48]. Early pilot studies showed that this therapy offered a potential for long-term survival in a limited number of patients thought to be incurable with conventional therapy [6-8]. Moreover, relapsing patients who experienced a complete response or a good partial response to salvage conventional therapy demonstrated a significantly better outcome after transplantation compared to those refractory to salvage therapy [7,49,50]. Several questions remain unanswered regarding the real place of this treatment in lymphoma patients.

First, the optimal source of haematopoietic stem cells used for rescue has not yet been determined. The majority of bone marrow transplant regimens utilized in lymphoma patients included autologous bone marrow reinfusion. The use of allogenic bone marrow has been hampered by high graft-versus-host-disease related toxicity and the lack of clinical evidence for a graft-versus-lymphoma effect [6,51]. For this reason, allogenic transplants have been reserved for patients with high-grade lymphomas (particularly LBL), or with massive bone marrow involvement, or with severe impairment of bone marrow reserve. In patients in whom the bone marrow cannot be used as a source of stem cells, autologous peripheral blood stem cells (PBSC) have been utilized as an alternative source of support for high-dose therapy [52, 53]. The optimal methods for stimulating and collecting circulating haematopoietic progenitor cells are still being determined [54]. Whether or not PBSC should be preferred to autologous bone marrow also remains unclear.

Secondly, several high-dose regimens have been developed including diverse combinations of drugs (mostly cyclophosphamide, etoposide, carmustine, cytarabine, melphalan) with or without total body irradiation (TBI). Limited patient series, heterogeneity of patient selection, and lack of long-term follow-up preclude any comparison regarding the respective efficacy of these regimens for achieving CR and long-term survival. Several of the earlier regimens were very toxic, with mortality rates approaching 20% in the initial studies in which heavily pre-treated patients with poor prognosis were transplanted [7]. However, with improved support and patient selection, the toxicity of the procedure has decreased. For example, the morbidity in two large recent series was quite low: 2% in 100 selected patients with sensitive relapse receiving cyclophosphamide/TBI and purged bone marrow [55], and less than 1% in 180 patients transplanted in first CR with cyclophosphamide/carmustine/etoposide [43]. However, the optimal conditioning regimen before rescue has yet to be determined, as well as the need for TBI. As high-dose therapy with BM or PBSC rescue is being developed and is becoming standard treatment for relapsing patients, randomized prospective trials will be needed to address these issues.

Finally, the possible impact of *in vitro* bone marrow manipulation deserves further attention. Bone marrow purging has been utilized to treat potential lymphoma cell contamination prior to reinfusion. Pharmacological agents (4-hydroperoxy-cyclophosphamide or etoposide) and

immunological methods (complement-mediated monoclonal antibody (MoAb) lysis, toxin- or drug-conjugated MoAbs, or MoAb-mediated physical depletion) have been used, separately or in combination. Comparison of earlier results from different centres obtained with either purged [8,50,56,57] or unpurged [7,49,58] bone marrow did not indicate an advantage for bone marrow purging. Since DLCL patients receiving BMT often relapse after treatment at their prior sites of disease [7], it has been claimed that bone marrow purging is not a major determinant for the outcome. However, recent data suggest that efficient immunological purging may significantly decrease relapse rates after BMT in *bcl-2* positive lymphoid malignancies [59]. Another study reports that the frequency of relapse after BMT is correlated with the presence of lymphoma cells in the bone marrow that will grow in appropriate *in vitro* assays [60]. Although these results need to be confirmed in prospective studies, they suggest that the use of purged bone marrow (and perhaps PBSC which may not be contaminated with tumour cells) may prove to be beneficial.
Given the lack of valid comparisons between multiple small series of patients with various histories of lymphoma disease, these issues deserve to be addressed in prospective trials in some subsets of patients when the therapeutic advantage of high-dose therapy will become more apparent.

Can High-Dose Therapy with Stem Cell Transplantation be Proposed as Upfront Therapy in DLCL Patients?

Several studies have attempted to intensify therapy in patients with a predictable poor outcome early in their disease course. Seventeen patients who achieved only a partial response (PR) after induction therapy were treated with high-dose therapy supported with BMT [45]. Two-year overall survival was 75%, markedly higher that what could have been expected with conventional therapy [45]. Fourteen other patients with adverse prognostic factors (elevated LDH or bulky disease) were transplanted after achieving PR or CR on induction therapy and 79% of them were alive at 5 years [42,61]. These results were reproduced by others [49,55,56] and the European BMT register reported 135 selected patients who were transplanted in first CR with an expected DFS of 70% at 5 years [62].
To address the role of high-dose therapy with stem cell rescue as consolidation therapy in poor prognosis patients, the GELA conducted a randomized study including 727 poor prognosis patients (with at least one of the following characteristics: performance status >1, >1 extranodal sites, bulky tumour ≥10 cm, bone marrow infiltration, lymphoblastic or Burkitt subtype) from 1987 to 1991 [43]. After an ACVB regimen induction (LNH-84) therapy, 67% of the patients achieved CR and were randomized to receive either high-dose therapy (CBV regimen: cyclophosphamide, carmustine, etoposide) supported with ABMT or the sequential LNH-84 consolidation chemotherapy [43]. Preliminary results (with a 24-month median follow-up) in the first 370 randomized patients showed a 58% disease-free survival in both arms of the study [43]. A longer follow-up of these patients is necessary to assess if high-dose therapy with ABMT will provide any benefit. Other studies addressing the same therapeutic approach are currently under way (EORTC, Medical Research Council [MRC]). Until the final results of these studies are available, early intensification of poor prognosis patients must be an experimental approach reserved for well designed studies.

Conclusions and Practical Recommendations for Treating a New Patient

All these results indicate that no outstanding therapeutic improvement has been achieved in the last 10 years. Regimens more intensive than CHOP were initially reported to potentially cure more patients than CHOP but preliminary reports from randomized trials comparing these so-called modern chemotherapy regimens to CHOP do not support the initial findings [21,63]. However, the results of more intensive regimens should be compared to CHOP (or other regimens) in all subgroups of patients. Elderly patients with advanced DLCL do not tolerate intensive regimens well [38,64, 65] and may not benefit by such treatment. Furthermore, it is difficult to demonstrate any statistically significant improvement in the outcome of patients with a favourable prognosis. Finally, only some high-risk patients are likely to benefit from such intensive treatments. The introduction of an International Index for determining patient prognosis will facilitate the reproducible identification of patient subgroups with predictable outcomes [9]. Again, only prospective randomized trials can establish the superiority of any therapeutic regimen and the classical CHOP remains a good standard treatment to be compared to new approaches.

Therefore, the first suggestion regarding the treatment of DLCL patients would be to keep including these patients in prospective randomized trials. Such trials should be well designed and should include enough patients to adequately address a single important question, with stratification of patients according to one of the major prognostic indices. If participation in prospective randomized trials is impossible, patients may be treated with one of the modern chemotherapy regimens known to be effective and reproducible (Table 2) as long as physicians have some experience with the regimen(s) and deliver full drug doses on the appropriate schedule. Therapeutic innovations based upon small modifications of previous regimens are unlikely to result in significant differences in outcome and may actually turn out to be less efficient than the original regimen.

Therapeutic Approaches to Specific Patient Subgroups

Patients with Localized Disease

Five to 10% of DLCL patients are found to have extremely localized disease (Ann Arbor stage I or IE) and no adverse prognostic factors after diagnosis and staging. Isolated radiation therapy in such patients is associated with a high relapse risk [66,67]. For these reasons, most patients with localized disease are currently treated with systemic chemotherapy. Three to 6 courses of CHOP or a CHOP-like regimen followed by involved field radiotherapy is associated with a 95% CR rate with a 80 to 90% probability of cure at 5 years [68-71]. The long-term survival in patients with either stage I disease and adverse prognostic factors or stage II disease is not so favourable (only 60 to 80% of the patients survive at 5 years) and more intensive approaches should be prospectively tested in such patients [70-72].

The use of radiotherapy and combined modality treatments in patients with aggressive lymphoma may increase the risk of secondary malignancies [73,74], as already observed in Hodgkin's disease patients. In addition, radiotherapy may generate discomfort and sequelae when specific locations such as the head and neck or gastrointestinal tract are treated [67,75]. For these reasons, it is important to define the possible benefit associated with radiation therapy when full doses of CHOP or a more intensive regimen are used, by comparing the combination of chemotherapy/radiotherapy to chemotherapy alone in a randomized trial. However, given the excellent prognosis of these patients, it will be difficult to demonstrate the superiority of one (combined modality) or the other (chemotherapy alone) treatment in patients with localized disease.

The Role of Radiotherapy in Patients with Bulky Tumours

Lymphoma patients presenting with bulky tumours (>10 cm) in the mediastinum, retroperitoneum or any other lymphoid area comprise 25 to 30% of all DLCL patients. The negative prognostic value of bulky disease has been well established in patients with either advanced disease [76-79] or localized disease (stage I or II) [70,71]. Radiotherapy is often delivered to the site(s) of bulky disease after completion of the chemotherapy regimen. However, the patterns of relapse in bulky disease patients indicate that the majority of patients do not relapse solely at their site(s) of prior bulky disease [80,81]. Several studies in which patients received "adjuvant" radiation therapy or no radiation therapy failed to demonstrate any advantage for this treatment [10, 81]. For these reasons, "adjuvant" radiotherapy to sites of prior bulky disease cannot be considered as a standard treatment in advanced aggressive lymphoma patients. Prospective randomized regimens have to address the role of radiotherapy in responding patients with persistent localized masses that may contain some residual viable lymphoma cells.

Specific Extranodal Disease Sites

The gastrointestinal tract is the most frequent extranodal site of lymphomatous involvement [82]. The possibility of chemotherapy-associated gastrointestinal haemorrhages has resulted in a recommendation of surgical debulking prior to chemotherapy [75,83]. No randomized studies have demonstrated a benefit for surgery, which has its own risks of short and long-term complications [84,85]. In fact, recent studies suggest that the risk of haemorrhages may have been overstated in patients responding to intensive combination chemotherapy [84-86]. Retrospective analysis of 56 patients with localized gastrointestinal lymphomas (stage IE bulky and stage IIE) treated with the LNH-84 regimen indicated that complete surgical resection did not influence survival [85]. The overall 5-year survival of patients with localized aggressive gastric lymphoma treated with chemotherapy alone was superior to 75% in several recent reports [84-86].

Patients with central nervous system (CNS) disease have a very poor prognosis. However, isolated leptomeningeal infiltration can be cured and some patients achieve long-term survival with intensive combination chemotherapy [10,87]. Primary CNS lymphomas are infrequent in non-immunocompromised patients although an increased incidence has recently been reported [88]. The respective roles of radiotherapy and chemotherapy have recently been reconsidered in several studies [89-91]. Radiotherapy alone was associated with a median survival of less than 2 years, whereas combined modalities incorporating intensive chemotherapy regimens appeared to improve survival by 1 or 2 years. High-dose i.v. methotrexate is an important element of the therapy in these patients [89,92].

T-Cell Lymphoma Subtypes

The prognostic value of immunological phenotype in DLCL is somewhat controversial [93-95]. T-cell peripheral lymphomas represent a heterogeneous group with different histological subtypes, the majority being classified as diffuse mixed, large cell and immunoblastic lymphomas [96,97]. Peripheral T-cell lymphoma patients often present with more adverse prognostic features at diagnosis than B-cell lymphoma patients [96]. Multivariate analysis conducted in a large series of 361 patients homogeneously treated with the LNH-84 regimen clearly demonstrated that T-cell phenotype was an adverse independent prognostic factor for FFR survival and overall survival [98]. In this study, patients with T-cell lymphomas progressed more rapidly than those with B-cell lymphomas (43% versus 29% progressed, $p < 0.001$) and had a shorter overall survival (median 42 versus 50 months) [98].

Elderly Patients

A recent population-based registry of lymphoma patients in Denmark established the median age of lymphoma patients to be 65 years and indicated that patients over 70 may represent up to 38% of the patients with DLCL [99]. The proportion of diffuse large cell lymphomas was also found to be significantly higher in patients over 70 [99]. Older DLCL patients have the same adverse prognostic factors as younger patients, but they appear to have a worse outcome [65,99,100]. In early studies, this shorter survival was associated with the reduced doses of active drugs that the elderly patients received [37,38,64,101]. However, more recent studies specifically directed at assessing the outcome of older patients indicate that age *per se* is an important and independent prognostic factor for response and survival [65,76,102,103]. Even when the higher rates of death from unrelated causes were taken into account, elderly patients had a higher incidence of adverse outcomes than younger patients [100]. Specific causes of death were found to be related to lymphoma progression or treatment toxicity, particularly infectious and cardiac problems [65].

Recently, a few prospective studies have addressed the therapeutic approaches in these patients [104-107]. In one study, 72 patients between 65 and 85 years were prospectively treated with two successive protocols, low-dose ACOP-B and VABE [105]. More than two-thirds of the patients responded to these treatments (70% and 91% overall response rates) with an acceptable lethal toxicity (5% and 6% of toxic deaths), but grade 4 toxicity (mainly haematological) was observed in 58% of the patients receiving the VABE regimen [105]. Overall survival was 28% at 6 years with LD-ACOP and 36% at 4 years with VABE with a relatively low number (2 and 4, respectively) of deaths unrelated to the lymphoma [105]. Another study of 38 previously untreated patients showed a high percentage of responders (89% of overall response) with a VMP regimen (etoposide, mitoxantrone, prednimustine) and a median survival of 14 months [107]. Again, in the large majority of cases the cause of death was attributed to lymphoma [107].

Taken together, these results suggest that elderly patients have aggressive disease and an associated high probability of relapse and death from lymphoma. The use of aggressive chemotherapy regimens is, however, limited by their substantial toxicity. New regimens with low cardiotoxicity and additional administration of haematopoietic growth factors may improve the current results and must be compared to standard regimens in randomized studies.

Conclusions

With an optimal therapeutic regimen that is carefully administered, approximately half of the DLCL patients under 70 years of age can achieve a complete remission and become long-term survivors. There is substantial room for improvement of these results, particularly in younger patients with adverse prognostic factors and elderly patients in general. Well designed prospective studies can address the possible benefit of chemotherapy intensification. The necessity to conduct prospective randomized trials is not only scientific but also relates to ethical and economic considerations. However, small improvements in the therapy of certain subsets of patients are unlikely to dramatically change the outcome in aggressive lymphoma patients treated with current approaches. For these reasons, new therapeutic approaches based upon an improved understanding of the molecular mechanisms of malignant transformation and of the host reaction need to be developed.

Acknowledgement

Gilles Salles and Bertrand Coiffier are supported in part by grants from the "Programme National de Recherche Clinique Lyon 004".

REFERENCES

1 DeVita V, Canellos GP, Chabner B et al: Advanced diffuse histiocytic lymphoma, a potentially curable disease. Results with combination chemotherapy. Lancet 1975 (1):248-250

2 Coiffier B, Bryon PA, Ffrench M et al: Intensive chemotherapy in aggressive lymphomas: updated results of LNH-80 protocol and prognostic factors affecting response and survival. Blood 1987 (70): 1394-1399

3 Klimo P and Connors JM: MACOP-B chemotherapy for the treatment of diffuse large-cell lymphoma. Ann Intern Med 1985 (102):596-602

4 Longo DL, Duffey PL, Devita VT et al: The calculation of actual or received dose intensity: A comparison of published methods. J Clin Oncol 1991 (9):2042-2051

5 Skarin AT, Canellos GP, Rosenthal DS et al: Improved prognosis of diffuse histiocytic and undifferentiated lymphoma by use of high dose methotrexate alternating with standard agents (M-BACOD). J Clin Oncol 1983 (1):91-98

6 Appelbaum FR, Sullivan KM, Buckner CD: Treatment of malignant lymphoma in 100 patients with chemotherapy, total body irradiation, and marrow transplantation. J Clin Oncol 1987 (5):1340-1347

7 Philip T, Armitage JO, Spitzer G et al: High-dose therapy and autologous bone marrow transplantation after failure of conventional chemotherapy in adults with intermediate-grade or high-grade non-Hodgkin's lymphoma. N Engl J Med 1987 (316): 1493-1498

8 Takvorian T, Canellos GP, Ritz J et al: Prolonged disease-free survival after autologous bone marrow transplantation in patients with non-Hodgkin's lymphoma with a poor prognosis. N Engl J Med 1987 (316):1499-1505

9 The International Non-Hodgkin's Lymphoma Prognostic Factors Project: A predictive model for aggressive non-Hodgkin's lymphoma. N Engl J Med 1993 (329):987-994

10 Coiffier B, Gisselbrecht C, Herbrecht R et al: LNH-84: a multicenter study of intensive chemotherapy in 737 patients with aggressive malignant lymphoma. J Clin Oncol 1989 (7):1018-1026

11 Kwak LW, Wilson M, Weiss LM et al: Clinical significance of morphologic subdivision in diffuse large cell lymphoma. Cancer 1991 (68):1988-1993

12 Surbone A, Longo DL, DeVita VT et al: Residual abdominal masses in aggressive non-Hodgkin's lymphoma after combination chemotherapy: significance and management. J Clin Oncol 1988 (6):1832-1837

13 Hryniuk WM and Goodyear M: The calculation of received dose intensity. J Clin Oncol 1990 (8): 1935-1937

14 Armitage JO and Cheson BD: Interpretation of clinical trials in diffuse large-cell lymphoma. J Clin Oncol 1988 (6):1335-1347

15 McKelvey EM, Gottlieb JA, Wilson HE et al: Hydroxyldaunomycin (adriamycin) combination chemotherapy in malignant lymphoma. Cancer 1976 (38):1484-1493

16 Brown MJ, Hubbard SM, Longo DL et al: Excess prevalence of pneumocystis carinii pneumonia in patients treated for lymphoma with combination chemotherapy. Ann Intern Med 1986 (104):338-344

17 Coltman CA, Dahlberg S, Jones SE: CHOP is curative in thirty percent of patients with large cell lymphoma: a twelve-year Southwest Oncology Group follow-up. In: Skarin AT (ed) Update on Treatment for Diffuse Large Cell Lymphoma. Projects in Medicine, Park Row Publishers 1986 pp 71-77

18 Shipp MA, Yeap BY, Harrington DP et al: The m-BACOD combination chemotherapy regimen in large-cell lymphoma: Analysis of the completed trial and comparison with the M-BACOD regimen. J Clin Oncol 1990 (8):84-93

19 Hoskins PJ, Ng V, Spinelli JJ et al: Prognostic variables in patients with diffuse large-cell lymphoma treated with MACOP-B. J Clin Oncol 1991 (9):220-226

20 Dumontet C, Bastion Y, Felman P et al: Long-term outcome and sequelae in aggressive lymphoma patients treated with the LNH-80 regimen. Ann Oncol 1992 (3):639-644

21 Fisher RI, Gaynor ER, Dahlberg S et al: Comparison of a standard regimen (CHOP) with three intensive chemotherapy regimens for advanced non-Hodgkin's lymphoma. N Engl J Med 1993 (328):1002-1006

22 Simon R and Friedman MA: The design and interpretation of clinical trials. In: Perry MC (ed) The Chemotherapy Source Book. Williams & Wilkins, Baltimore 1992 p 130

23 Cabanillas F, Velasquez WS, Hagemeister FB et al: Clinical, biological, and histologic features of late relapses in diffuse large cell lymphoma. Blood 1992 (79):1024-1028

24 Gams RA, Rainey M , Dandy M et al: Phase III study of BCOP v CHOP in unfavorable categories of malignant lymphoma: a Southeastern Cancer Study Group trial. J Clin Onocl 1985 (3):1188-1195

25 Jones SE, Grozea PN, Metz EN et al: Superiority of adriamycin-containing combination chemotherapy in the treatment of diffuse lymphoma. A Southwest Oncology Group study. Cancer 1979 (43):417-425

26 Carde P, Meerwaldt JH, van Glabbeke M et al: Superiority of second over first generation chemotherapy in a randomized trial for stage III-IV intermediate and high-grade non-Hodgkin's lymphoma (NHL): the 1980-1985 EORTC trial. Ann Oncol 1991 (2):431-435

27 DeVita VT, Hubbard SM, Longo DL: The chemotherapy of lymphomas: Looking back, moving forward. The Richard and Hinda Rosenthal Foundation Award lecture. Cancer Res 1987 (47): 5810-5824

28 Lee R, Cabanillas F, Bodey GP, Freireich EJ: A 10-year update of CHOP-Bleo in the treatment of diffuse large-cell lymphoma. J Clin Oncol 1986 (4):1455-1461

29 Zuckerman KS, LoBuglio AF, Reeves JA: Chemotherapy of intermediate grade and high grade non-Hodgkin's lymphomas with a high-dose doxorubicin-containing regimen. J Clin Oncol 1990 (8):248-256

30 Longo DL, Devita VT, Duffey PL: Superiority of ProMACE-CytaBOM over ProMACE-MOPP in the treatment of advanced diffuse aggressive lymphoma - Results of a prospective randomized trial. J Clin Oncol 1991 (9):25-38

31 Gottlieb AJ, Anderson JR, Ginsberg SJ: A randomized comparison of methotrexate dose and the addition of bleomycin to CHOP therapy for diffuse large cell lymphoma and other non-Hodgkin's lymphomas. Cancer and Leukemia Group B Study 7851. Cancer 1990 (66):1888-1896

32 Harding M, Mcnulty L, Paul J et al: An alternating chemotherapy combination (MACOBLE) for intermediate and high-grade non-Hodgkin's lymphoma. Hematological Oncology 1991 (9):93-102

33 Koppler H, Pfluger KH, Eschenbach I et al: CHOP-VP16 chemotherapy and involved field irradiation for high grade non-Hodgkin's lymphomas: A phase II multicentre study. Br J Cancer 1989 (60):79-82

34 Sweetenham JW, Mead GM, Whitehouse JMA: Intensive weekly combination chemotherapy for patients with intermediate-grade and high-grade non-Hodgkin's lymphoma. J Clin Oncol 1991 (9): 2202-2209

35 Meyer RM, Hryniuk WM, Goodyear MDE: The role of dose intensity in determining outcome in intermediate-grade non-Hodgkin's lymphoma. J Clin Oncol 1991 (9):339-347

36 Gelman R and Neuberg D: Making cocktails versus making soup. J Clin Oncol 1991 (9):200-203

37 Dana BW, Dahlberg S, Miller TP et al: m-BACOD treatment for intermediate-grade and high-grade malignant lymphomas: A Southwest Oncology Group phase II trial. J Clin Oncol 1990 (8):1155-1162

38 Dixon DO, Neilan B, Jones SE et al: Effect of age on therapeutic outcome in advanced diffuse histiocytic lymphoma: the Southwest Oncology Group experience. J Clin Oncol 1986 (4):295-305

39 Epelbaum R, Faraggi D, Ben-Arie Y et al: Survival of diffuse large cell lymphoma. A multivariate analysis including dose intensity variables. Cancer 1990 (66):1124-1129

40 Kwak LW, Halpern J, Olshen RA, Horning SJ: Prognostic significance of actual dose intensity in diffuse large cell lymphoma: Results of a tree structured survival analysis. J Clin Oncol 1990 (8): 963-977

41 Dahlberg S, Miller TP, Dana B et al: Dose intensity is not associated with subsequent survival after adjustment for known prognostic factors in non-Hodgkin's lymphoma patients treated with m-BACOD, ProMACE-CytaBOM, and MACOP-B in Southwest Oncology Group studies. Proc Amer Soc Clin Oncol 1990 (9):255

42 Gulati SC, Shank B, Black P et al: Autologous bone marrow transplantation for patients with poor-prognosis lymphoma. J Clin Oncol 1988 (6):1303-1313

43 Haïoun C, Lepage E, Gisselbrecht C et al: Autologous bone marrow transplantation versus sequential chemotherapy in first complete remission aggressive non-Hodgkin's lymphoma: first interim analysis on 370 patients (LNH87 Protocol). In: 28th Meeting of the American Society of Clinical Oncology. San Diego, CA 1992 (11):316 (Abst # 1071)

44 McMaster ML, Greer JP, Wolff SN et al: Results of treatment with high intensity, brief duration chemotherapy in poor prognosis non-Hodgkin's lymphoma. Cancer 1991 (68):233-241

45 Philip T, Hartmann O, Biron P et al: High-dose therapy and autologous bone marrow transplantation in partial remission after first-line induction therapy for diffuse non-Hodgkin's lymphoma. J Clin Oncol 1988 (6):1118-1124

46 Gianni AM, Bregni M, Siena S: Recombinant human granulocyte-macrophage colony-stimulating factor reduces hematologic toxicity and widens clinical applicability of high-dose cyclophosphamide treatment in breast cancer and non-Hodgkin's lymphoma. J Clin Oncol 1990 (8):768-778

47 Ho AD, Del Valle F, Haas R: Sequential studies on the role of mitoxantrone, high-dose cytarabine, and recombinant human granulocyte-macrophage colony-stimulating factor in the treatment of refractory non-Hodgkin's lymphoma. Sem Oncol 1990 (17):14-19

48 Appelbaum FR, Herzig GP, Ziegler JL et al: Successful engrafment of cryopreserved autologous bone marrow in patients with malignant lymphoma. Blood 1978 (52):85-95

49 Gribben JG, Goldstone AH, Linch DC et al: Effectiveness of high-dose combination chemotherapy and autologous bone marrow transplantation for patients with non-Hodgkin's lymphomas who are still responsive to conventional-dose therapy. J Clin Oncol 1989 (7):1621-1629

50 Petersen FB, Appelbaum FR, Hill R et al: Autologous marrow transplantation for malignant lymphoma - a report of 101 cases from Seattle. J Clin Oncol 1990 (8):638-647

51 Jones RJ, Ambinder RF, Piantadosi S, Santos GW: Evidence of a graft-versus-lymphoma effect associated with allogeneic bone marrow transplantation. Blood 1991 (77):649-653

52 Campos L, Bastion Y, Roubi N et al: Peripheral blood stem cells harvested after chemotherapy and GM-CSF for treatment intensification in patients with advanced lymphoproliferative diseases. Leukemia 1993 (7):1409-1415

53 Kessinger A, Armitage JO, Smith DM et al: High-dose therapy and autologous peripheral blood stem cell transplantation for patients with lymphoma. Blood 1989 (74):1260-1265

54 Kessinger A and Armitage JO: The evolving role of autologous peripheral stem cell transplantation following high-dose therapy for malignancies. Blood 1991 (77):211-213

55 Freedman AS, Takvorian T, Anderson KC et al: Autologous bone marrow transplantation in B-cell non-Hodgkin's lymphoma: Very low treatment-related mortality in 100 patients in sensitive relapse. J Clin Oncol 1990 (8):784-791

56 Colombat P, Gorin NC, Lemonnier MP: The role of autologous bone marrow transplantation in 46 adult patients with non-Hodgkin's lymphomas. J Clin Oncol 1990 (8):630-637

57 Weisdorf DJ, Haake R, Miller WJ: Autologous bone marrow transplantation for progressive non-

Hodgkin's lymphoma - Clinical impact of immunophenotype and in vitro purging. Bone Marrow Transplant 1991 (8):135-142

58 Vose JM, Peterson C, Bierman PJ et al: Comparison of high-dose therapy and autologous bone marrow transplantation for T-cell and B-cell non-Hodgkin's lymphomas. Blood 1990 (76):424-431

59 Gribben JG, Freedman AS, Neuberg D: Immunologic purging of marrow assessed by PCR before autologous bone marrow transplantation for B-cell lymphoma. N Engl J Med 1991 (325):1525-1533

60 Sharp JG, Joshi SS, Armitage JO et al: Significance of detection of occult non-Hodgkin's lymphoma in histologically uninvolved bone marrow by a culture technique. Blood 1992 (79):1074-1080

61 Gulati SC, Yahalom J, Whitmarsh K et al: Factors affecting the outcome of autologous bone marrow transplantation. Ann Oncol 1991 (2):51-55

62 Goldstone AH, Singer CRJ, Gribben JC et al: Fifth report of EBMTG experience of ABMT in malignant lymphoma. Bone Marrow Transplant 1988 (3):33-36

63 Gordon LI, Harrington D, Andersen J et al: Comparison of a second generation combination chemotherapeutic regimen (m-BACOD) with a standard regimen (CHOP) for advanced diffuse non-Hodgkin's lymphoma. N Engl J Med 1992 (327): 1342-1349

64 Tirelli U, Zagonel V, Serraino D et al: Non-Hodgkin's lymphomas in 137 patients aged 70 years or older: A retrospective European Organization for Research and Treatment of Cancer Lymphoma Group study. J Clin Oncol 1988 (6):1708-1713

65 Vose JM, Armitage JO, Weisenburger DD et al: The importance of age in survival of patients treated with chemotherapy for aggressive non-Hodgkin's lymphoma. J Clin Oncol 1988 (6):1838-1844

66 Mauch P, Leonard R, Skarin AT et al: Improved survival following combined radiation therapy and chemotherapy for unfavorable prognosis stage I-II non-Hodgkin's lymphomas. J Clin Oncol 1985 (3):1301-1308

67 Tsutsui K, Shibamoto Y, Yamabe H: A radiotherapeutic experience for localized extranodal non-Hodgkin's lymphoma - Prognostic factors and re-evaluation of treatment modality. Radiotherapy and Oncology 1991 (21):83-90

68 Jones SE, Miller TP, Connors JM: Long-term follow-up and analysis for prognostic factors for patients with limited-stage diffuse large-cell lymphoma treated with initial chemotherapy with or without adjuvant radiotherapy. J Clin Oncol 1989 (7):1186-1191

69 Longo DL, Glatstein E, Duffey PL et al: Treatment of localized aggressive lymphomas with combination chemotherapy followed by involved-field radiation therapy. J Clin Oncol 1989 (7):1295-1302

70 Prestidge BR, Horning SJ, Hoppe RT: Combined modality therapy for stage I-II large cell lymphoma. Int J Radiat Biol Phys 1988 (15):633-639

71 Velasquez WS, Fuller LM, Jagannath S: Stages I and II diffuse large cell lymphomas: Prognostic factors and long-term results with CHOP-Bleo and radiotherapy. Blood 1991 (77):942-947

72 O'Connell MJ, Harrington DP, Earle JD et al: Chemotherapy followed by consolidation radiation therapy for the treatment of clinical stage II aggressive histologic type non-Hodgkin's lymphoma. Cancer 1988 (61):1754-1758

73 Travis LB, Curtis RE, Hankey BF, Fraumeni JF: Second cancers in patients with chronic lymphocytic leukemia. JNCI 1992 (84):1422-1427

74 Zarrabi MH: Association of non-Hodgkins lymphoma and second neoplasms. Sem Oncol 1990 (17):120-132

75 Shiu MH, Nisce LZ, Pinna A et al: Recent results of multimodal therapy of gastric lymphoma. Cancer 1986 (58):1389-1399

76 Coiffier B, Gisselbrecht C, Vose JM et al: Prognostic factors in aggressive malignant lymphomas. Description and validation of a prognostic index that could identify patients requiring a more intensive therapy. J Clin Oncol 1991 (9):211-219

77 Cowan RA, Jones M, Harris M et al: Prognostic factors in high and intermediate grade non-Hodgkin's lymphoma. Br J Cancer 1989 (59):276-282

78 Jagannath S, Velasquez WS, Tucker SL et al: Tumor burden assessment and its implication for a prognostic model in advanced diffuse large-cell lymphoma. J Clin Oncol 1986 (4):859-865

79 Shipp MA, Harrington DP, Klatt MM et al: Identification of major prognostic subgroups of patients with large-cell lymphoma treated with m-BACOD or M-BACOD. Ann Inter Med 1986 (104):757-765

80 Guglielmi C, Amadori S, Martelli M et al: The F-MACHOP sequential combination chemotherapy regimen in advanced diffuse aggressive lymphomas: long-term results. Ann Oncol 1991 (2):365-371

81 Engelhard M, Meusers P, Brittinger G et al: Prospective multicenter trial for the response-adapted treatment of high-grade malignant non-Hodgkin's lymphoma: Updated results of the COP-BLAM/IMVP-16 protocol with randomized adjuvant radiotherapy. Ann Oncol 1991 (2):177-180

82 Otter R, Gerrits WBJ, Sandt MMVD et al: Primary extranodal and nodal non-Hodgkin's lymphoma. A survey of a population-based registry. Eur J Cancer Clin Oncol 1989 (25):1203-1210

83 List AF, Greer JP, Cousaz JC et al: Non-Hodgkin's lymphoma of the gastrointestinal tract: an analysis of clinical and pathologic features affecting outcome. J Clin Oncol 1988 (6):1125-1133

84 Gobbi PG, Dionigi P, Barbieri F et al: The role of surgery in the multimodal treatment of primary gastric non-Hodgkin's lymphomas. A report of 76 cases and review of the literature. Cancer 1990 (65):2528-2536

85 Salles G, Herbrecht R, Tilly H et al: Aggressive primary gastrointestinal lymphomas. Review of 91 patients treated with the LNH-84 regimen. A study of the Groupe d'Etude des Lymphomes Agressifs. Amer J Med 1991 (90):77-84

86 Maor MH, Velasquez WS, Fuller LM, Silvermintz KB: Stomach conservation in stage IE and stage IIE gastric non-Hodgkin's lymphoma. J Clin Oncol 1990 (8):266-271

87 Haddy TB, Adde MA, Magrath IT: CNS involvement in small noncleaved-cell lymphoma: Is CNS disease per se a poor prognostic sign? J Clin Oncol 1991 (9):1973-1982

88 O'Sullivan MG, Whittle IR, Gregor A, Ironside JW: Increasing incidence of CNS primary lymphoma in South-East Scotland. Lancet 1991 (338):895-896

89 DeAngelis LM, Yahalom J, Thaler HT, Kher U: Combined modality therapy for primary CNS lymphoma. J Clin Oncol 1992 (10):635-643

90 Neuwelt EA, Goldman DL, Dahlborg SA: Primary CNS lymphoma treated with osmotic blood-brain barrier disruption - prolonged survival and preservation of cognitive function. J Clin Oncol 1991 (9): 1580-1590

91 Shibamoto Y, Tsutsui K, Dodo Y: Improved survival rate in primary intracranial lymphoma treated by high-dose radiation and systemic vincristine-doxorubicin-cyclophosphamide-prednisolone chemotherapy. Cancer 1990 (65):1907-1912

92 Blay JY, Lasset C, Carrie C et al: Multivariate analysis of prognostic factors in patients with non HIV-related primary cerebral lymphoma. A proposal for a prognostic scoring. Br J Cancer 1993 (67): 1136-1141

93 Armitage JO, Vose JM, Linder J et al: Clinical significance of immunophenotype in diffuse aggressive non-Hodgkin's lymphoma. J Clin Oncol 1989 (7):1783-1790

94 Cheng AL, Chen YC, Wang CH et al: Direct comparisons of peripheral T-cell lymphoma with diffuse B-cell lymphoma of comparable histological grades. Should peripheral T-cell lymphoma be considered separately? J Clin Oncol 1989 (7):725-731

95 Kwak LW, Wilson M, Weiss LM et al: Similar outcome of treatment of B-cell and T-cell diffuse large-cell lymphomas: The Stanford experience. J Clin Oncol 1991 (9):1426-1431

96 Coiffier B, Berger F, Bryon PA, Magaud JP: T-cell lymphomas: immunologic, histologic, clinical, and therapeutic analysis of 63 cases. J Clin Oncol 1988 (6):1584-1589

97 Horning SJ, Weis LM, Crabtree GS, Waruke RA: Clinical and phenotypic diversity of T cell lymphomas. Blood 1986 (67):1578-1582

98 Coiffier B, Brousse N, Peuchmaur M et al: Peripheral T-cell lymphomas have a worse prognosis than B-cell lymphomas: a prospective study of 361 immunophenotyped patients treated with the LNH-84 regimen. Ann Oncol 1990 (1):45-50

99 d'Amore F, Brincker H, Christensen BE: Non-Hodgkin's lymphoma in the elderly. A study of 602 patients aged 70 or older from a Danish population-based registry. Ann Oncol 1992 (3):379-386

100 Dumontet C, Anderson JR, Sebban C et al: Elderly non-Hodgkin lymphoma patients have comparable prognostic factors but a poorer outcome than younger patients. In: 11th American Society of Clinical Oncology Meeting. San Diego, CA 1992 (11):328 (abstract 1118)

101 Hoerni B, Sotto JJ, Eghbali H et al: Non-Hodgkin's malignant lymphomas in patients older than 80. 70 cases. Cancer 1988 (61):2057-2059

102 Danieu L, Wong G, Koziner B, Clarkson B: Predictive model for prognosis in advanced diffuse histiocytic lymphoma. Cancer Res 1986 (46):5372-5379

103 Velasquez WS, Jagannath S, Tucker SL et al: Risk classification as the basis for clinical staging of diffuse large-cell lymphoma derived from 10-year survival data. Blood 1989 (74):551-557

104 McMaster ML, Johnson DH, Greer JP et al: A brief duration combination chemotherapy for elderly patients with poor-prognosis non-Hodgkin's lymphoma. Cancer 1991 (67):1487-1492

105 O'Reilly SE, Klimo P, Connors JM: Low-dose ACOP-B and VABE - weekly chemotherapy for elderly patients with advanced-stage diffuse large-cell lymphoma. J Clin Oncol 1991 (9):741-747

106 Sonneveld P and Michiels JJ: Full dose chemotherapy in elderly patients with non-Hodgkin's lymphoma - a feasibility study using a mitoxantrone containing regimen. Br J Cancer 1990 (62):105-108

107 Tirelli U, Zagonel V, Errante D: A prospective study of a new combination chemotherapy regimen in patients older than 70 years with unfavorable non-Hodgkin's lymphoma. J Clin Oncol 1992 (10): 228-236

108 O'Connell MJ, Harrington DP, Earle JD et al: Prospectively randomized clinical trial of three intensive chemotherapy regimens for the treatment of advanced unfavorable histology non-Hodgkin's lymphoma. J Clin Oncol 1987 (5):1329-1339

109 Heinz R: Long-term follow-up of CHOP-treated non-Hodgkin lymphoma of high-grade malignancy. Blut 1990 (60):68-75

110 Banavali SD, Advani SH, Gopal R et al: Continuous cyclophosphamide, doxorubicin, vincristine, and prednisolone. A new, innovative protocol for diffuse aggressive lymphomas. Cancer 1990 (65): 1704-1710

111 Boyd DB, Coleman M, Papish SW et al: COPBLAM III: infusional combination chemotherapy for diffuse large-cell lymphoma. J Clin Oncol 1988 (6):425-433

112 Liang R, Chiu E, Chan TK et al: m-BACOD chemotherapy for intermediate-grade and high-grade non-Hodgkin's lymphoma. Cancer Chemother Pharmacol 1991 (28):135-138

113 Schneider AM, Straus DJ, Schluger AE et al: Treatment results with an aggressive chemotherapeutic regimen (MACOP-B) for intermediate-grade and some high-grade non-Hodgkin's lymphomas. J Clin Oncol 1990 (8):94-102

114 Weick JK, Dahlberg S, Fisher RI et al: Combination chemotherapy of intermediate-grade and high-grade non-Hodgkin's lymphoma with MACOP-B - A Southwest Oncology Group study. J Clin Oncol 1991 (9):748-753

115 Vitolo U, Bertini M, Brusamolino E: MACOP-B treatment in diffuse large-cell lymphoma: Identification of prognostic groups in an Italian multicenter study. J Clin Oncol 1992 (10):219-227

116 Miller TP, Dahlberg S, Weick JK et al: Unfavorable histologies of non-Hodgkin's lymphoma treated with ProMACE-CytaBOM: A groupwide Southwest

Oncology Group study. J Clin Oncol 1990 (8):1951-1958
117 Steinke B, Bross K, Reinold HM et al: Cyclic alternating chemotherapy of high-grade malignant non-Hodgkin lymphomas with VIM-Bleo and CHOP. Eur J Cancer 1992 (28):100-104
118 Fisher RI, DeVita VT, Hubbard SM et al: Diffuse aggressive lymphomas: Increased survival after alternating flexible sequences of ProMACE and MOPP chemotherapy. Ann Intern Med 1983 (98): 304-309
119 Coiffier B, Bryon PA, Berger F et al: Intensive and sequential combination chemotherapy for aggressive malignant lymphomas (Protocol LNH-80). J Clin Oncol 1986 (4):147-153

Mantle Cell Lymphoma. Clinical Features, Diagnosis, Biology, Treatment and Prognosis

Maria K. Angelopoulou, Flora N. Kontopidou and Gerassimos A. Pangalis

Leukaemia and Lymphoma Clinic, 1st Department of Internal Medicine, National and Kapodistrian University of Greece, School of Medicine, Laikon General Hospital, Athens 11527, Greece

Mantle cell lymphoma (MCL) has been described under the names of mantle zone lymphoma [1], intermediate lymphoma [2-5], centrocytic lymphoma [6,7] and diffuse small cleaved cell lymphoma [8]. It is a type of lymphoma that requires special attention because its histological diagnosis is not always easy to be made, particularly by unexperienced pathologists. Its clinical behaviour is usually aggressive and in a considerable percentage of cases (~25%) it may present with a leukaemic picture, mimicking other chronic lymphoproliferative disorders. Therefore its differential diagnosis from the latter is considered crucial, particularly for therapeutic purposes.

Clinical Features

MCL affects elderly patients (median age 60 years; rare below 30 years) and its male to female ratio is approximately 3:1 [9]. Its frequency among the non-Hodgkin's lymphomas varies from 2.5-4% in the United States to 6-9% in Europe [7,10-14]. Patients present with advanced stage disease (III and IV >80%), B symptoms (~40%), bulky tumour mass (~25%), rapid tumour growth (~50%) and poor performance status (≥20%) [10-16]. Lymphadenopathy is usually generalized (~90% of the patients) with splenomegaly in ~55%, hepatomegaly in ~35%, bone marrow involvement in 65-80%, blood involvement in 25-40%, gastrointestinal location in 10-30% and Waldeyer's ring involvement in 10-20% [10-16].

Histological Diagnosis

The criteria for establishing the histological diagnosis of MCL have been extensively discussed in the literature [4-11]. Recently, these criteria were reviewed by an expert pannel of pathologists during two workshops on MCL organized in Toronto (Canada) and Annecy (France) [17], and the histological diagnosis of the disease was formulated as shown in Table 1. Experts recognize two groups of MCL: the typical (tMCL) and the variant type (vMCL). In both categories emphasis is placed on the cell cytology and the growth pattern of the disease [17]. It is of interest that in tMCL the growth pattern indicates a category of diffuse histology without residual germinal centres (GC), while in vMCL the cytology indicates a category with a predominance of blastoid cells with lymphoblastic features [17].
From the morphological description it is evident that for a secure diagnosis of MCL further support of immunological and molecular markers is required [17].

Immunophenotype of MCL

For the immunophenotyping of MCL formalin-fixed material, frozen tissue, flow cytometry and cytospin preparations can be used. The most simple and efficient way is immunohistochemistry on formalin-fixed and paraffin-embedded material [8-10,18-25]. The available

Table 1. Histological consensus criteria for the diagnosis of mantle cell lymphoma+

Typical Form	Variant Form
Cytology	
Small to medium-sized cells Irregular or mixed irregular and round nuclei Fine condensed not clumped chromatin Small inconspicuous nucleoli Pale indistinct scant cytoplasm Centroblasts and immunoblasts absent or rare Mitotic rate usually low	Predominance of small to medium-sized round cells Abundant pale cytoplasm Mixture of small to medium-sized blastoid* cells Predominance of blastoid cells*
Growth Pattern	
Nodular with residual GC (mantle zone pattern) Nodular without residual GC and loosely structured FDC-meshwork Nodular without residual GC and tight FDC clusters (GC colonization or induction of tight FDC clusters) Diffuse with/without residual GC	Same features as in typical forms (nodular, mixed, diffuse)

+ Based on data analysed during the 1994 MCL Workshop, Annecy, France [17]
* Blastoid cells: cells with morphological features of lymphoblasts
GC: germinal centres; FDC: follicular dendritic cells

data from immunological studies on tMCL and vMCL are given in Table 2. Cells of tMCL are always CD5+, CD20++, CD10-, CD23-, CD25-, sIgM+D+ (strong expression) and *bcl*-2+, while cells of vMCL are CD20++, CD5+, CD10-/(+), CD23-/(+), and *bcl*-2+.

Table 2. Immunophenotype consensus criteria for the diagnosis of mantle cell lymphoma*,**

Typical Form	Variant Form
B-cell antigens+ (CD19, 20, 22, 45RA, 79A)	CD20++
CD20++	CD5±
CD5+	CD10-/(+)?
CD10-	CD23-/(+)
CD23-	sIgM and IgD high
CD25-	CD43±
sIgM and IgD high	Bcl-2+
λ or κ clonality	no FDC meshwork or FDC features as tMCL (more common)
CD11c/CD18-	
CD43+	
Bcl-2+	
FDC meshwork loosely organised	

* Atypical morphology requires typical immunology and *vice versa*
** Based on data presented during the 1994 MCL Workshop, Annecy, France [17]

These data are significant because immunophenotyping is the most important and reliable way of differentiating MCL from other forms of lymphoproliferative disease, either on tissue sections or in the blood, if this is involved (Tables 2 and 3). However, even with the best possible immunological support it may remain difficult in certain cases to establish an accurate diagnosis. In such cases the molecular biology of the tumour cells can be of help.

Molecular Biology

Of the molecular markers described to date the chromosomal aberration t(11;14) (q13;q32) is the most important, although not characteristic, for the diagnosis of MCL [9,26-28]. This translocation is very frequently found in MCL (see Table 4 by Dr Leroux) and therefore it may be used as a diagnostic marker [29]. The breakpoint of chromosome 11 is found in the region of the *bcl*-1 gene. Whether this could be used as a marker remains to be seen, although there is convincing evidence that it could [30-37].
The *bcl*-1/PRAD-1 oncogene is considered as one entity since it has been found to be juxtaposed to the Ig heavy-chain gene in the

Table 3. Immunophenotype of mantle cell lymphoma and its differential diagnosis from other lymphoproliferative diseases*

	Disease Entity								
Marker	MCL	B-CLL	PLL	SLL	LPL	MonoL	MALT	FL	LBL/ALL
sIg M ± D	strong	weak	strong	weak	weak	+	+	strong	
CD19,20	+	+	+	+	+	+	+	+	
CD5	+	+	-	+	-	-	-	-	
CD23	-	+	-	-	-	-	-	-	
CD25	-	+	-	-/+	-	-	NA	-	
CD22	+	+	+	+	+	+	+	+	
CD11α/18	-	-	+	-	+	-	NA		
CD38	-	-	-	-	+	-	NA	-	
CD10	-	-	-	-	-	-	-	+	+**

* Based on data presented during the 1993 Toronto Workshop on small mature B-cell lymphoid malignancies including MCL, and the 1994 Annecy MCL Workshop [17]
** Mainly for the differential diagnosis of the blastoid (lymphoblastoid) form from the lymphoblasts of LBL/ALL
MCL= mantle cell lymphoma; B-CLL=B-chronic lymphocytic leukaemia; PLL=prolymphocytic leukaemia; SLL=small lymphocytic lymphoma; LPL=lymphoplasmacytic lymphoma; MonoL=monocytoid lymphoma; MALT=mucus-associated lymphoid tissue lymphoma; FL=follicular lymphoma; LBL/ALL=lymphoblastic lymphoma/acute lymphoblastic leukaemia
NA: not available

t(11;14) chromosomal translocation. This gene is overexpressed in MCL, as has been shown by mRNA analysis, and this overexpression is considered characteristic of MCL. It is of interest that the CCND-1 nuclear protein (cyclin-D1) encoded by *bcl*-1/PRAD-1 is also overexpressed in MCL [36,38]. This nuclear protein is required for cell cycle progression to the G1 phase. Cyclin-D1 is inhibited by *p53* and *p16*. Cyclin-D1 is not expressed in other lymphoproliferative disorders including B-CLL, large cell lymphomas and myelomas. Interestingly, cyclin-D1 is not expressed in normal lymphoid tissue either.

Laboratory Features

Patients with MCL may present with a leukaemic picture (~25%). Cytologically the leukaemic cells may express all morphological variations described in histological material. Care should be taken not to make a rash diag-

Table 4. Chromosomal anomalities in MCL*. Data on 37 patients from the Grenoble Group

t(11;14) positive	29	
negative	8	
del (1) (p21 p32)	12	
t/del/7q	6	[5 among the 8 t(11;14) negative]
del/6q	10	[2 among the 8 t(11;14) negative]
-13/del13q	8	
-8/del/8q	9	[3 among the 8 t(11;14) negative]
t/del/9p	9	[2 among the 8 t(11;14) negative]
del 9q22	4	[2 among the 8 t(11;14) negative]
del 10q	4	
-17/del 17p	4	

* Data presented by Leroux et al. at the 1994 MCL Workshop, Annecy, France [17]

nosis of acute lymphoblastic leukaemia if the clinical picture of the patient is more consistent with MCL. In such cases the diagnosis should be confirmed by immunological and molecular studies. Anaemia (Hb <12g/dl) may be present in 20% of patients, thrombocytopenia (<100 x 10^9/l) in 10%, monoclonal gammopathy in <10%, high LDH level in ~30% and increased ß2-microglobulin levels in >50%. Hypergammaglobulinaemia and Coombs-positive haemolytic anaemia are rare.

Differential Diagnosis

The differential diagnosis of MCL from other lymphoproliferative disorders is important because a considerable number of diseases such as B-chronic lymphocytic/prolymphocytic leukaemia, follicular small cleaved or mixed cell lymphoma, lymphoplasmacytic lymphoma, monocytoid B-cell lymphoma, MALT lymphoma, and lymphoblastic lymphoma may be confused with MCL. The criteria for the differential diagnosis may be morphological, immunological or molecular. For the morphological criteria the picture described above (see Table 1) should be considered, including the parameters of mitotic figures (frequently increased in most forms of MCL), the growth fraction of the tumour as determined by Ki-67 antibody positivity (also increased in most cases of MCL), and the number and growth pattern of development (solid sheets) of blastoid cells, findings which are not frequent in the other forms of low grade B-cell proliferation. For the immunological criteria a pannel of monoclonal antibodies may be used either on paraffin or frozen sections when tissue material is available or in cell suspensions or cytospin preparations when a leukaemic picture is present. The data concerning the immunological profile of the various lymphoproliferative diseases compared to MCL are given in Tables 2 and 3. Support for the differential diagnosis of MCL from other lymphoid disorders may also derive from cytogenetic and molecular studies.

Prognostic Factors

Among the various parameters studied in relation to the prognosis of MCL, the age of the patient (>60 years), performance status (>2), the presence of more than one extranodal site of involvement, and increased serum LDH and ß2-microglobulin levels were found to be significant in univariate and multivariate analysis [12,16]. These parameters appear to be similar to those described for other forms of non-Hodgkin's lymphomas.

Treatment

The treatment of MCL varies according to published reports and institutional experience from the "watch-and-wait" policy to third-generation chemotherapy (ProMACE/MOPP) or megatherapy with peripheral stem cell support (PSCS) [17]. Monotherapy with oral alkylating agents (chlorambucil, cyclophosphamide) or administration of the newer purine analogues fludarabine or 2-chlorodeoxyadenosine are not effective [17]. Some groups believe that the anthracycline containing regimens (e.g. CHOP) give better results [17] while others do not share this view [39].

The overall complete remission (CR) rate varies from 20% to 50%, but these CRs are not durable and eventually all patients relapse. Therefore, some groups have started treatment with megatherapy and peripheral stem cell support in a small number of selected MCL patients. Of 5 patients treated in Lyon by professor Coiffier's group 2 achieved CR (36 months and 9 months) and 2 PR. Whether any of these patients will be cured remains to be seen.

Survival

The median survival of MCL patients varies from 30 to 40 months. Only a very small proportion survive at 5 years. The survival of complete responders is longer [17].

Comments

The histological diagnosis of MCL (particularly the variant form) may be difficult, even among expert morphologists. Therefore, in every case where the morphology is not convincing, tissue immunophenotyping and molecular biology are necessary to rule out entities that may mimic MCL on tissue sections. The ultimate goal in MCL, like in the other forms of aggressive lymphomas, is the achievement of complete remission. How this can be attained successfully remains to be seen. Younger patients (the minority of those affected) may be considered candidates for megatherapy and PSCS as upfront therapy; patients with limited disease may be treated aggressively from the start with third-generation combination chemotherapy. For the time being, however, MCL is considered an incurable disease with a poor prognosis. Novel treatments, including radiolabelled monoclonal antibodies, may be investigated in the near future in an attempt to change its dismal outcome.

REFERENCES

1 Weisenburger DD, Kim H, Rappaport H: Mantle-zone lymphoma. A follicular variant of intermediate lymphocytic lymphoma. Cancer 1982 (49):1429-1438

2 Berard CW: Reticuloendothelial system: an overview of neoplasia. In: Rebuck JW, Berard CW, Abell MR (eds) The Reticuloendothelial System. International Academy of Pathology Monograph No. 16. Williams and Wilkins, Baltimore 1975 pp 301-317

3 Jaffe ES, Braylan RC, Namba K, Frank MM, Berard CW: Functional markers: a new perspective on malignant lymphomas. Cancer Treat Rep 1977 (61): 1953-1962

4 Namba K, Jaffe ES, Braylan RC, Soban EJ, Berard CW: Alkaline phosphatase-positive malignant lymphoma. A subtype of B-cell lymphomas. Am J Clin Pathol 1977 (68):535-542

5 Weisenburger DD, Nathwani BN, Diamond LW et al: Malignant lymphoma, intermediate lymphocytic type. A clinicopathologic study of 42 cases. Cancer 1981 (48):1415-1425

6 Lennert K: Malignant lymphomas other than Hodgkin's disease. Springer-Verlag, Berlin 1978 pp 284-302

7 Swerdlow SH, Habeshaw JA, Murray LJ, Dhaliwal HS, Lister TA, Stansfeld AG: Centrocytic lymphoma. A distinct clinicopathologic and immunologic entity. A multiparameter study of 18 cases at diagnosis and relapse. Am J Pathol 1983 (113):181-197

8 Palutke M, Eisenberg L, Mirchandani I, Tabaczka P, Husain M: Malignant lymphoma of small cleaved lymphocytes of the follicular mantle zone. Blood 1982 (59):181-197

9 Weisenburger DD: Mantle cell lymphoma. In: Knowles DM (ed) Neoplastic Hematopathology. Williams and Wilkins, Baltimore 1992 pp 617-628

10 Lardelli P, Bookman MA, Sundeen J, Longo DL, Jaffe ES: Lymphocytic lymphoma of intermediate differentiation. Morphologic and immunophenotypic spectrum and clinical correlations. Am J Surg Pathol 1990 (14):752-763

11 Weisenburger DD, Duggan MJ, Perry DA, Sanger WG, Armitage JO: Non-Hodgkin's lymphomas of mantle-zone origin. In: Rosen PP, Fechner RE (eds) Pathology Annual. Appleton and Lange, East Norwalk 1990 pp 139-158

12 Brittinger G, Bartels H, Common H et al (Kiel Lymphoma Study Group): Clinical and prognostic relevance of the Kiel classification of non-Hodgkin's lymphomas. Results of a prospective multicenter study by the Kiel Lymphoma Study Group. Hematol Oncol 1984 (2):269-306

13 Richards MA, Hall PA, Gregory WM et al: Lymphoplasmacytoid and small cell centrocytic non-Hodgkin's lymphoma. A retrospective analysis from St. Bartholomew's Hospital, 1972-1986. Hematol Oncol 1989 (7):19-35

14 Barbone A, Poletti A, Manconi R et al: Intermediate lymphocytic lymphoma encompassing diffuse and mantle zone variants. A distinct entity among low-grade lymphomas? Eur J Clin Oncol 1989 (25):113-121

15 Duggan MJ, Weisenburger DD, Ye YL et al: Mantle zone lymphoma. A clinicopathologic study of 22 cases. Cancer 1990 (66):522-529

16 Bookman MA, Lardelli P, Jaffe ES, Duffey PL, Longo DL: Lymphocytic lymphoma of intermediate differentiation. Morphologic, immunophenotypic and prognostic factors. JNCI 1990 (82):742-748

17 Zucca E, Stain H, Coiffier B: European Lymphoma Task Force (ELTF): Report of the workshop on mantle cell lymphoma (MCL). Ann Oncol 1994 (5):507-511

18 Samoszk MK, Epstein AL, Said J, Lukes RJ, Nathwani BN: Sensitivity and specificity of immunostaining in the diagnosis of mantle zone lymphoma. Am J Clin Pathol 1986 (85):557-563

19 Stein H, Lennert K, Feller AC, Mason DY: Immunohistological analysis of human lymphoma: correlation of histological and immunological categories. Adv Cancer Res 1984 (67):67-147

20 Harris NL, Nadler LM, Bhan AK: Immunohistologic characterization of two malignant lymphomas of germinal center type (centroblastic/centrocytic and centrocytic) with monoclonal antibodies. Follicular and diffuse lymphomas of small-cleaved cell type are related but distinct entities. Am J Pathol 1984 (117):262-272

21 Van den Oord JJ, de Wolf-Peeters C, Pulford KAP, Mason DY, Desmet VJ: Mantle-zone lymphoma. Immuno and enzyme-histological studies on the cell of origin. Am J Surg Pathol 1986 (10):789-788

22 Strickler JG, Medeiros LJ, Copenhaver CM, Weiss LM, Weiss RA: Intermediate lymphocytic lymphoma. An immunophenotypic study with comparison to small lymphocytic lymphoma and diffuse small cleaved cell lymphoma. Hum Pathol 1988 (19):550-554

23 Abe M, Ono N, Nazawa Y, Hojo H, Wakasa H: A histogenesis of malignant lymphoma, small cleaved cell of the B cell type and intermediate lymphocytic lymphoma (mantle zone lymphoma). An immuno- and enzyme-histochemical study. Virch Archiv A Pathol Anat 1988 (413):205-213

24 Hollema H and Poppema S: Immunophenotypes of malignant lymphoma centroblastic-centrocytic and malignant lymphoma centrocytic. An immunohistologic study indicating derivation from different stages of B cell differentiation. Hum Pathol 1988 (19):1053-1059

25 Salter DM, Krajewski AS, Cunningham S: Activation and differentiation antigen expression on B-cell non-Hodgkin's lymphomas. J Pathol 1988 (154):209-222

26 Daibata M, Kubonishi I, Eguchi T, Yano S, Ohtsuki Y, Miyoshi I: The establishment of Epstein-Barr virus nuclear antigen-positive (SP-50B) and Epstein-Barr virus nuclear antigen-negative (SP-53) cells with t(11;14) (q13;q32) chromosome abnormality from an intermediate lymphocytic lymphoma. Cancer 1989 (64):1248-1253

27 Frizzera G, Masaharu S, Notohara K, Konishi T: t(11;14)(q13;q32) in B cell lymphomas (intermediately differentiated and follicular). A report of four cases. Am J Clin Pathol 1991 (95):684-691

28 Vandenberghe E, de Wolfe-Peeters C, Van den Oord J et al: Translocation (11;14): a cytogenetic anomaly associated with B-cell lymphomas of non-

follicle center cell lineage. J Pathol 1991 (163):13-18
29 Leroux D, Le Marc Hadour F, Gressin R et al: Non-Hodgkin's lymphomas with t(11;14) (q13;q32): a subset of mantle zone/intermediate lymphocytic lymphoma? Br J Haematol 1991 (77):346-353
30 Raffeld M, Jaffe ES: bcl-1 t(11;14) and mantle cell derived lymphomas. Blood 1991 (78):259-263
31 Williams ME, Meeker TC, Swerdlow SH: Rearrangements of chromosome 11 bcl-1 locus in centrocytic lymphomas: Analysis with multiple breakpoint probes. Blood 1991 (78):493-498
32 Brito-Bapapulle Y, Ellis J, Matutes E, Oscier D, Khokhnar T, MacLennan K, Catovsky D: Chromosome translocation t(11;14) (q13;q32) in chronic lymphoid disorders. Genes, Chromosomes and Cancer 1994 (in press)
33 Ince C, Blick M, Lee M et al: Bcl-1 gene rearrangements in B cell lymphoma. Leukemia 1988 (2):343-346
34 Williams ME, Westermann CD, Swerdlow SH: Genotypic characterization of centrocytic lymphoma: frequent rearrangement of the chromosome 11 bcl-1 locus. Blood 1990 (76):1387-1391
35 Vanderberghe E, De Wolf-Peeters C, Van den Oord J et al: Translocation (11;14): a cytogenetic anomaly associated with B-cell lymphomas of non-follicle centre cell lineage. J Pathol 1991 (163):13-18
36 Motokura T, Bloom T, Kim HG et al: A novel cyclin encoded by a bcl-1 linked candidate oncogene. Nature 1991 (350):512-515
37 Rimokh R, Berger F, Delsol G et al: Rearrangement and overexpression of the Bcl-1/PRAD-1 gene in intermediate lymphocytic lymphomas and in t(11q13) bearing leukemias. Blood 1993 (81):3063-3067
38 Withers DA, Harvey RC, Faust JB, Melny KO, Carey K, Meeker TC: Characterization of a candidate bcl-1 gene. Mol Cell Biol 1991 (11):4846-4853
39 Meusers P, Engelhard M, Martels H et al: Multicentre randomized therapeutic trial for advanced centrocytic lymphoma. Anthracycline does not improve prognosis. Hematol Oncol 1989 (7):365-380

Fludarabine Monophosphate, an Effective New Agent in Leukaemias and Lymphomas

Gerassimos A. Pangalis [1], Maria K. Angelopoulou [1], Christos Poziopoulos [1], Aaron Polliack [2] and Shamuel Gillis [2]

1 Lymphoma Clinic, 1st Department of Internal Medicine, National and Kapodistrian University of Greece, School of Medicine, Laikon General Hospital, Athens 11527, Greece
2 Lymphoma-Leukaemia Unit, Department of Haematology, Hadassah University Hospital, Jerusalem, Israel

Chronic lymphocytic leukaemia and low-grade non-Hodgkin's lymphomas are diseases for which until recently no treatment leading to long lasting complete remission or cure existed. Fludarabine monophosphate, a purine analogue, was recently introduced into clinical trials for chronic lymphocytic leukaemia and low-grade non-Hodgkin's lymphomas and found to be very effective. In this report we review the available data relating to fludarabine monophosphate and present our experience with fludarabine administration in refractory B-chronic lymphocytic leukaemia and low-grade lymphocytic lymphoma in Athens and Jerusalem.

Pharmacodynamics and Pharmacokinetics

After the success of cytarabine (ara-C), efforts have been made to identify other purine analogues with antineoplastic activity. The first of these nucleosides was ara-A which is inactivated by adenosine deaminase and therefore its biovailability is limited [1]. After some structural modifications, the soluble and adenosine deaminase-resistant fluorinated purine analogue F-ara-A monophosphate (fludarabine) was developed by Montgomery and Hewson [2]. Its structural formula (9-B-D-arabinosyl-2-fluoroadenine) is presented in Figure 1.

Mechanism of Action

After 5 minutes of systemic administration fludarabine monophosphate is dephosphorylated to F-ara-A [3] phosphorylation to obtain cytotoxic activity. The enzyme responsible for this phosphorylation is intracellular deoxycytidine kinase [4,5], although adenosine kinase has been proposed as an alternative [6]. F-ara-A is thus converted to its active form F-ara-ATP.
Many models of the mechanisms of action have been proposed (Table 1). However, the major mechanism is inhibition of DNA synthesis in two ways: 1) F-ara-ATP directly competes with dATP for utilization by DNA polymerases [7], and 2) F-ara-ATP is incorporated into DNA [7,8], resulting in disturbance of the DNA replication machinery. Thus whenever F-ara-ATP is incorporated into DNA, DNA strand elongation is terminated at the incorporated sites. F-ara ATP acts as a DNA chain termination [7], may cause deletion of genetic material and may be responsible for mutagenicity and cytoxicity [9].

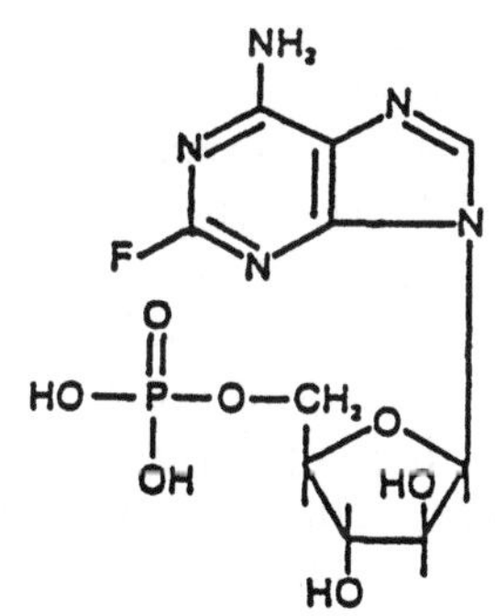

Fig. 1. Structural formula of fludarabine

Table 1. Mechanisms of action of fludarabine

1. Inhibition of DNA synthesis
   a. Competition with dATP for utilization by DNA polymerases
   b. Incorporation into DNA
2. Termination of RNA synthesis
3. Inhibition of DNA repair
4. Depletion of NAD pools
5. Inhibition of several enzymes: DNA polymerases, DNA primase, ribonucleoside diphosphate reductase, DNA ligase, topoisomerase II and deoxycytidine kinase

Clinical trials have demonstrated the therapeutic efficacy of fludarabine in B-chronic lymphocytic leukaemia (B-CLL). It is known that peripheral lymphocytes are not actively replicating so that inhibition of DNA synthesis may not be the major mechanism of fludarabine action in B-CLL and related disorders. Termination of RNA synthesis may in fact contribute to the cytotoxic effect of fludarabine in these malignancies. In this respect it has been shown that F-ara-ATP is also incorporated into RNA [8,10] - although not as strongly as into DNA - and might thereby interfere with the termination of protein translation [11]. Two other mechanisms have been postulated especially for lymphoid tissues. The first is inhibition of DNA repair [12]. Lymphoid tissues have the lowest levels of deoxynucleotide and the highest activity of deoxycytidine kinase whereas in other tissues the reverse is observed [13,14]. DNA repair directly correlates with the level of deoxynucleotide. The second possible mechanism is that F-ara-ATP may induce increased poly (ADP) ribosylation and depletion of NAD pools, which may lead to decreased cellular anergy and thereby to cell death [15].

Fludarabine also appears to inhibit the activity of several enzymes which interfere with DNA and RNA synthesis such as DNA polymerases and DNA primase and ribonucleoside diphosphate reductase [16]. Other possible enzyme targets are DNA ligase and topoisomerase II [17]. The above-mentioned increased deoxycytidine kinase activity in lymphoid tissues, which is of great importance for fludarabine-induced toxicity, may be due to a direct effect on the enzyme itself [18]. Recent studies by Robertson and Plunkett have shown that there is enhanced apoptosis in B-CLL cells when fludarabine is used. Thus cell death due to apoptosis is yet another possible mechanism for the effect of fludarabine in CLL [18].

Fludarabine acts as a modulator of the metabolism of ara-C and other purine analogues such as 2-CdA. It has been shown that there is a two-fold increase in the rate of intracellular ara-CTP accumulation if fludarabine is administered before incubation of human lymphocytes with ara-C [19]. It has been demonstrated that *in vitro* synergy takes place between fludarabine and other chemotherapeutic agents such as gallium nitrate, cytarabine plus cisplatinum and mitoxanthrone. Pre-exposure of human leukaemic cells to fludarabine, followed by cytarabine, resulted in a 2.2 times higher accumulation of cytarabine triphosphate. The simultaneous incubation of B-CLL cells with fludarabine and mitoxanthrone resulted in additive cytotoxicity. Dose and schedule-dependent radiosensitization has also been proved with fludarabine administered 1 hour before irradiation.

Competitive intracellular interaction takes place between the natural and fraudulent nucleotides [4]. Decrease of the cellular pools of dATP is crucial for the development of combination chemotherapy regimens containing fludarabine [20].

Effects of Fludarabine on Healthy Cells

Treatment with fludarabine results in reversible lymphocytopenia [22]. In fact, B cell counts increased after two treatment cycles. Lymphocytopenia developed rapidly within 6 days and was generally reversible within 3 weeks. A decrease of only 18% was observed in absolute neutrophil counts. A relation between white blood cell toxicity and fludarabine dosage has not been demonstrated. Potential mechanisms of fludarabine toxicity in leukaemic lymphocytes versus healthy tissues are more efficient intracellular transport and enhanced phosphorylation of F-ara-A [23]. The effect on CD4+ cells is quite strong and results in relatively long lasting immunosuppression with a tendency to infections which is troublesome [23].

Pharmacokinetics and Metabolism

As already mentioned, fludarabine is rapidly dephosphorylated to F-ara-A after intravenous infusion [3]. All pharmacokinetic data are therefore related to F-ara-A rather than to fludarabine itself. Fludarabine shows linear pharmacokinetics [3,24] and accumulation after multiple dose administration has not been demonstrated. High performance liquid chromatography separation and fluorescence detection for F-ara-A have been used for these studies [25] and a biphasic decline in plasma F-ara-A concentration has been described with the distribution half-lives ranging between 0.9 and 1.7 hours [24].

Studies indicate that fludarabine enters the peripheral leukaemic blood cells as well as leukaemic infiltrated bone marrow, whereas the F-ara-ATP concentration in normal marrow is significantly lower [26]. As regards the elimination of intracellular F-ara-ATP, a single-phase elimination has been reported, its rate being independent of the dose. Terminal elimination half-lives range between 6.9 and 12.4 hours [24,26].

The clearance of F-ara-A is strongly related to serum creatinine levels ($p=0.029$), indicating the importance of renal excretion of the drug. The total body clearance of F-ara-A is significantly decreased in patients with renal failure (serum creatinine >15 mg/l, BUN >250 mg/l, creatinine clearance <4.2 l/h) [27]. It has also been noted that neutropenia directly correlates with fludarabine clearance <3l/h in patients receiving the drug [25]. The bioavailability of F-ara-A after oral administration is quite acceptable with an intracellular exposure of 57% when compared with the intravenous route [28].

Dosage and Route of Administration

Fludarabine is administered intravenously at a dose of 25-30 mg/m^2 in a 30-minute infusion on days 1-5, repeated every 4 to 5 weeks. This dose schedule was found to be effective for CLL and LGNHL [29]. The optimal treatment duration for these diseases has not been established and it appears that 6 cycles usually result in a maximum response, while administration of 3 additional cycles is recommended for responding patients. Other treatment schedules have also been tried, including a weekly low-dose schedule of 30 mg/m^2 once a week [30] or 30 mg/m^2 for 3 days every 4 weeks [31].

Therapeutic Results

Fludarabine has been administered in several low-grade lymphoproliferative malignancies including chronic lymphocytic leukaemia (B or T), prolymphocytic leukaemia (B or T), hairy cell leukaemia, low-grade non-Hodgkin's lymphomas, Waldenström's macroglobulinaemia, mycosis fungoides and also in acute myelogenous leukaemia [29]. Fludarabine has been shown to be effective in these diseases but not equally in all of them.

Chronic Lymphocytic Leukaemia

The median survival of B-chronic lymphocytic leukaemia (B-CLL) patients who require treatment because of advanced stage or presence of risk factors, remains the same (approx. 48 months) [32]. All CLL patients will eventually become refractory to conventional therapy and will therefore need alternative treatment. Fludarabine was found to be effective in such patients. Review of the literature indicates that fludarabine monophosphate is highly effective in B-CLL, with a response rate of >50% in refractory cases [13,14,33-41] (Table 2). Similar or even better results were produced when the drug was given to untreated patients [38]. The addition of prednisone to fludarabine has not altered the results in CLL patients [23] and there is no justification for its use. As a matter of fact, listeriosis is a much more frequent complication in CLL patients when prednisone is added to fludarabine [23]. In this study logistic regression analysis selected 4 factors that were significantly associated with a worse response, namely Rai stage 3 and 4 disease, prior therapy, older age and low albumin levels. Using this regression equation once can derive data on the probability of response based on these 4 characteristics. When this equation/model was applied to CLL patients various outcomes could be predicted. In the

Table 2. Studies of fludarabine in patients with chronic lymphocytic leukaemias*

Reference	CLL subtype/ No. pts	Fludarabine dosage [a] (mg/m²/day)	Clinical response (%) CR	nPR	PR	Duration of response (months)
Fenchel et al. 1991 [33]	B/11 T/1	25	0 (0)	NA	6 (50)	> 3-14
Grever et al. 1988 [14]	NR/32	20	1 (3)	NA	3 (9)	CR >12, PR 5-8
Hiddeman et al. 1991 [34]	B/20	25	4 (25)	NA	7 (30)	
Johnson et al. 1993 [35]	NR/14	25	3 (12)			
Kantarjian et al. 1991 [36]	PLL/13 CLL-Pro/4	30 [b]	3 (18)	NA	3 (18)	>5 - >23
Keating et al. 1989 [37]	B/68	25-30	9 (13)	11 (16)	19 (28)	CR 21, PR 43
Knauf et al. 1992 [38]	B/9	25	1 (11)	NA	2 (22)	
O'Brien et al. 1992 [39]	B/95 [c] B/169	30 [d]	30 (32) 12 (7)	32 (34) 26 (15)	19 (20) 14 (8)	CR >22, PR 26 CR >28, PR 21
Puccio et al. 1991 [40]	B/40	20 mg/m² + 30 [e]	0 (0)	1 (2)	21 (50)	1-24
Pangalis et al. (1995) [41]	B/20	25	7 (33)	0	5 (25)	> 5-28

[a] Unless otherwise specified, fludarabine was administered daily for 5 days repeated every 4 weeks
[b] Five of 17 patients received prednisone 60 mg/m²/day for 5 days every 4 weeks simultaneously with fludarabine
[c] Previously untreated patients
[d] Patients received prednosine 30 mg/m²/day for 5 days every 4 weeks simultaneously with fludarabine
[e] Fludarabine administered as a 20 mg/m² intravenous bolus followed by a 30 mg/m²/day continuous infusion for 48 hours

Abbreviations: CLL = chronic lymphocytic leukaemia; CLL-Pro = prolymphocytoid variant of leukaemia; PLL = prolymphocytic leukaemia; CR = complete response; NA = category of response not applied in this study; PR = partial response; nPR = nodular partial response; NR = not reported

* Modified from Ross et al. [29]

group which had 3 or more unfavourable factors the response rate was only 22%.

At the Lymphoma Unit in Athens, we have had the opportunity of using fludarabine monophosphate to treat 20 B-CLL patients refractory to conventional chemotherapy. Fourteen were males and 6 females, with a median age of 38 years (range 44-70); 8 were International Stage B and 12 Stage C; all had been heavily pretreated with chlorambucil, prednisone, COP, mini-CHOP and irradiation, with a mean disease duration prior to fludarabine administration of 49 months (range 7-180).

Fludarabine was given at a dose of 25 mg/m² daily intravenously as a 30-min infusion for 5 consecutive days, repeated every month. The induction phase was scheduled for 6 months and when a response occurred treatment was continued for up to 12 months. All patients underwent clinical and laboratory investigation at monthly intervals or more frequently if necessary. Complete restaging of the responding patients including bone marrow aspiration and biopsy was performed at 6 and 12 months.

For the interpretation of response the criteria introduced by the IWCLL were used [42]. Our patients were classified into complete responders (CR), partial responders (PR), stable disease (SD) and progressive disease (PD). Based on these criteria 7 patients (33%) entered CR, 5 (25%) PR, 3 (15%) had SD and 5 (25%) PD (Table 2). Of the 7 CRs 5 were males and 2 females with a median age of 60 years (range 55-68); 3 had stage B and 4

Table 3. Studies of fludarabine in patients with non-Hodgkin's lymphoma*

Reference	Number of evaluable pts	Fludarabine dosage [a] (mg/m²/day)	Clinical response (%) CR	PR	Duration of response (months)
Hochster et al. 1992 [48]	60	18	9 (15)	9 (15)	
Leiby et al. 1987 [49]	25	20 mg/m² + 30 [b]	1 (4)	7 (28)	CR >9, PR 2-20
Redman et al. 1992 [50]	60 [c]	20-30	5 (8)	18 (30)	CR 8 - >27
Whelan et al. 1991 [51]	34	25	6 (18)	7 (20)	

a Unless otherwise indicated fludarabine was administered daily for 5 days, repeated every 4 weeks
b Fludarabine administered as an intravenous loading dose followed by a continuous infusion for 48 hours
c This study included 76 patients, 16 of whom had transformed lymphoma, mycosis fungoides, or Hodgkin's disease and are not included in this table
Abbreviations: CR = complete response; PR = partial response
* modified from Ross et al. [29]

stage C disease; their median disease duration prior to fludarabine was 47 months (24-180); the mean number of fludarabine cycles necessary to achieve CR was 3 (2-5) and all patients but one tolerated treatment fairly well. Among the CRs one patient died due to a severe hypersensitivity reaction with Stevens-Johnson syndrome. All complete responders relapsed subsequent to discontinuation of fludarabine therapy. Three of them remained leukopenic in spite of the fact that their disease reappeared with mild lymphadenopathy and splenomegaly. Because of the leukopenia fludarabine was administered every 3-4 months and the disease was very well controlled in this manner, the patients enjoying a very good PR. In all CRs a monoclonal CD5-positive blood lymphocytic population and residual bone marrow disease were present. Toxicity was mainly related to infection, with the exception of one patient who died due to the Stevens-Johnson syndrome. In 8 patients (40%) infections developed, mainly pulmonary, which required hospitalization [41].

Low-Grade Non-Hodgkin's Lymphomas

Treatment of low-grade non-Hodgkin's lymphomas (LGNHL), be it with a single modality, first-generation combination or aggressive chemotherapy, rarely changes the natural history of the disease, particularly when advanced disease is present at diagnosis [44-46]. Therefore in most cases salvage therapy is needed [47].

Fludarabine is considered as an effective drug for the treatment of LGNHL, producing responses (CR+PR) in about 30-40% of previously treated patients [48-51] (Table 3). Pigaditou and Lister recently reported response rates (CR+PR) of 45% (10/45) for previously treated patients, 45% (9/20) for patients with minimal residual disease and 69% (11/16) for newly diagnosed LGNHL patients [52].

Jerusalem experience - 24 patients with CLL and lymphocytic lymphoma (Tables 4a-4c)

Twenty-four patients were entered into this study and their characteristics are listed in Table 4a. There were 18 male and 6 female patients with a mean age of 52.2 years (range 26-71). All these patients had been heavily treated previously; 6 of them (25%) had received prior radiation therapy. All patients had advanced disease refractory to previous treatment and 10 of the LGL cases were in a leukaemic phase.

Patients were treated with 25 mg/m² of fludarabine, administered by slow intravenous infusion daily for 5 days every 28 days. The 24 patients received a total of 122 5-day cycles of fludarabine and the mean number of cycles received was 5.1 (range 1-9).

Objective responses were observed in 14 patients (58%) - 4 with CLL (40%) and 10 with LGL (71%). Four patients (17%) (1 with CLL

Table 4a. Patients' characteristics - Jerusalem cases

	No. pts.	%	
Sex			
Male	18	75	
Female	6	25	
Median age, years (range)			52.2 (26-71)
Median disease duration, years (range)			4.5 (0.5-13)
Prior chemotherapy			
1 regimen	5	21	
2 regimens	11	46	
3 regimens or more	8	33	
Prior radiotherapy	6	25	
Stage of CLL (Rai)			
Progressive stage 2	4	40	
stage 3	2	20	
stage 4	4	40	
Stage of LGL			
stage 4	14	100	
leukaemic phase	10	71	

and 3 with LGL) entered complete remission. Two relapsed after 13 and 25 months while another 2 are still in CR 23 and 25 months after treatment. One also underwent autologous bone marrow transplantation (ABMT). Ten patients (42%) (3 with CLL and 7 with LGL) had partial responses lasting a mean of 9.7 months (range 3-30 months) while the other 10 patients (42%) had progressive disease while receiving fludarabine therapy (Tables 4b and 4c).

Of the 10 patients with PR, 4 are alive a mean of 21.5 months (range 12-29 months) following termination of fludarabine therapy. One young 24-year-old CLL patient successfully underwent allogeneic bone marrow transplantation and currently has no evidence of CLL 13 months after BMT.

Only one of the 10 patients whose disease progressed while receiving fludarabine is still alive 12 months after cessation of therapy. The other 9 all died within 6 months of disease progression on fludarabine. In general the treatment was well tolerated. Patients were admitted to hospital with fever following 9 of the 122 courses (7.4%); they all rapidly recovered. Four patients developed Herpes zoster infections, but there were no cases of acute neurological toxicity. One patient developed listeriosis one year after receiving 5 courses of fludarabine and this was the only instance of the complication so frequently described by others [23].

In conclusion, our results are similar to those reported in larger series. Four patients (17%) in this heavily pretreated group achieved a complete remission. One of them underwent successful ABMT while two others have had their remission marrow cryopreserved and are candidates for myeloablative chemotherapy and subsequent ABMT if their disease progresses. The 10 patients who had partial responses lasting up to 30 months showed a marked improvement in their clinical status and in their quality of life. These responses are highly significant in patients with advanced heavily treated resistant disease.

The toxicity of the drug was relatively low and patients tolerated the treatment well. In particular there were no cases of acute neurological toxicity, which has been reported even at the relatively low doses used recently. Among our patients there was only one case of listeriosis, which occurred long after cessation of fludarabine treatment and while the patient was receiving an alternative regimen including mitoxanthrone, vinblastine, prednisone and etoposide. Listeriosis has been reported in up to

Table 4b. Results in 14 low-grade lymphoma patients (Jerusalem)

Complete remission	3	(21%)
Partial remission	7	(50%)
Stable disease	2	(14%)
Progression	2	(14%)
Mean duration of response		
CR	24+ months	(23+ - 25+)
PR	10+ months	(3 - 30+)

Table 4c. Results in 10 CLL patients (Jerusalem)

Complete remission	1	Response rate	40%
Partial remission	3		
Stable disease	3	Failure rate	60%
Progressive disease	3		
Mean duration of response			
CR	13 months		
PR	8 months (5-11)		

1.7% of patients receiving both fludarabine and prednisone but only rarely in patients like ours who received fludarabine alone.

Waldenström's macroglobulinaemia (WM) resistant to treatment also responds to fludarabine administration with a response rate of 45% (5/11) including a >50% decrease in tumour load and serum IgM levels [53]. According to updated results from Houston, Texas, of all cases of lymphoma, the best results with fludarabine have been achieved in this disorder [54]. Recently 68 patients with WM were treated with either fludarabine or 2-chlorodeoxyadenosine (2-CdA) with excellent results. Overall, 93% of previously treated patients, 93% of relapsing patients off-therapy and 48% of primary refractory patients responded, with only a few late relapses [54].

Mycosis Fungoides

Mycosis fungoides (MF) is a chronic T-cell malignancy of the skin which was also found to respond to fludarabine monophosphate. Von Hoff et al. reported a response rate (CR+PR) of 19% (6/31) in MF patients [55] while Foss et al. observed that this response was much better when the drug was combined with interferon-α (46%) [56].

Hairy Cell Leukaemia

Also in hairy cell leukaemia (HCL) patients resistant to conventional therapies a response to fludarabine has been reported [36,57]. Of course HCL is now effectively treated with interferon-α, deoxycoformycin and 2-chlorodeoxyadenosine, so there is no place for fludarabine in the near future.

Acute Leukaemias

Fludarabine monotherapy in acute leukaemias failed to produce complete remission in phase I/II trials [58]. Subsequent studies indicated a synergistic action of fludarabine with cytarabine. In these studies infusion of fludarabine 4 hours prior to cytarabine administration increased the rate of cytarabine triphosphate accumulation in acute myelogenous leukaemia (AML) cells by 1.8 to 2.2 fold [59]. Some reports in the literature indicate responses (12 out of 36) in relapsed or refractory AML after administration of fludarabine (30 mg/m^2/day) with cytarabine (1 g/m^2/day) 4 hours later for 5 days and cytarabine alone on day 6. However, this combination needs further investigation [60].

Non-Haematological Malignancies

After extensive studies performed in several non-haematopoietic malignancies, fludarabine is considered virtually inactive against solid tumours [29].

Toxicity

The major adverse effect of fludarabine is myelosuppression. This was severe even with the 25 mg/m^2/d for 5 days schedule repeated every 4 weeks. Severe neutropenia (<.5x10^9/l) was observed in 59% of the patients and a haemoglobin and platelet decrease from the baseline of 60% and 55%, respec-

Table 5. Incidence of non-haematological side-effects in 101 chronic lymphocytic leukaemia patients treated with fludarabine

Side-effect	%
Fever	60
Nausea/vomiting	36
Infection	33
Pain	20
Pneumonia	16
Diarrhoea	15
Rash	15

Modified from [29]

tively. This suppression appeared not to be cumulative in B-CLL [13,37], although it was reported to be so in LGNHL [50]. A depletion of CD4+ lymphocytes leading to a high incidence of infections is a frequent finding [61-63]. The CD4+ lymphocyte depletion phenomenon is further enhanced by simultaneous administration of prednisone [23,64]. The incidence of non-haematological toxicity of fludarabine is given in Table 5. Fever, nausea, vomiting and infections are the most frequent side-effects while interstitial pneumonitis consistent with drug-induced lung injury [65-67], tumour lysis syndrome [68] and severe autoimmune haemolytic anaemia [69,70] have also been reported. Severe neurological complications with CNS demyelination have been reported in patients receiving high-dose fludarabine >90 mg/m^2/day for 5 days [71], but this is extremely rare in patients receiving the 25 mg/m^2/day for 5 days schedule [48,72].

Conclusions

Fludarabine monophosphate is a new purine analogue derivative which is very active in both untreated and pretreated CLL and LGNHL patients. Efficacy has also been observed in hairy cell leukaemia, mycosis fungoides and acute myelogenous leukaemia. In the latter disease combination with cytarabine appears promising. At a dose of 25 mg/m^2/day for 5 days the drug is well tolerated and its major toxicity affects the bone marrow with varying degrees of reversible myelosuppression. CD4+ lymphocyte depletion has been documented and side-effects require further investigation. Non-haematological adverse events such as fever, nausea, vomiting and infection occur but are generally well controlled with supportive therapy.

REFERENCES

1 Le Page GA, Khalil A, Guttleib JA: Studies of 9-B-D-arabinofuranosyl adenine in man. Drug Metab Dispos 1973 (1):756-759
2 Montgomery JA and Hewson K: Synthesis of potential anticancer agents: Part XX - 2 - Fluoropurines. J Am Chem Soc 1960 (82):463-468
3 Hersh MR, Kuhn JG, Phillips JL, Clark G, Ludden TM, Von Hoff DD: Pharmacokinetic study of fludarabine phosphate (NSC 312887). Cancer Chemother Pharmacol 1986 (17):277-280
4 Tseng WC, Derse D, Cheng YC, Brockman RW, Benett LL Jr: In vitro activity of 9-B-D-arabinofuranose-2-fluoroadenine and the biochemical actions of its triphosphate on DNA polymerase and ribonuclease reductase from HeLa cells. Mol Pharmacol 1982 (21):474-479
5 Gandhi V and Plunkett W: Interaction of arabinosyl nucleotides in K562 human leukemia cells. Biochem Pharmacol 1989 (38):3551-3558
6 Chang CH, Brockman RW, Benett LL Jr: Adenosine kinase from L1210 cells: Purification and some properties of the enzyme. J Biol Chem 1980 (255): 2366-2371
7 Hang P, Chubb S, Plunkett W: Termination of DNA synthesis by 9-B-D-arabinofuranosyl-2-fluoroadenine. A mechanism for cytotoxicity. J Biol Chem 1990 (265):16617-16625
8 Spriggs D, Robbins G, Mitchell T, Kufe D: Incorporation of 9-B-D-arabinofuranosyl-2-fluoroadenine into HL-60 cellular RNA and DNA. Biochem Pharmacol 1986 (35):247-252
9 Huang P, Siciliano MS, Plunkett W: Gene deletion, a mechanism of induced mutation by arabinosyl nucleotides. Mutat Res 1989 (210):291-301
10 Plunkett W and Chubb S: Toxicity, metabolism and incorporation into DNA and RNA of arabinosyl-2-fluoroadenine (F-ara-A). Proc Am Assoc Cancer Res 1985 (26):19
11 Huang P and Plunkett W: Preferential incorporation of arabinosyl-2-fluoroadenine into poly(A+) RNA and in inhibitory effects on transcription and transplantation. Proc Am Assoc Cancer Res 1986 (27):21
12 Durhan JP and Ives DH: Deoxycytidine kinase. Part I. Distribution in normal and neoplastic tissues and interrelationships of deoxycytidine and 1-B-D arabinofuranosyl etosine phosphorylation. Mol Pharmacol 1969 (5):358-375
13 Keating MJ, Kantarjian H, Talpaz M, Redman J, Koller C: Fludarabine: A new agent with major activity against chronic lymphocytic leukemia. Blood 1989 (74):19-25
14 Grever MR, Kopecky KJ, Coltman CA, Files JC, Greenberg VR: Fludarabine monophosphate: A potentially useful agent in chronic lymphocytic leukemia. Nouv Rev Fr Hematol 1988 (30):457-459
15 Brager PM and Grever MR: 9-B-D-arabinofuranosyl-2-fluoroadenine reduced NAD in normal lymphocytes and neoplastic cells in CLL. Proc Am Assoc Cancer Res 1986 (27):21
16 Parker WB, Bapat AR, Shen JX, Townsend AJ, Cheng YC: Interaction of 2-halogenated dATP analogs (F, Cl and Br) with human DNA polymerases. DNA primase and ribonucleotide reductase. Mol Pharmacol 1988 (34):485-491
17 Lin SY, Hwang BD, Liu ZC, Cheng YC: Interaction of several nucleoside triphosphate analogues and 10-hydroxycamptothecin with human DNA topoisomerases. Cancer Res 1989 (49):1366-1370
18 Robertson LE and Plunkett W: Apoptotic cell death in chronic lymphocytic leukemia. Leukemia and Lymphoma 1993 (11 suppl 2):71-74
19 Gandhi V, Nowak B, Keating MJ, Plunkett W: Modulation of arabinosylcytosine metabolism by arabinosyl-2-fluoroadenine in lymphocytes from patients with chronic lymphocytic leukemia: Implications for combination therapy. Blood 1989 (74): 2070-2075
20 Plunkett W, Huang P, Gandhi V: Metabolism and action of fludarabine phosphate. Sem Oncol 1990 (5 suppl 8):3-17
21 Brockman RW, Cheng YC, Schobel FM Jr, Montgomery JA: Metabolism and chemotherapeutic activity of 9-B-D-arabinofuranosyl-2-fluoroadenine against murine leukemia L1210 and evidence for its phosphorylation by deoxycytidine kinase. Cancer Res 1980 (40):3610-3615
22 Boldt DH, Von Hoff DD, Kuhn JC, Hersh M: Effects on human peripheral lymphocytes of in vivo administration of 9-B-D-arabinofuranosyl-2-fluoroadenine-5-monophosphate (NSC 312887), a new purine antimetabolite. Cancer Res 1984 (44):4661-4666
23 O'Brien S, Kantarjian H, Beran M et al: Results of fludarabine and prednisone therapy in 264 patients with CLL and multivariate analysis derived prognostic model for response to treatment. Blood 1993 (82):1695-1700
24 Avramis VI, Champagne J, Sato J et al: Pharmacology of fludarabine phosphate after a phase I/II trial by a loading bolus and continuous infusion in pediatric patients. Cancer Res 1990 (50):7226-7231
25 Kemena A, Fernandez M, Bauman J, Keating M, Plunkett HW: A sensitive fluorescence assay for quantitation of fludarabine and metabolites in biological fluids. Clin Chim Acta 1991 (200):95-106
26 Danhauser L, Plunkett W, Keating M, Cabanillas F: 9-B-D-arabinofuranosyl-2-fluoroadenine-5-monophosphate pharmacokinetics in plasma and tumor cells of patients with relapsed leukemia and lymphoma. Cancer Chemother Pharmacol 1986 (18): 145-152
27 Malpeus L, Grever MR, Stanbus AC, Young D: Pharmacokinetics of 2-F-ara-A in cancer patients during the phase I clinical investigation of fludarabine phospate. Sem Oncol 1990 (17 suppl 8):18-32
28 Kemena A, Keating M, Plunkett W: Oral bioavailability of plasma fludarabine and fludarabine triphosphate (F-ara-ATP) in peripheral CLL cells. Onkologie 1991 (14 suppl 2):83
29 Ross SR, McTavish D, Faulds D: Fludarabine. A review of its pharmacological properties and therapeutic potential in malignancy. Drugs 1993 (45):737-759
30 Kemena A, O'Brien S, Kantarjian H et al: Phase 2 clinical trial of fludarabine in CLL on a weekly low-dose schedule. Leukemia and Lymphoma 1993 (10):187-193

31 Robertson LE, O'Brien S, Koller C et al: A three-day schedule of fludarabine in CLL. Blood 1992 (80 suppl 1):47a (abstract)
32 Boussiotis VA, Panayitodis PG, Pangalis GA: Prolonged intermittent chlorambucil administration in B-chronic lymphocytic leukemia: Experience from a single Hematology Unit. Leukemia and Lymphoma 1991 (5 suppl):113-118
33 Fenchel K, Bergman L, Jahn B, Mitrou P, Hoelzer D: Fludarabine phosphate in refractory chronic lymphocytic leukemia. Onkologie 1991 (14 suppl 2):190
34 Hiddemann W, Rottmann R, Warmann TA et al: Treatment of advanced chronic lymphocytic leukemia by fludarabine: Results of a clinical phase II study. Ann Hematol 1991 (63):1-4
35 Johnson SA, Richardon D, Hopkins J, Howe D, Phillips MJ: Complete remission after fludarabine for chronic lymphocytic leukemia. Correspondence. Blood 1993 (81):560-566
36 Kantarjian HM, Schachner J, Keating MJ: Fludarabine therapy in hairy cell leukemia. Cancer 1991 (67):1291-1293
37 Keating MJ, Kantarjian H, O'Brien S et al: Fludarabine: a new agent with marked cytoreductive activity in untreated chronic lymphocytic leukemia. J Clin Oncol 1991 (9):44-49
38 Knauf WU, Kreuser ED, Pottgiesser E, Thielk E: In vitro and in vivo effectiveness of fludarabine in B-cell chronic lymphocytic leukemia (B-CLL). Ann Hematol 1992 (65 suppl):A80 (abstract # 203)
39 O'Brien S, Kantarjian H, Koller C et al: Fludarabine-prednisone: a highly effective regimen in chronic lymphocytic leukemia (CLL). Proc Am Soc Clin Oncol 1992 (11):260 (abstract # 850)
40 Puccio CA, Mittelman A, Lichtman SM et al: A loading dose/continuous infusion schedule of fludarabine phosphate in chronic lymphocytic leukemia. J Clin Oncol 1991 (9):1562-1569
41 Angelopoulou MK, Poziopoulos Ch, Boussiotis VA, Pangalis GA: Fludarabine monophosphate in refractory to chemotherapy B-chronic lymphocytic leukemia. Leukemia and Lymphoma 1995 (in press)
42 International Working Group on CLL: Chronic lymphocytic leukemia: Recommendations for diagnosis, staging and response criteria. Ann Intern Med 1989 (110):236-238
43 Gillis S, Dann E, Gass Y, Polliack A: Activity of fludarabine in refractory chronic lymphocytic leukemia and low grade non-Hodgkin's lymphoma. The Jerusalem experience. Leukemia and Lymphoma 1994 (in press)
44 Portlock CS: Management of the indolent non-Hodgkin's lymphomas. Sem Oncol 1980 (7):292-301
45 Hoppe RT, Kughlan P, Kaplan HS, Rosenberg SA, Brown BW: The treatment of advanced stage favorable histology non-Hodgkin's lymphoma: A preliminary report of a randomized trial comparing single agent chemotherapy, combination chemotherapy and whole body irradiation. Blood 1981 (58): 592-598
46 Pangalis GA, Roussou PA, Kokkinou S, Anagnostopoulos N, Fessas Ph: Treatment of low grade non-Hodgkin's lymphomas. Chemiotherapia 1985 (suppl 2):1118-1119
47 Angelopoulou MK, Lafioniatis SN, Pangalis GA: Low grade non-Hodgkin's lymphomas: Disease control with mitoxanthrone monotherapy in patients refractory to conventional therapy. Leukemia and Lymphoma 1994 (12):253-258
48 Hochster HS, Kim K, Green MD et al: Activity of fludarabine in previously treated non-Hodgkin's low grade lymphoma. Results of an Eastern Cooperative Oncology Group Study. J Clin Oncol 1992 (10):28-32
49 Leiby JM, Snider KM, Kraut EH, Metz EN, Malspeis L: Phase II trial of 9-B-D-arabinosyl-2-fluoroadenine 5'-monophosphate in non-Hodgkin's lymphoma: prospective comparison of response with deoxycytidine kinase activity. Cancer Res 1987 (47): 2719-2722
50 Redman JR, Cabanillas F, Velasquez WS, McLaughlin P, Hagemeister FB: Phase II trial of fludarabine phosphate in lymphoma. J Clin Oncol 1992 (10):970-974
51 Whelan JS, Davis CL, Rule S et al: Fludarabine phosphate for the treatment of low grade lymphoid malignancy. Br J Cancer 1991 (64):120-123
52 Pigaditou A and Lister A (personal communication)
53 Kantarjian HM, Alexian R, Koller CA, Kurzrock R, Keating MJ: Fludarabine therapy in macroglobulinemic lymphoma. Blood 1990 (75):1928-1931
54 Dimopoulos M, O'Brien S, Kantarjian H, Estey EE, Keating MJ, Alexanian R: Treatment of Waldenström's macroglobulinemia with nucleoside analogues. Leukemia and Lymphoma 1993 (11 suppl 2):1005-1008
55 Von Hoff DD, Green S, Surwit EA, Hannigan EV, Alberts DS: Phase II study of fludarabine phosphate (NSC 312887) in patients with advanced cervical cancer. A Southwest Oncology Group Study. American J Clin Oncol 1990 (13):433-435
56 Foss F, Ihde D, Phelps R, Fischmann A et al: Phase II study of fludarabine and interferon-alfa-2a in advanced mycosis fungoides/Sezary syndrome (MF/SS). Proc Am Soc Clin Oncol 1992 (11):315 (abstract # 1065)
57 Kraut EH, Crowley JJ, Grever MK, Keppen MD, Bonnet JD: Phase II study of fludarabine phosphate in multiple myeloma. A Southwest Oncology Group Study. Invest New Drugs 1990 (8):199-200
58 Warrell RP Jr and Berman E: Phase I and II study of fludarabine phosphate in leukemia: therapeutic efficacy with delayed central nervous system toxicity. J Clin Oncol 1986 (4):74-79
59 Gandhi V, Estey E, Keating MJ, Plunkett W: Fludarabine potentiates metabolism of cytarabine in patients with acute myelogenous leukemia during therapy. J Clin Oncol 1993 (11):116-124
60 Gandhi V: Fludarabine for treatment of adult acute myelogenous leukemia. Leukemia and Lymphoma 1993 (11 suppl 2):7-14
61 Wijermans PW, Van der Linden JSM, Gerritis WBJ, Haak HL: Severe immunodeficiency and opportunistic infections seen in patients treated with fludarabine monophosphate. Blood 1992 (80 suppl 1):46a
62 Reis Borges R, Zylberait D, Broquie G, Veyssier P: Pneumocystose, keratite herpetique, meningite a cryptocoques chez un patient VIH negatif atteint

d'une LLC et traité par fludarabine. Revue de Medicine Interne 1992 (13):S436

63 Sanders C, Perez EA, Lawrence HJ: Opportunistic infections in patients with chronic lymphocytic leukemia following treatment with fludarabine. Correspondence. Am J Hematol 1992 (39):314-315

64 Anaissie E, Kontoyiannis DP, Kantarjian H, Elting L, Robertson LE, Keating M: Listerosis in patients with chronic lymphocytic leukemia who were treated with fludarabine and prednisone. Ann Int Med 1992 (117):466-469

65 Cervantes F, Salgado C, Montserrat E, Rozman C: Fludarabine for prolymphocytic leukemia and risk of interstitial pneumonitis. Lancet 1990 (336):1130

66 Hurst PG, Habib MP, Garewal H et al: Pulmonary toxicity associated with fludarabine monophosphate. Invest New Drugs 1987 (5):207-210

67 Kane GC, McMichael AJ, Patrick H, Erslev AJ: Pulmonary toxicity and acute respiratory failure associated with fludarabine monophosphate. Resp Med 1992 (86):221-263

68 List AF, Kummet TD, Adams JD, Chun HG: Tumor lysis syndrome complicating treatment of chronic lymphocytic leukemia. Ann Oncol 1992 (3):171-173

69 Bastion Y, Coiffier B, Dumontet C, Espinouse D, Bryon PA: Severe autoimmune hemolytic anemia in two patients treated with fludarabine for chronic lymphocytic leukemia. Ann Oncol 1992 (3):171-173

70 Tosti S, Caruso R, D'Adamo F et al: Severe autoimmune hemolytic anemia in a patient with chronic lymphocytic leukemia responsive to fludarabine-based treatment. Ann Hematol 1992 (65):238-239

71 Chung HG, Leyland-Jones B, Cheson BD: Fludarabine phosphate: a synthetic purine antimetabolite with significant activity against lymphoid malignancies. J Clin Oncol 1991 (9):175-188

72 Cohen RB, Abdallan JM, Gray JR, Foss F: Reversible neurologic toxicity in patients treated with standard-dose fludarabine phosphate for mycosis fungoides and chronic lymphocytic leukemia. Ann Int Med 1993 (118):114-116

Role of Haemopoietic Growth Factors in Lymphoma Therapy

George P. Canellos

Division of Medical Oncology, Dana-Farber Cancer Institute, 44 Binney Street, Boston, MA 02115, U.S.A.

Recombinant haemopoietic growth factors are now well established in their efficacy as agents which can promote the growth and function of granulocytes and/or macrophages. These factors expand the number of dividing precursor cells and shorten the postmitotic maturation time of maturing granulocytes in the bone marrow. They have proved to be an important addition to the supportive care armamentarium in patients treated with myelosuppressive chemotherapeutic agents. Pilot and phase II trials have shown that the recovery of maturing granulocytes is hastened following myelosuppression, especially after high-dose chemotherapy programmes [1-4]. The duration of severe neutropenia (≤1000 ANC x 10^9/l) is clearly shortened from 5.4 days to 1 day with conventional dose therapy and from 30 days to 16 days with high-dose therapy plus autologous bone marrow transplantation (ABMT). "Full" doses of chemotherapy appeared to be delivered on time; with high-dose therapy, shortened periods of hospitalization were seen. These growth factors were surprisingly well tolerated with G-CSF and recombinant (yeast) GM-CSF being the least toxic. Thus, they could be safely administered to the majority of patients without regard for serious organ toxicity. Mild fever or medullary bone pain may occur with G-CSF that can be controlled by analgesics. The recovery of platelets and red cells was not enhanced.

The schedule of administration has varied in early clinical trials from twice daily subcutaneous dosing to 24-hour continuous infusion to short infusions of 2-4 hours. The doses of GM-CSF used varied greatly from 2 μg/kg/d up to 60 μg/kg/d. Most trials of GM-CSF utilized 250 μg/m^2/day given as either a 24-hour continuous infusion or a subcutaneous bolus dose or even a 2-hour infusion i.v. Earlier trials with bacterial recombinant GM-CSF gave 10 μg/kg/d by 4-6 hour infusion. The neutrophilia following GM-CSF or G-CSF is dose dependent. If the dose is held constant at a level of 5 μg/kg/d with G-CSF, the neutrophils will rise by the second day and maximize at about day 4 without further change if the same dose level is maintained in a patient who is not pretreated with chemotherapy.

Because of the uncertainty as to the optimal dose and schedule, there is some variation in dose/schedule amongst the more recent trials which are controlled with placebo only. The ultimate value of these agents is the amelioration of the morbidity and potential mortality associated with severe myelosuppression and, if possible, to increase the benefit of chemotherapy by allowing higher doses. These issues are important if for no other reason than that the costs of these factors are considerable. If hospitalization time can actually be reduced, then the cost savings is obvious and could easily justify their use. However, in order to demonstrate an improvement in progression-free (and more importantly overall) survival, a very "dose-responsive" disease should be investigated.

The malignant lymphomas are probably the most drug responsive adult tumours with the possible exception of germ-cell tumours of the testis. Because the latter have such a high cure rate with conventional-dose chemotherapy, the concept of growth factors and chemotherapy is better tested in the malignant lymphomas where the more advanced-age patients on average as well as higher-risk patients have a considerably lower likelihood of a drug-induced cure.

Table 1. Prospective randomized trials with recombinant growth factors

Trial	No. pts.	Disease	Recombinant GM-CSF	Dose	Shortened duration of hospitalization	Reduced infection	Relapse-free survival
Gulati et al. 1992 [5]	24	HD	*E. coli*	10 μg/kg/d over 6 hrs	yes	no	unchanged
Advani et al. 1992 [6]	69	HD, NHL	*E. coli*	10 μg/kg/d 4-6 hrs infusion	no	yes	unchanged
Nemunaitis et al. 1991 [7]	128	NHL, ALL	yeast	250 μg/m^2/d over two hrs	yes	yes	unchanged
Link et al. 1992 [8]	81	NHL, ALL	*E. coli*	250 μg/m^2/d ci over 24 hrs	no	yes	unchanged
Khwaja et al. 1992 [9]	61	HD, NHL	*E. coli*	250 μg/m^2/d once daily sc	no	no	unchanged
Gorin et al. 1992 [10]	91	NHL	*E. coli*	250 mg/m^2/d ci over 24 hrs	yes	yes	unchanged

HD = Hodgkin's disease; NHL = non-Hodgkin's lymphoma; ALL = acute lymphoblastic leukaemia

This chapter will examine the scientific data derived from prospective randomized trials in malignant lymphoma. The initial prospective trials entailed the use of high-dose chemotherapy or chemo-radiotherapy with or without recombinant growth factors - in most trials recombinant GM-CSF derived from bacterial or yeast sources. Six prospective trials are outlined on Table 1. All studies examined the duration of hospitalization, incidence of serious infections or positive blood cultures and response to therapy for lymphoma. The results are quite interesting because in all instances neutrophil dose recovery was enhanced, but in 3/6 trials the duration of hospitalization was unchanged compared to placebo and in 3/6 there was no difference in the occurrence of serious infections. Relapse-free or progression-free survival was unchanged. Clearly there are institutional differences in discharge policy and institutional capacity for maintaining an ambulatory platelet transfusion capacity which may also affect the likelihood of early discharge, even if the ANC has reached 5 x 10^9/l. The recovery time to that level of mature neutrophils averaged about 14 days after ABMT (12-19 range) and GM-CSF compared to about 20 days (16-28) on the placebo. Infusions were continued until the neutrophil doses >0.5 x 10^9/μl were sustained for 7 days or to a total of 30 days of infusion. In only one of the 6 randomized trials comprising a total of 454 patients was both the duration of hospitalizations and the incidence of infections shown to be reduced [5-10]. Not surprisingly, since a fixed dose of high-dose therapy was given, there was no difference in relapse-free survival.

There are only two published randomized trials using conventional-dose chemotherapy for large cell lymphoma where GM-CSF or G-CSF were employed post therapy compared to placebo [11,12]. In the Manchester trial, patients were treated with VAPEC-B, an intensive regimen given over 11 weeks. Thus, each week some therapy was given which varied in content and myelosuppressive potential. The G-CSF was given at 230 mg/m^2 as daily subcutaneous injection for 13 weeks vs no G-CSF. This trial showed a higher frequency of dose reduction and/or dose delay in the control group compared to the G-CSF treated group. Doses were reduced in 1/3 of the control patients but the dose intensity of the G-CSF group was higher without increasing the incidence of drug toxicity, except for mucositis which was dose-limiting. Despite the relatively higher dose intensity, the relapse-free survival did not differ between the two arms of the trial.

The second trial randomized 182 patients between placebo or GM-CSF (400 mg total dose) following COP-BLAM chemotherapy for large cell lymphoma. The GM-CSF was given for 7 days following each chemotherapy cycle. Neutropenia and the incidence of infection and hospitalization for infectious complications were reduced. The complete response rates were 79% in the GM-CSF arm vs 95% in the control in low-risk (low volume of disease) patients. These differences were not statistically significant. There was a difference in favour of GM-CSF for high-risk patients with a complete response rate of 69% vs 48% in the controls (p=0.04). After one year, there was no difference in overall survival. There was no calculation of total dose delivered or dose intensity. Thus, the impact of growth factors with high-dose or conventional dose chemotherapy is that infectious complications are reduced in most but not all instances. The outcome in terms of surviving the tumour was not affected, although perhaps high-risk patients may achieve a higher complete response rate.

These trials were not tests of dose intensity and its value in the treatment of lymphoma. This could best be achieved by identifying high-risk or poor-prognosis drug-sensitive tumours, such as advanced stage large cell lymphoma with elevated LDH, poor performance status or advanced Hodgkin's disease with multiple extranodal sites, and prospectively comparing conventional doses to escalated doses with haemopoietic growth factor support. The higher-dose patients clearly will benefit by an enhanced recovery of neutrophils. If growth factors allow for the cycles of higher-dose therapy, then a comparison in poor prognosis patients to conventional-dose therapy is justified since the long-term disease-free survival in such patients is only 25-35% with standard therapy. Unquestionably, these agents have a role in the treatment of lymphoma. Certainly recovery from high-dose (ABMT) regimens is enhanced but whether their use in the less-than-transplant-dose setting will increase the cure rate remains to be investigated.

REFERENCES

1 Nemunaitis J, Singer JW, Buckner CD et al: Use of recombinant human granulocyte-macrophage colony-stimulating factor in autologous marrow transplantation for lymphoid malignancies. Blood 1988 (72):834-836

2 Sheridan WP, Begley CG, Juttner CA et al: Effect of peripheral-blood progenitor cells mobilised by filgrastim (G-CSF) on platelet recovery after high-dose chemotherapy. Lancet 1992 (339):640-644

3 Taylor KM, Jagannath S, Spitzer G et al: Recombinant human granulocyte colony-stimulating factor hastens granulocyte recovery after high-dose chemotherapy and autologous bone marrow transplantation in Hodgkin's disease. J Clin Oncol 1989 (7):1791-1799

4 Lazarus HM, Andersen J, Chen MG et al: Recombinant granulocyte-macrophage colony-stimulating factor after autologous bone marrow transplantation for relapsed non-Hodgkin's lymphoma: Blood and bone marrow progenitor growth studies. A phase II Eastern Cooperative Oncology Group Trial. Blood 1991 (78):830-837

5 Gulati SC and Bennett CL: Granulocyte-macrophage colony-stimulating factor (GM-CSF) as adjunct therapy in relapsed Hodgkin disease. Ann Intern Med 1992 (116):177-182

6 Advani R, Chao NJ, Horning SJ et al: Granulocyte-macrophage colony-stimulating factor (GM-CSF) as an adjunct to autologous hemopoietic stem cell transplantation for lymphoma. Ann Intern Med 1992 (116):183-189

7 Nemunaitis J, Rabinowe SN, Singer JW et al: Recombinant granulocyte-macrophage colony-stimulating factor after autologous bone marrow transplantation for lymphoid cancer. N Engl J Med 1991 (324):1773-1778

8 Link H, Boogaerts MC, Carella AM et al: A controlled trial of recombinant human granulocyte-macrophage colony-stimulating factor after total body irradiation, high-dose chemotherapy, and autologous bone marrow transplantation for acute lymphoblastic leukemia or malignant lymphoma. Blood 1992 (80): 2188-2195

9 Khwaja A, Linch DC, Goldstone AH et al: Recombinant human granulocyte-macrophage colony-stimulating factor after autologous bone marrow transplantation for malignant lymphoma: a British National Lymphoma Investigation double-blind, placebo-controlled trial. Br J Haematol 1992 (82):317-323

10 Gorin NC, Coiffier B, Hayat M et al: Recombinant human granulocyte-macrophage colony-stimulating factor after high-dose chemotherapy and autologous bone marrow transplantation with unpurged and purged marrow in non-Hodgkin's lymphoma: a double-blind, placebo-controlled trial. Blood 1992 (80):1149-1157

11 Pettengell R, Gurney H, Radford JA et al: Granulocyte colony-stimulating factor to prevent dose-limiting neutropenia in non-Hodgkin's lymphoma: a randomized controlled trial. Blood 1992 (80):1430-1436

12 Gerhartz HH, Engelhard M, Meusers P et al: Randomized, double-blind, placebo-controlled, phase III study of recombinant human granulocyte-macrophage colony-stimulating factor as adjunct to induction treatment of high-grade malignant non-Hodgkin's lymphomas. Blood 1993 (82):2329-2339

High-Dose Therapy for the Malignant Lymphomas

Wendy Mills and Anthony H. Goldstone

University College Hospitals, Gower Street, London WC1 6AU, United Kingdom

Hodgkin's Disease comprises several related malignancies of the reticuloendothelial system, characterized by the presence of the Reed-Sternberg cell, which are now generally associated with a good prognosis. Since the turn of the century [1], patients with localized disease have been cured by extended-field radiotherapy alone, at a dose of not less than 40 Gy, and the alkylating agents were introduced in 1946 [2] as treatment for patients with more extensive disease. Long-term disease-free survival was initially reported in the 1960s with MOPP chemotherapy (mechlorethamine, vincristine, procarbazine and prednisone) [3,4]. More recent non-crossresistant oncolytic regimens such as ABVD (adriamycin, bleomycin, vinblastine and dacarbazine) probably provide a failure-free advantage over MOPP [5]. Non-crossresistant protocols may be used sequentially, as alternating therapy, or as multi-drug hybrid programmes intended to minimize the emergence of drug resistance.

Current combination chemotherapy protocols cure a high proportion of those presenting with extensive disease, but despite these advances in therapy, at least one third of patients with advanced Hodgkin's Disease do not achieve complete remission or will relapse from remission within 12 months [6]. The outlook for such patients is poor; conventional-dose salvage therapy may achieve responses in up to 80%, but remissions are seldom durable and the long-term survival is less than 10% [7-9]. Contemporary management strategies aim to minimize the toxicity of curative therapy for patients with good prognostic features, and to improve the disease-free survival of those with poor-risk disease.

The non-Hodgkin's lymphomas represent a diverse group of lymphoproliferative disorders for which management depends on patient status, histological characteristics, and disease extent. Patients with localized disease may be cured with radiotherapy alone, but most present with more advanced disease and require chemotherapy [10].

The use of aggressive multi-agent combination chemotherapy for the treatment of advanced diffuse aggressive lymphomas has resulted in a dramatic change in the overall prognosis for patients with these malignancies. Once rarely curable or even controllable, the high and intermediate-grade lymphomas have become amongst the most curable of disseminated malignancies. Sustained disease-free survival rates have risen from 5% in the 1960s to greater than 65% in the 1990s [11]. Nevertheless, the one third of patients who do not attain complete response, and those who relapse from complete remission, generally experience a fulminating course and rarely survive more than 2 years [12]. Current protocols aim to minimize the toxicity of curative treatment modalities for patients with favourable prognostic features, and to improve salvage therapy for those with refractory or relapsed malignancy.

Low-grade malignant follicular lymphomas are characterized by their indolent course, with a median survival of 4 to 8 years. Remissions may be readily achieved with single-agent or multi-agent chemotherapy protocols, but few patients will be cured. Most low-grade lymphomas may be effectively palliated for many years, but eventually transform to aggressive diffuse large cell lymphomas or become increasingly resistant to chemotherapy [13]. Ongoing investigation with intensive chemoradiotherapy and bone marrow or peripheral stem cell transplantation is towards the development of curative therapy.

The Concept of High-Dose Therapy

Pioneering work by Skipper and colleagues in the 1960s showed, in an animal model, that the log kill rate of chemotherapy was dependent on dose and not the population size of the malignant cells, and confirmed the importance of dose in cure [14]. The concept of dose intensity was first elaborated by de Vita and coworkers [15], who documented decreased cure rates in patients requiring dose reduction or increased intervals between courses of MOPP chemotherapy. Goldie and Coldman, in their monograph predicting the rate of emergence of drug-resistant malignant clones [16], provided further evidence in favour of early dose-intensive chemotherapy in the treatment of malignant lymphomas. Non-crossresistant combination regimens were initially introduced as rapidly alternating or hybrid programmes to increase treatment intensity and eliminate resistant clones [17], and observations that the major toxicity of combination chemotherapy protocols is haemopoietic led to the investigation of autologous bone marrow support as a means of avoiding fatal myeloablation with high-dose chemotherapy. The first reports of successful outcome after transplantation in end-stage patients were published as early as 1959 and the 1960s [18,19], but it was only in the 1980s that the technique became widely accepted as a salvage modality for patients with refractory lymphoma. By the end of 1990, nearly 2000 autografts for lymphoma had been reported to the European Bone Marrow Transplant Group (EBMT) registry [16], and high-dose therapy is increasingly utilized earlier in the course of the disease.

Dose Intensification for Hodgkin's Disease

High-dose therapy is associated with an inevitable substantial morbidity and mortality. Toxicity considerations determine patient selection, and hitherto bone marrow transplantation has been reserved for those failing conventional treatment. The eligibility criteria for dose intensification have become increasingly refined with experience, and vary according to treatment centre. Table 1 summarizes the current consensus regarding acceptability criteria for high-dose therapy for Hodgkin's Disease [20], based on subgroups of patients identified from the BNLI database as having a poor prognosis with conventional therapy.

The role of transplantation for patients with poor prognostic Hodgkin's disease in first complete remission (1CR) is more controversial. Carella and his coworkers [21] identified patient characteristics at presentation which were associated with significantly decreased survival rates after alternating therapy. These include age greater than 40 years, bulky mediastinal disease, B symptoms, more than one extranodal site of disease, serum lactate dehydrogenase greater than 400 IU/l, bone marrow involvement, and anaemia. At 5 years, patients with no adverse prognostic factors are all alive; with one, 94%; with two, 60%; and those with three or more adverse features have a 5-year survival of less than 20%. These authors suggest that patients with two

Table 1. Eligibility criteria for high-dose therapy for Hodgkin's disease

Patients younger than 65, with no clinically significant cardiac, respiratory, renal or hepatic dysfunction

1. Patients relapsing from, or not attaining CR after MOPP-type chemotherapy, if grade 2 histology, or ESR > 59 mm/hr
2. Patients relapsing from, or not attaining CR after alternating chemotherapy (e.g. MOPP/ABVD) or hybrid chemotherapy
3. Those relapsing from, or not attaining CR after one line of chemotherapy plus radiotherapy, if the refractory disease is within the irradiated field

or more poor prognostic characteristics should receive high-dose therapy as consolidation in first remission. However, 30% of these patients are likely to have been cured with alternating therapy, and the risk of procedure-related mortality associated with transplantation may be unacceptable.

Unlike the situation with NHL, chemosensitivity of the tumour to conventional-dose chemotherapy at the time of transplantation is not necessary for eligibility to high-dose therapy. Several groups have shown that chemosensitivity status predicts for outcome post transplant [22,23], and analysis of the EBMT registry data confirms a survival advantage for patients with chemosensitive disease, but it is nevertheless true that a significant proportion of patients not responding to the relatively intensive mini-BEAM (BcNU, etoposide, cytarabine and melphalan) salvage protocol will achieve prolonged disease-free survival after BEAM and autologous bone marrow transplantation [24]. This experience demonstrates that the dose-intensity relationship for treatment of Hodgkin's Disease does not plateau even at the extreme end of the spectrum.

Although both chemotherapy and total body irradiation (TBI) have been used as conditioning therapy for transplantation for the lymphomas, the toxicity of TBI is unacceptably high in patients who have previously received extended-field radiotherapy for Hodgkin's Disease [26,27], and thus combination chemotherapy has become the mainstay of high-dose treatment in this disease. The most widely utilized protocols are BEAM and CBV (cyclophosphamide, BcNU and VP16), although many different regimens have evolved (Table 2).

The outcome of high-dose therapy depends not only on the ability of the intensive chemotherapy to ablate the malignant clone, but also the possibility of reinfusing contaminated marrow. Patients with histological evidence of marrow infiltration are usually excluded from bone marrow transplantation programmes as, because of the elusive immunological nature of the Reed-Sternberg cell, *in vitro* purging of contaminated marrow is not feasible. The prognostic implication of occult marrow disease is, however, not fully elucidated; in a small blinded study of bilateral trephine assessment of marrow infiltration at the time of harvest in patients with previous negative biopsies, it was demonstrated that durable remissions could be obtained in some patients with extensive marrow infiltration [25]. Patients with histological evidence of marrow infiltration are frequently subjected to conventional-dose salvage therapy in an attempt to clear the marrow prior to harvest, but may be offered high-dose therapy with peripheral blood precursor support instead. The outcome of peripheral stem cell transplantation in those with chemorefractory marrow infiltration is likely to be poor.

Table 2. High-dose chemotherapy protocols

BEAM:	
BcNU (Carmustine) 300 mg/m^2 IV	day -6
Etoposide 200 to 400 mg/m^2 IV	days -5 to -2
Ara C (Cytarabine) 200 mg/m^2 bd IV	days -5 to -2
Melphalan 140 mg/m^2 IV	day -1
Followed by infusion of >1x10^8 nucleated cells/ ↑ kg bone marrow (or peripheral blood precursor cells)	day 0
CBV:	
Cyclophosphamide 1.5 g/m^2 IV	days -5 to -2
VP16 (Etoposide) 250 mg/m^2 IV	days -5 to -2
BcNU (Carmustine) 150 mg/m^2 IV	days -4 to -2
Infusion of bone marrow or peripheral blood stem cells	day 0

Following bone marrow transplantation, the median time to recovery of neutrophils to >0.5 x10^9/l is 22 days, and to platelets >20 x10^9/l unsupported, 27 days [28]. This prolonged period of neutropenia and thrombocytopenia results in a substantial risk of infection and haemorrhage, which contribute to the mortality and morbidity of high-dose therapy. The immediate non-haematological toxicity of high-dose chemotherapy includes pneumonitis, which may prove fatal, and renal, cardiac, and hepatic damage. Mucositis, which may involve the entire gastrointestinal tract, usually causes painful stomatitis, dysphagia, epigastric pain, nausea, diarrhoea and vomiting, but may result in life-threatening colitis. With increasing experience and intensive support, the procedure-related mortality for bone marrow transplantation has gradually declined, and now averages about 5% [6,29].

Results of High-Dose Therapy in Hodgkin's Disease

Prognostic factors predicting for long-term disease-free survival following high-dose therapy have been identified as chemosensitivity status at the time of transplantation, disease extent, age, sex, and performance status [30]. Patients with primary refractory disease, defined as those never attaining complete or good partial remission, those with bulky disease (>5 cm in diameter), female patients, those older than 40 years or with a Karnofsky rating of 70 or less, have a worse outcome than those without these characteristics. Overall long-term disease-free survival rates from large series of patients are in the order of 40 to 60% [6,29-31], which is clearly superior to the results of conventional-dose salvage therapy in patients with relapsed or refractory disease. The survival of patients transplanted in first complete remission is projected to be higher; in a small study [21] 13 of 15 patients (87%) were in sustained remission at a median follow-up of 36 months but two of these potentially cured patients (13%) suffered procedure-associated mortality. A survival advantage was unequivocal compared with a control group of patients matched for prognostic indicators, not treated with dose intensification in 1CR, in whom only 33% maintained remission for a median of 42 months; the remainder relapsed and died within 34 months of completing first-line therapy.

Patients undergoing high-dose therapy are inevitably a selected subgroup, and proof of the value of transplantation can only accrue from randomized controlled trials, although such trials are difficult to execute as patients are increasingly reluctant to be randomized to non-transplant therapy. Linch and colleagues at the British National Lymphoma Investigation Group have recently published results of a randomized trial of BEAM and autologous transplantation compared with 3 courses of the relatively less intensive mini-BEAM protocol, which uses the same drug combination in lower doses not requiring stem cell support [32]. Forty patients with refractory or recurrent Hodgkin's Disease entered the study; there were 2 deaths in the BEAM arm compared with none in the mini-BEAM group, but 53% of patients randomized to receive BEAM were alive without disease progression at 3 years compared to only 10% for mini-BEAM. This confirms results from previous non-randomized studies and, as the same drug combination was used at different intensities, further reinforces the relationship between dose intensity and potential for cure in Hodgkin's Disease.

High-Dose Therapy for Non-Hodgkin's Lymphoma

The high and intermediate-grade non-Hodgkin's lymphomas, excluding lymphoblastic lymphoma and Burkitt's lymphoma, encompass the diffuse small cleaved cell, diffuse large cell, diffuse mixed small and large cell, and immunoblastic lymphomas. The conventional treatment for these is radiotherapy or chemotherapy for stage I disease, and combination chemotherapy for more extensive disease. The standard CHOP chemotherapy (cyclophosphamide, adriamycin, vincristine and prednisone) results in complete remission in about 60% of patients with stage II to IV disease, of whom approximately two thirds will be cured [33]. There is no evidence that second and third-generation protocols, such as MACOP-B (methotrexate, adriamycin, cyclophosphamide, vincristine, prednisone and bleomycin), offer significant disease-free survival advantage over CHOP [34]. Thus 60% of patients presenting with advanced disease will not attain complete remission on first-line chemotherapy, or will relapse from remission, and the prognosis for such patients with conventional-dose salvage therapy is poor. Although 30% may obtain complete response with ifosfamide or cisplatin-based regimens, responses are seldom durable, and the survival is less than 10% at 3 years [35-38]. That there is a correlation between relative dose intensity and disease control in non-Hodgkin's lymphoma has been confirmed from clinical studies [39], and high-dose therapy is readily justified in this group.

Lymphoblastic lymphomas and small non-cleaved cell lymphomas are more aggressive diseases than the other high-grade lymphomas, and despite intensive chemotherapy protocols, including programmes similar to those used for acute lymphoblastic leukaemia, with central nervous system prophylaxis, patients with these malignancies have a projected 5-year survival of less than 50%. Those with stage IV disease, bone marrow or central nervous system involvement, or elevated serum lactate dehydrogenase level at presentation have a prognosis of less than 20% at 5 years [40], and high-dose treatment with autologous stem cell support in first remission undoubtedly improves survival in patients with these poor prognostic indicators.

Despite the indolent nature of the disease, patients with low-grade NHL are probably incurable with traditional chemotherapy and have a median survival of only 4 to 8 years. Analysis of the Eastern Cooperative Oncology Group data [41] identified age greater than 60 years, failure to attain complete remission with initial chemotherapy, and duration of response of less than 1 year, as independent poor prognostic variables. Patients younger than 60 with an initial CR of more than 1 year had a median survival of 5.9 years, whilst those showing short-lived partial response survive for only 2 years with conventional treatment. High-dose chemoradiotherapy and bone marrow transplantation with curative intent is now favoured by many oncologists for young patients with low-grade lymphoma beyond first remission, but it is possible that dose intensification in first complete remission will improve survival. Salvage therapy after histological transformation of follicular lymphomas is unlikely to succeed; even bone marrow transplantation seldom results in prolonged survival [42].

The criteria for selection of NHL patients for high-dose therapy are summarized in Table 3. Chemoresponsiveness of the malignancy at the time of transplantation is the most significant prognostic indicator predicting for survival after high-dose therapy [43,44] and, moreover, correlates with procedure-related mortality rates [43]. Patients with disease refractory to conventional-dose salvage chemotherapy have an increased risk of perishing from complications of transplantation, and are unlikely to obtain lasting benefit, the projected long-term survival being around 10%. The demonstration of chemosensitivity is thus a requisite for acceptance to most transplantation programmes.

Combination chemotherapy protocols such as those used for Hodgkin's Disease are commonly used for high-dose therapy for intermediate and high-grade NHL, excluding the small non-cleaved cell and lymphoblastic lymphomas, for which total body irradiation is usually advocated in addition to high-dose chemotherapy, particularly cyclophosphamide for Burkitt's lymphoma. Treatment for low-grade lymphomas is more controversial; preliminary studies have mostly used low-dose total body irradiation.

Purging of marrow, using monoclonal antibodies, heat, or *ex vivo* chemotherapeutic agents in an attempt to remove residual malignant cells, is widely practised, but the efficacy of purging methods and benefit remain unproven [46]. However, review of the EBMT registry data shows no advantage in relapse-free survival for purging in low-grade NHL, or intermediate and high-grade NHL. Only in Burkitt's lymphoma, with patients closely matched for all prognostic factors, could a trend towards significant (p=0.06) survival advantage be demonstrated [47].

Table 3. Indications for high-dose therapy for NHL

Patients younger than 65 years with no clinically significant cardiac, renal or pulmonary dysfunction

HIGH AND INTERMEDIATE-GRADE MALIGNANCY:

1. Patients with partial response to first-line therapy
2. Patients relapsing from CR

but still responsive to conventional-dose chemotherapy

3. Adults with high-risk lymphoblastic lymphoma or Burkitt's lymphoma in 1CR
4. Other high-risk patients in 1CR or as part of initial therapy

LOW-GRADE MALIGNANCY:

1. Patients beyond 1 CR with chemosensitive disease

Outcome of High-Dose Therapy for NHL

The results of transplantation in large series of patients with advanced high and intermediate-grade NHL have been published [44,48]. Chemosensitivity status, extent and bulk of disease, sex and performance status have emerged as predicting for outcome of high-dose therapy [49]. Patients transplanted in first remission have a projected long-term disease-free survival of 75 to 80%; those in first partial response approximately 60%; those with chemosensitive relapse 40 to 50%; with resistant relapse 20 to 30%; and patients with tumours progressing on conventional chemotherapy 10%. Despite concerns that T-cell histology in NHL confers a worse prognosis than B-cell disease, Vose et al. [50] demonstrated equivalent survival after transplantation. Preliminary results for high-dose therapy for low-grade lymphomas suggest that about half of these patients will achieve prolonged remission, but the indolent nature of this disease mandates prolonged follow-up for accurate assessment of the benefit of transplantation.

Patients who do not respond to high-dose therapy and those with recurrent disease after transplantation usually respond poorly to palliation, and succumb within months [49].

As with Hodgkin's Disease, incontrovertible evidence favouring high-dose therapy in comparison with traditional-dose salvage therapy will only be possible with randomized trials in patients with similar disease parameters. Such trials are starting to emerge in the literature. Two large muticentre studies have compared high-dose chemotherapy and autologous bone marrow transplantation for patients with refractory or recurrent high and intermediate-grade non-Hodgkin's lymphoma with a cisplatin-based salvage regimen, DHAP (dexamethasone, cytarabine and cisplatin). In the Italian analysis [51] 25 patients with residual or relapsed disease after F-MACHOP (5-fluorouracil, methotrexate, adriamycin, cyclophosphamide, cytarabine, vincristine and dexamethasone) or MACOP-B were randomized to receive DHAP, and 22 were transplanted, using BAVC (BcNU, cytarabine, VP-16 and cyclophosphamide) as conditioning therapy. The progression-free survival at 40 months was 74% for the high-dose group, and only 22% for the conventional-dose group. A similar favourable advantage was shown for transplantation with BEAC (BcNU, etoposide, cytarabine and cyclophosphamide) (40 patients) compared with DHAP (44 patients) in the PARMA international randomized prospective study [52] in patients with relapsed aggressive lymphoma, with a 3-year follow-up. Although these series are relatively small and the observation period limited, the outcome is convincingly in favour of dose intensification.

Allogeneic Transplantation for Lymphoma

Whether a graft-versus-lymphoma effect exists has been a contentious subject. Analysis of the EBMT registry data [53], matching patients with lymphoma treated by allogeneic transplantation to patients with similar prognostic characteristics undergoing autologous bone marrow transplantation, failed to show a survival advantage for allografted patients (49% versus 46%); although the relapse rate was 23% compared to 38%, this was not statistically significant. For those with lymphoblastic lymphoma, however, allogeneic transplantation conferred a considerable relapse-free survival advantage. Jones et al. [54] confirmed that a freedom-from-progression advantage in NHL, similar in magnitude to the graft-versus-leukaemia effect, may exist, but is countered by the increased procedure-related toxicity of allogeneic transplantation.

Clinical Application of Growth Factors

The proliferation and differentiation of bone marrow progenitor cells is controlled by cytokines released from stromal cells and T lymphocytes. Mixed myeloid precursors arise from pluripotent stem cells under the influence of interleukin (IL)-1, 3 and 6. Granulocyte-macrophage colony stimulating factor (GM-CSF) increases commitment to granulocyte and monocyte production, granulocyte colony stimulating factor (G-CSF) to neutrophils, IL-5 to eosinophils, and macrophage colony stimulating factor (M-CSF) to monocytes. These cytokines also affect function, membrane integrity and surface adhesion properties of their mature target cells. The availability of recombinant human growth

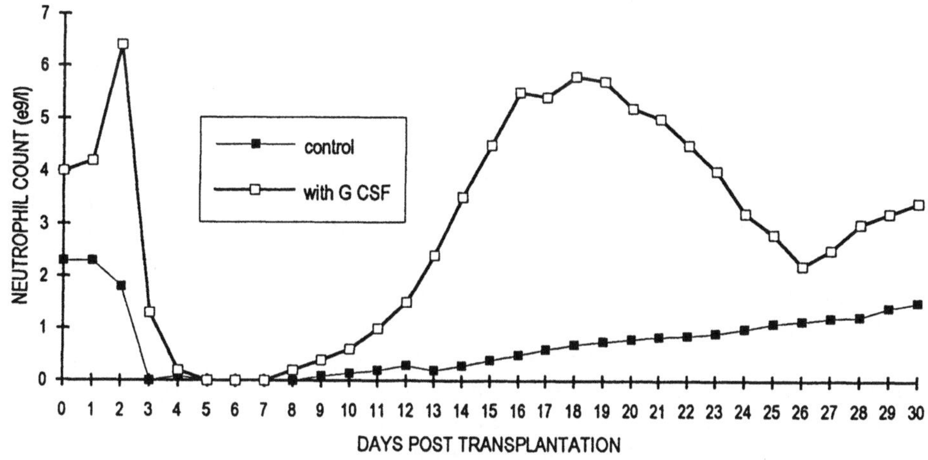

Fig. 1. Neutrophil recovery with G-CSF

factors, manufactured in *E. coli*, has had tremendous impact on therapy for malignancy. Both G-CSF and GM-CSF significantly accelerate neutrophil recovery following high-dose therapy and bone marrow transplantation, to around 14 days as compared with 22 without growth factors (see Fig. 1) [55], and IL-3 also enhances platelet recovery. Myalgias, bone pains, fevers, fluid retention, rashes and serositis may prove dose-limiting for GM-CSF; headaches, fevers and rashes occur frequently with IL-3; G-CSF appears well tolerated with bone pain occurring in approximately 10%.

Several studies have shown decreased hospital inpatient stay, infective episodes and antibiotic use [55-57], and the use of cytokines in this setting is clearly cost effective despite their price [61]. Growth factors have also been used with conventional-dose chemotherapy protocols, and have been shown to minimize dose reductions and delays in administration of chemotherapy, and thus to improve remission rates and possibly survival. Use of growth factors may allow increased intensity of treatment, the impact of which is as yet conjectural.

Peripheral Blood Precursor Support

Precursor cells capable of reconstituting haematopoiesis after high-dose therapy are found not only in the marrow, but also in small numbers in circulating peripheral blood. Enrichment of these precursors occurs after conventional combination chemotherapy, low-dose single agent chemotherapy, and with the use of haematopoietic growth factors such as G-CSF and GM-CSF, allowing collection of adequate numbers of precursor cells by apheresis of the buffy coat from peripheral blood. Several studies have demonstrated accelerated and durable trilineage engraftment after high-dose chemotherapy utilizing peripheral blood precursors (PBP) alone, with a median time to achieve a neutrophil count of >0.5 x10^{9}/l and platelet count of >50 x10^{9}/l of around 12 days post transplantation [59,60]. Data are emerging to show a significant advantage in total inpatient stay [61], infective complications, antibiotic use [62], as well as erythrocyte and platelet transfusion requirement [61] after PBP support compared with marrow transplantation, with obvious implications regarding cost and the use of resources (Table 4).

Furthermore, peripheral stem cell harvesting obviates the need for a general anaesthetic and the discomfort involved in bone marrow harvesting, and may allow high-dose therapy to be offered to patients whose marrow has been rendered hypocellular following previous extensive chemotherapy or pelvic irradiation, or is infiltrated with lymphoma. Contamination of

Table 4. Advantages of peripheral progenitors over marrow

1. Accelerated haematological reconstitution; decreased hospital stay
2. Allows high-dose therapy despite hypocellular marrow
3. No anaesthesia required for harvest
4. Postulated lower tumour burden in peripheral progenitor population

the peripheral blood apheresis product by malignant cells is nevertheless a possibility; Reed-Sternberg cells have been found in circulating blood, and Hardingham and coworkers [63] have demonstrated the presence of a molecular marker of disease (immunoglobin heavy chain or T cell receptor rearrangement, or the *bcl*-2/JH fusion product) in the peripheral blood stem cell collection of 5 of 11 patients.

Patients undergoing high-dose therapy with PBP support after conventional-dose therapy has failed to clear marrow infiltration are unlikely to have a good outcome, due to the chemoresistant nature of the malignancy. Relapses associated with occult marrow contamination, moreover, tend to occur at sites of prior bulky disease, rather than at new sites, suggesting that the ability to detect occult lymphoma cells in marrow (or peripheral blood apheresis product) is a marker of biologic aggressiveness or resistance to therapy, or that reinfused cells can only grow in previously involved areas [49].

Purification of peripheral blood stem cells allows removal of contaminating malignant cells, manipulation for gene therapy, and *ex vivo* expansion using growth factors [65]. Culture with G-CSF and CM-CSF yields approximately 60-fold expansion of stem cells; using gamma interferon a 260-fold enrichment is possible, which would enable collection of 350 ml of whole blood as starting material and obviate the need for apheresis [66]. The facilities for *in vitro* stem cell expansion are, however, obviously limited.

Biological Response Modifying Agents

The realisation that some patients with malignant lymphomas have a poor response to chemotherapy from the outset, and that relapse continues to occur after high-dose therapy, has led to the investigation of biological response modifying agents as adjuvant therapy. These range from calcium channel blockers to inhibit the multi-drug resistance p-glycoprotein [63], to immune stimulation of the host defences against residual malignant cells. Interferon alpha, which has shown antiproliferative activity in several haematopoietic malignancies, is undergoing trials in NHL, particularly of low-grade malignancy [64]. Low-dose interferon alpha is reported to induce tumour regression in up to 70% of previously untreated patients with low-grade lymphoma [65], and disease control may be enhanced by the simultaneous administration of conventional chemotherapeutic drugs. Interleukin 2, with or without *ex vivo* generated lymphokine-activated killer cells, may enhance immune eradication of residual malignancy, and preliminary results are encouraging. Monoclonal antibodies directed against antigens on the malignant cell, and conjugated to growth factors, may stimulate natural killer cells. Other cytokines may have direct or indirect antitumour activity, and research into the natural function and clinical application of the cytokines holds enormous promise.

Conclusions

High-dose therapy clearly improves disease-free survival for patients with relapsed and refractory malignant lymphoma, and may benefit patients at high risk of relapse if utilized as consolidation for first remission. The growth factors limit the duration of cytopenia, and thus inpatient stay, following bone marrow transplantation, but peripheral blood stem cell transplantation offers significant advantages and is likely to replace bone marrow as support for high-dose therapy. Disease-modifying cytokines are being explored and may offer alternative or adjuvant treatment strategies in the fight against the lymphomas.

REFERENCES

1 Pusey WA: Cases of sarcoma and of Hodgkin's disease treated by exposure to X rays: A preliminary report. JAMA 1902 (38):166
2 Goodman LS, Wintrobe MM, Damershek W et al: Nitrogen mustard therapy: Use of methyl-bis (B chloroethyl) amine hydrochloride on neoplastic disorders of the haematopoeitic system. JAMA 1946 (132):126
3 Rosenberg SA: Report of the committee on the staging of Hodgkin's disease. Cancer Res 1966 (26):1310
4 De Vita VT, Simon RM, Hubbard SM et al: Curability of advanced Hodgkin's disease with chemotherapy: Long term follow up of MOPP treated patients at the NCI. Ann Intern Med 1980 (92):587-595
5 Santoro A and Bonadonna G: Prolonged disease free survival in MOPP resistant Hodgkin's disease after treatment with adriamycin, bleomycin, vinblastine and dacarbazine (ABVD). Cancer Chemother Pharmacol 1979 (2):101
6 Goldstone AH and Linch DC: Bone marrow transplantation in the malignant lymphomas. In: Hoffbrand AV and Brenner MK (eds) Recent Advances in Haematology. Churchill Livingstone, London 1992
7 Longo DL, Duffey PL, Young RC et al: Conventional dose salvage chemotherapy in patients relapsing with Hodgkin's disease after combination chemotherapy: The low probability for cure. J Clin Oncol 1991 (10):210
8 Klimo P and Connors JM: An update of the Vancouver experience in the management of advanced Hodgkin's disease treated with the MOPP/ABVD hybrid program. Sem in Haematol 1988 (25):34
9 Viviani S, Santoro A, Negretti E et al: Salvage chemotherapy in Hodgkin's disease. Ann Oncol 1990 (1):123
10 Vose JM and Armitage JO: The present status of therapy for patients with aggressive non-Hodgkin's lymphoma. Ann Oncol 1991 (2 suppl 2):171-176
11 Jones JM: Advances in the treatment of non Hodgkin's lymphoma. J Med Assoc Ga 1989 (78):105-108
12 Armitage JO, Vose JM, Bierman PJ: Salvage therapy for patients with non Hodgkin's lymphoma. NCI Monogr 1990 (10):39-43
13 Diaz-Pavon JR and Cabinillas F: Treatment of non Hodgkin's lymphomas. Curr Opin Oncol 1991 (3): 830-835
14 Skipper HE: Criteria associated with the destruction of leukaemia and solid tumor cells in animals. Cancer Res 1967 (27):2636-2645
15 De Vita VT, Serpick AA, Carbone PP: Combination chemotherapy in the treatment of advanced Hodgkin's disease. Ann Intern Med 1970 (78):881
16 Goldie JH and Coldman AJ: A mathematical model for relating the drug sensitivity of tumours to their spontaneous mutation rate. Cancer Treat Rep 1979 (63):1727-1733
17 De Vita VT: The influence of information on drug resistance on protocol designs. Ann Oncol 1991 (2): 93-106
18 McFarland W, Granville NB, Damashek W: Autologous bone marrow infusion as an adjunct in therapy of malignant disease. Blood 1959 (14):503
19 Stewert JW: The treatment of malignant disease by irradiation and cytotoxic drugs followed by bone marrow transfusion. Nucleonics 1960:251-256
20 Gribben JG, Vaughan-Hudson B, Linch DC: The potential value of therapy with autologous bone marrow rescue in the treatment of the malignant lymphomas. Haematol Oncol 1987 (5):281-286
21 Carella AM, Carlier P, Congui A et al: Autologous bone marrow transplantation as an adjuvant therapy of high risk Hodgkin's disease patients in first complete remission after MOPP/ABVD protocol. Bone Marrow Transplant 1991 (8):31-35
22 Jones RJ, Piantadosi S, Mann RB et al: High dose cytotoxic therapy and bone marrow transplantation for relapsed Hodgkin's Disease. J Clin Oncol 1990 (8):527-537
23 Jaganath S, Armitage JO, Dicke KA et al: Prognostic indicators after high dose cyclophoshamide, carmustine and etoposide with autologous bone marrow transplantation for relapsed Hodgkin's disease. J Clin Oncol 1989 (7):179-185
24 Chopra R, Linch DC, McMillan AK et al: MiniBEAM plus BEAM ABMT as salvage treatment for very poor prognosis Hodgkin's Disease. Br J Haem 1991 (77 suppl 1):20
25 Chopra R, Wotherspoon A et al: The significance of occult bone marrow infiltration for high dose chemotherapy and autologous bone marrow transplantation in Hodgkin's Disease. J Clin Oncol 1994 (in press)
26 Phillips GL, Wolf SN, Herzig RH et al: Treatment of progressive Hodgkin's disease with intensive chemoradiotherapy and autologous bone marrow transplantation. Blood 1989 (73):2086
27 Peterson FB, Appelbaum FR, Hill R et al: Autologous bone marrow transplantation for malignant lymphoma: A report of one hundred and one cases from Seattle. J Clin Oncol 1990 (8):638
28 McMillan AK, Goldstone AH, Linch DC: One hundred cases of relapsed Hodgkin's disease treated with BEAM chemotherapy in a single centre. In: Proceedings of the Fourth International Conference on Malignant Lymphomas, June 6-9 1990, Lugano, Switzerland, p 22
29 Desch CE, Lasala M, Smith TJ et al: The optimal timing of autologous bone marrow transplantation in Hodgkin's disease patients after a chemotherapy relapse. J Clin Oncol 1992 (10):200
30 Jagganath S, Armitage JO, Dicke KA et al: Prognostic indicators for response and survival after high dose cyclophosphamide, carmustine and etoposide with autologous bone marrow transplantation for relapsed Hodgkin's disease. J Clin Oncol 1989 (7):179
31 Zulian GB, Selby P, Milan S: High dose melphalan, BCNU and etoposide with autologous bone marrow transplantation for Hodgkin's disease. Br J Cancer 1989 (59): 631
32 Linch DC, Winfield D, Goldstone AH et al: Dose intensification is effective in relapsed or resistant Hodgkin's Disease: Results of the BNLI randomised study. Lancet 1994 (in press)

33 Gore ME and McElwain TJ: Lymphomas: the impact of chemotherapy on survival. Cancer Surv 1989 (8):647-670
34 Weick J, Dahlberg S, Miller T et al: The treatment of Non Hodgkin's lymphoma with m-BACOD, ProMACE-CytaBOM and MACOP-B: The Southwest Oncology Group (SWOG) Experience. Proceedings of ASCO, San Francisco 1989 (8):254 (abstract 990)
35 Vose JM and Armitage JO: The present status of therapy for patients with aggressive Non Hodgkin's Lymphoma. Ann Oncol 1991 (2 suppl 2):171-176
36 De Lord C, Newland AC, Linch DC, Vaughan-Hudson B, Vaughan-Hudson G: Failure of IM VP16 as second line treatment for relapsed or refractory high grade non Hodgkin's lymphoma. Haemat. Oncol 1992 (10):81-86
37 Velasquez WS, Cabinillas F, Salvador P: Effective salvage therapy for lymphoma with cisplatin in combination with high dose Ara C and dexamethasone (DHAP). Blood 1988 (71):117-122
38 Cabinillas F: Experience with iphosphamide combinations in malignant lymphomas. Sem Oncol 1989 (16):78-81
39 Lepage E, Gisselbrecht C, Haioun C et al: Relative received dose intensity in poor risk lymphoma patients: higher DI correlates with longer survival. Blood 1992 (80 suppl 1):158
40 Santini G, Coser P, Chiseri T et al: Autologous bone marrow transplantation for advanced stage adult lymphoblastic lymphoma in first complete remission: report of the Non Hodgkin's Lymphoma Cooperative Study Group. Ann Oncol 1991 (2 suppl 2):181-185
41 Weisdorf DJ, Andersen JW, Glick JH and Oken MM: Survival after relapse of low grade non Hodgkin's lymphoma: implications for transplantation. J Clin Oncol (10):942-947
42 Schouten HC, Bierman PJ, Vaughan WP et al: Autologous bone marrow transplantation in follicular non Hodgkin's lymphoma before and after histological transformation. Blood 1989 (15):2579-2584
43 Armitage JO: Autologous bone marrow transplantation for patients with aggressive non Hodgkin's lymphoma. Bone Marrow Transplant 1992 (10 suppl 1):62-63
44 Vose JM, Armitage JO, Bierman PJ et al: Salvage therapy for relapsed or refractory non Hodgkin's lymphoma utilising autologous bone marrow transplantation. Am J Med 1989 (87):285-288
45 Freedman AS, Takvorian T, Anderson KC et al: Autologous bone marrow transplantation in B-cell non Hodgkin's lymphoma: very low treatment related mortality in 100 patients in sensitive relapse. J Clin Oncol 1990 (8):784-791
46 Sharp J G, Joshi SS, Armitage JO et al: Significance of detection of occult non Hodgkin's lymphoma in histologically uninvolved bone marrow by a culture technique. Blood 1992 (79):1074-1080
47 Favrot M, Philip T, Pavone E: Ex vivo purging is efficient in Burkitt's lymphoma but high dose chemotherapy is ineffective in patients with active disease in the bone marrow. In: Dicke KA, Spitzer G, Jaganath S et al (eds) Proceedings of the IVth International Symposium of Autologous Bone Marrow Transplantation, University of Texas, 1989
48 Coser P, Santini G, Rizzoli V et al: Autologous bone marrow transplantation (ABMT) in poor prognosis diffuse non Hodgkin's lymphoma: Report of the Non Hodgkin's Lymphoma Cooperative Study Group. Bone Marrow Transplant 1989 (4 suppl 4):164-175
49 Vose JM, Bierman PJ, Anderson JR et al: Progressive disease after high dose therapy and autologous transplantation for lymphoid malignancy: clinical course and patient follow up. Blood 1992 (80):2142-2148
50 Vose JM, Peterson C, Bierman PJ et al: Comparison of high dose therapy and autologous bone marrow transplantation for T-cell and B-cell non Hodgkin's lymphoma. Blood 1990 (76):424-431
51 Tura S, Zinzani PL, Mazza P et al: ABMT vs DHAP in residual disease following third generation regimens for aggressive non Hodgkin's lymphomas. Blood 1992 (80 suppl 1):157
52 Phillip T, Chauvin F, Bron D et al: PARMA international protocol: pilot study on 50 patients and preliminary analysis of the ongoing randomised study. Ann Oncol 1991 (2 suppl 1):57-64
53 Chopra R, Goldstone AH, Pearce R et al: Autologous versus allogeneic bone marrow transplantation for non Hodgkin's lymphoma: a case controlled analysis of the European Bone Marrow Transplant Registry Goup data. J Clin Oncol 1992 (10):1690-1695
54 Jones R J, Ambinder RF, Piantadosi S, Santos GW: Evidence of a graft versus lymphoma effect associated with allogeneic bone marrow transplantation. Blood 1991 (77):649-653
55 Goldstone AH and Kwaja AK: The role of haematopoietic growth factors in bone marrow transplantation. Leuk Res 1990 (14):721
56 Sheridan WP, Morstyn G, Wolf et al: Granulocyte colony stinulating factor and recovery after high dose chemotherapy and autologous bone marrow transplantation. Lancet 1989 (2):891-895
57 Kwaja A, Mills W, Leveridge K et al: Efficacy of delayed granulocyte colony stimulating factor after autologous bone marrow transplantation. Bone Marrow Transplant 1994 (in press)
58 Leveridge K, Mills W, Kwaja A et al: Cost effectiveness of delayed granulocyte colony stimulating factor after autologous bone marrow transplantation. Meeting of the European Bone Marrow Transplant Registry Group, Stockholm 1992
59 Gianni AM, Bregni M, Sienna S et al: Rapid and complete haemopoietic reconstitution following combined transplantation of autologous blood and marrow stem cells: a changing role for high dose chemotherapy? Haemat. Oncol 1989 (7):139-148
60 Kessinger A and Armitage JO: The evolving role of peripheral blood stem cell transplantation following high dose chemotherapy for malignancies. Blood 1991 (77):211-213
61 Kessinger A, Armitage JO, Smith DM, Landmark JD, Bierman PJ, Weisenberger DD: High dose chemotherapy and autologous peripheral blood stem cell transplantation for patients with lymphoma. Blood 1989 (74):1260-1265
62 Phillip T, Hartman O, Biron P et al: High dose therapy and autologous bone marrow transplantation in partial remission after first line induction

therapy for diffuse non Hodgkin's lymphoma. J Clin Oncol 1988 (6):1118-1124
63 Hardingham JE, Kotasek D, Sage RE, Dobovic A, Gooley T, Dale BM: Molecular detection of residual lymphoma cells in peripheral blood stem cell harvests and following autologous transplantation. Bone Marrow Transplant 1993 (11):15-20
64 Klingeman HG, Grigg AP, Wilkie-Boyd K et al: Treatment with recombinant interferon (alpha 2b) early after bone marrow transplantation in patients at high risk of relapse. Blood 1991 (78):3306-3311
65 Wagstaff J, Loynds P, Crowther D: A phase II study of human rDNA alpha-2 interferon in patients with low grade non Hodgkin's lymphoma. Cancer Chemother Pharmacol 1986 (18):54-58
66 Krants JP: Peripheral stem cell recruitment for transplantation following high dose therapy. Meeting of the European Bone Marrow Transplant Registry Group, Stockholm 1991
67 Brice P, Marolleau JP, Dombret H et al: Autologous peripheral blood stem cell transplantation after high dose chemotherapy in patients with advanced lymphoma. Bone Marrow Transplant 1992 (9):337-342

Malignant Lymphomas in Immunocompromised Hosts, in Particular with AIDS

Umberto Tirelli and Emanuela Vaccher

Division of Medical Oncology and AIDS, Centro di Riferimento Oncologico, via Pedemontana 12, 33081 Aviano, Italy

Prior to the AIDS epidemic, malignant lymphomas, in particular non-Hodgkin's lymphoma (NHL), were described in up to 30% of the patients with primary immunodeficiency disorders such as the X-linked lymphoproliferative syndrome or the Wiscott Aldrich syndrome. Moreover, patients with immune deficiency secondary to cytostatic anticancer therapy and also following organ transplantation, autoimmune diseases and connective tissue disorders are at increased risk of NHL. The lymphomas which arise in all these settings and in patients with HIV infection have certain features in common, including 1) prevalence of high-grade pathological types, predominantly large cell and immunoblastic lymphomas, or small noncleaved cell; 2) restriction to B-cell origin; 3) widely disseminated disease at presentation; 4) poor prognosis compared to patients with "common" lymphomas.

The aim of this chapter is to review the clinical and therapeutic aspects of HIV-related NHL.

Lymphoma in Aids

Since the beginning of the HIV epidemic, HIV-related NHLs have been associated with a poor outcome. This was mainly due to the adverse clinico-pathological features [1] and the underlying HIV disease with its opportunistic infections. HIV-related NHLs are distinguished from NHL in the general population by a high percentage of high-grade subtypes, frequent extranodal sites of disease and a high percentage of disease progression, therefore lower response rates to chemotherapy and higher mortality rates have been observed. Moreover, the toxicity of treatment is much higher also because of the immunosuppression caused by HIV. However, the availability of more efficacious agents anti HIV and anti opportunistic infections, the concomitant use of bone marrow growth factors, a better definition of prognostic risk factors associated with HIV infection and related NHL [2-9], seem to have improved the prognosis of systemic HIV-related NHL.

Overall, 1-2% of patients with AIDS present with primary CNS lymphoma and both systemic NHL and primary CNS lymphoma are recognized as AIDS-defining diseases by Centres for Disease Control. Although systemic and CNS NHL are different diseases with different primary sites, the general approaches for these diseases are similar and so are the reported survival rates.

The therapy of HIV-related NHL is quite controversial because it is not clear whether treatment with intensive chemotherapy can modify the natural history of these malignancies in the HIV setting. In fact, Levine et al., employing low-dose chemotherapy, observed the same results as with intensive chemotherapy [10]. On the other hand, the therapy of CNS lymphoma has not been investigated in larger trials, mainly because CNS lymphoma usually occurs in the later stages of HIV disease, rendering intensive chemotherapy quite difficult. In this setting palliative radiotherapy is the treatment of choice, with no impact on the overall survival. In order to improve the very poor survival of this disease, CNS lymphoma should be studied in prospective trials.

Clinical Findings

The increase in AIDS-related NHL concerns mostly high-grade B-cell types: large cell immunoblastic and small non-cleaved cell (SNC) lymphomas comprise about 70% of AIDS-related NHL. The intermediate-grade diffuse large cell lymphomas make up the remaining 30% [11-13]. Recent studies have shown that patients with SNC lymphoma had preserved immune function and better prognosis while those with large cell immunoblastic lymphoma had advanced immunodeficiency and poor prognosis [13,14].

The unusual clinical presentation of HIV-related NHL continues to be observed in recent case series and has also been seen in registry-based studies [15]. These lymphomas are clinically aggressive, with approximately 75% involving extralymphatic sites, particularly brain, bone marrow and gastrointestinal tract. Primary central nervous system lymphoma has been observed in 10% to 20% of all HIV-related NHL and many of these cases were diagnosed only at the time of autopsy [11,13, 16].

Recent molecular analysis of HIV-related NHL has disclosed 3 general patterns. Primary lymphomas of the brain tend to be monoclonal, immunoblastic, Epstein-Barr Virus (EBV) associated and lack c-*myc* rearrangements. "Peripheral" polyclonal NHLs tend to be immunoblastic, not associated with EBV, and also lack c-*myc* rearrangements. "Peripheral" monoclonal lymphomas are of varied high-grade histology, may be EBV-associated and tend to display c-*myc* rearrangements [17]. The clinical significance of these preliminary analyses awaits prospective studies.

Therapy

Retrospective Studies

Patients with HIV-related NHL have been treated with standard combination chemotherapy regimens known to be effective against aggressive non-HIV NHL. Unfortunately, the results of such therapies in the HIV setting have been poorer than those in "common" NHL. Overall, complete responses occurred in 17% to 56% of cases, all were of short duration and relapses within the CNS were a substantial problem. Survival was typically in the range of 4-11 months and deaths were most frequently due to recurrent lymphoma or opportunistic infections. These general observations were derived from retrospective studies (Table 1) describing patients with HIV-related NHL treated with standard chemotherapy regimens including CHOP (cyclophosphamide, adriamycin, vincristine, prednisone), CHOP-like regimens, proMACE/MOPP (prednisone, methotrexate, doxorubicin, cyclophosphamide, etoposide/mechlorethamine, vincristine, predni-

Table 1. HIV-related non-Hodgkin's lymphoma: Treatment results in retrospective studies

Reference	Evaluable pts.	Complete response (%)	OI [a] Follow-up (%)	Median Survival
Ziegle et al. 1984 [1]	66	53	33	6 mo
Kalte et al. 1985 [18]	14	43	?	?
Knowles et al. 1988 [2]	83 [b]	33	?	5 mo
Lowenthal et al. 1988 [3]	30	56	?	6 mo
Kaplan et al. 1989 [4]	26	46	48	11 mo
Bermudez et al. 1989 [19]	12	17	?	?
GICAT [c] 1990	44	23	?	4-5 mo [d]
Roithmann et al. 1991 [5]	100	37	?	5 mo
Pedersen et al. 1991 [7]	33	36	?	5 mo

[a] OI = Opportunistic infections; [b] only 44% were HIV seropositive; [c] GICAT = Italian Cooperative Study Group on AIDS and Tumours; [d] 5 mos for intravenous drug users and 4 for homosexual men - $p = 0.7$

sone, procarbazine), m-BACOD (methotrexate, bleomycin, adriamycin, cyclophosphamide, dexamethazone) and MACOP-B (methotrexate, adriamycin, cyclophosphamide, vincristine, bleomycin, prednisone). Important prognostic information has been obtained from these retrospective therapy studies. The most important predictor of survival, when available, was the total number of CD4-positive lymphocytes. In the absence of a CD4 count, no prior AIDS diagnosis was the best predictor of survival. Less important prognostic factors were Karnofsky Performance Status (PS), presence of extranodal disease and bone marrow involvement. The prognostic significance of histological subtype remains controversial; further studies are needed which should include large numbers of homogeneously treated patients with uniform pathological reviews [1-7,18-20].

Prospective Studies

The first prospective treatment trial was reported in 1987 by Gill et al. (Table 2). In this trial, AIDS-NHL patients were enrolled into two sequential phase II studies, the first using M-BACOD in 13 patients, and the second using a novel regimen of intensive induction therapy with high-dose cytarabine, vincristine, asparaginase, prednisone, cyclophosphamide and high-dose methotrexate with leucovorin rescue. Consolidation therapy was delivered as 3 cycles of CHOP alternated with 3 cycles of etoposide every 21 days. Prophylaxis of CNS with 2400 cGy to a helmet field was started on day 90. The first group achieved a complete response rate of 54%; 31% achieved disease-free survival for more than 1 year, and CNS progression occurred in 15%. In contrast, the complete response rate for the second group was 33%, whereas 11% achieved disease-free survival for longer than 1 year, and 67% experienced CNS progression, although the patients in this group had significantly more bone marrow involvement at presentation. The median survival for the first group was 11 months vs 6 months for the group treated with the intensive regimen. This new regimen was associated with development of opportunistic infections in 78% versus only 8% in the M-BACOD-treated patients, and led to early ter-

Table 2. Prospective treatment trials by Gill [8]

	M-BACOD [a] (No. pts. 13)	Novel regimen [b] (No. pts. 8)
KPS [c] median (range)	70 (55-100)	90 (35-100)
CD4 count/mm^3 median (range)	368 (9-2064)	173 (20-4820)
Pathologic type [d]:		
SNC	9	7
IB	4	2
Stage:		
III-IV	13 (100%)	8 (89%)
CNS [e] involvement	1 (8%)	2 (15%)
Response:		
CR [f]	7 (54%)	3 (33%)
OI [g] follow-up	1 (8%)	7 (78%)
CNS progression	1 (5%)	6 (32%)
Median survival (mo)	11	6

[a] M-BACOD = HD-MTX, bleomycin, adriamycin, cyclophosphamide, vincristine, dexametasone; [b] Novel regimen = HD-cytarabine, L-asparaginase, vincristine, prednisone, HD-cyclophosphamide, HD-methotrexate, CHOP/VP16 x 6 cycles; [c] KPS = Karnofsky Performance Status; [d] SNC = Small non-cleaved cell lymphoma, IB = Immunoblastic lymphoma; [e] CNS = Central Nervous System; [f] CR = Complete Remission; [g] OI = Opportunistic infections
(modified from [8])

mination of the trial. The investigators concluded that the novel intensive regimen was associated with a significant risk of early death due to opportunistic infections and haematologic toxicity; they therefore suggested that less intensive treatment strategies should be explored [8].

As part of a larger study on the clinical characteristics of patients with AIDS-NHL at San Francisco General Hospital, Kaplan et al. reported on the treatment of 33 patients in a prospective chemotherapy trial. A regimen (COMET-A) was devised that consisted of cyclophosphamide (1.4 g/m^2), vincristine, methotrexate with leucovorin rescue, etoposide and cytarabine. Patients also received CNS prophylaxis with intrathecal methotrexate and monthly *Pneumocystis carinii* prophylaxis with intravenous pentamidine (4 mg/kg/month). Complete responses were seen in 58% of patients treated with COMET-A, a percentage that was not statistically different from the 46% of patients with CR in a control group treated with a variety of standard regimens. In addition, the median survival time of the COMET-A group (5 months) was significantly shorter than that of the controls (11 months). In multivariate analysis, patients receiving greater dose intensity (as defined by a dose of cyclophosphamide >1g/m^2) showed a significantly shorter survival than patients treated less intensively [4].

On the basis of of these experiences, a prospective multicentre clinical trial was conducted by the AIDS Clinical Trials Group (ACTG) to evaluate the efficacy of lower-dose chemotherapy for HIV-related NHL. In this study, a modification of the standard M-BACOD regimen, with early CNS prophylaxis consisting of intrathecal cytarabine, and use of AZT at the completion of chemotherapy, was employed. Patients with poor prognostic indicators (history of AIDS, low CD4 count, poor PS) were not excluded. With 35 evaluable patients a complete remission rate of 46% was achieved, with long-term lymphoma survival in 75% of complete responders. Use of intrathecal prophylaxis was effective in that no patient experienced isolated CNS relapse.

Pneumocystis carinii pneumonia (PCP) developed in approximately 20% of the patients despite the use of prophylatic therapy. The median survival was 6.5 months for all evaluable subjects and 15 months for complete responders. Despite the low doses of chemotherapy used, approximately 60% of the subjects had a granulocyte nadir of less than 1000 x 10^6/l, while 21% showed granulocyte nadirs of 500 x 10^6/l or less. Clinical factors predictive of poor outcome included low CD4 count, history of AIDS, poor PS, stage IV disease and bone marrow involvement. Pathological subtype of disease was not found to be predictive of response or survival in this group of uniformly treated patients [10].

A phase I study with an intensive but short chemotherapy regimen was reported by Sawka et al. Thirty HIV-seropositive patients with intermediate-grade or SNC-NHL underwent a 12-week programme of weekly intravenous and oral chemotherapy consisting of etoposide, adriamycin, cyclophosphamide, bleomycin, vincristine, methotrexate and prednisone as well as biweekly intrathecal cytarabine. Prophylaxis against PCP and candida were given routinely. The 33% complete remission rate was similar to other published reports where conventional CT regimens were used, but a significant finding was the occurrence of leukopenia. The median survival was 8 months for all subjects evaluable, and 15 months for complete responders. Opportunistic infections occurred in 24% of patients, and NHL was the most common cause of death (59%) [21].

Based on some preclinical evidence suggesting a therapeutic advantage for the administration of cytotoxic agents via infusion compared to a bolus schedule [22], Sparano et al. conducted a pilot study of infusional CDE for patients with HIV or HTLV-I-related NHL. The new regimen consisted of cyclophosphamide, adriamycin and etoposide and was administered as a continuous intravenous infusion over 4 days to 16 patients. The treatment was repeated every 28 or more days for up to 6 cycles. Patients with SNC lymphoma or bone marrow involvement received CNS phrophylaxis consisting of intrathecal methotrexate and whole brain irradiation. All patients received prophylactic treatment against PCP during the chemotherapy. Complete remission occurred in 75% of HIV patients. The median survival for all patients (including 2 HTLV-I patients) was 17 months. CNS relapse occurred in 33% of patients receiving CNS prophylaxis therapy. Hospitalization was required after 19% of treatment cycles for neutropenic fever while

opportunistic infections occurred in 36% of patients. The encouraging results were not likely to be due to selection of favourable patients since all patients had at least one poor prognostic feature and the median CD4 count was low (87 cells/mm^3, range 2-484) [23].
Recently, Remick et al. reported on the treatment of 18 patients with a novel oral chemotherapy regimen consisting of lomustine, etoposide, cyclophosphamide and procarbazine. The overall objective response rate was 61%, with 7 complete remissions (39%) and a median survival of 7 months. Myelotoxicity was the most important toxic effect, with grade 3-4 leukopenia in 64% of cycles; opportunistic infections occurred in only 11% of patients. No change in quality of life scores over time were observed in this series. Interestingly, the overall cost of this novel regimen was considerably lower than that of other intravenous combination chemotherapy regimens [38].
Besides these prospective clinical trials of new chemotherapy regimens designed specifically for HIV-related NHL (Table 3), a "second generation" of HIV-NHL protocols has been developed in the last years. These trials were performed by stratification into "low or good" and "high or poor" risk categories according to the presence or not of prognostic factors (Tables 4 and 5).
In 1989, Bermudez et al. reported on a prospective series of 11 patients treated with MACOP-B (methotrexate, hydroxyldaunomycin, cyclophosphamide, vincristine, prednisone, bleomycin). Sixty-four percent (7 patients) obtained complete remission, with a median survival of 20 months. Six of the 7 complete responders had Karnofsky PS of 100% and none had a history of AIDS prior to developing the lymphoma [19].
Comparable results were obtained by Taillan et al. with the same CT regimen administered to 12 patients with HIV high-grade NHL, all with good prognostic factors (i.e., no prior AIDS diagnosis, high CD4 count, no bone marrow involvement). Complete remission was obtained in 58% of patients with a median duration of 15 months and a median survival of 16 months. The investigators concluded that a subgroup of patients with HIV-NHL may benefit from

Table 3. Prospective clinical trials of new chemotherapy regimens designed specifically for HIV-related NHL

Regimen	Evaluable pts.	Median CD4 count (cells/mm^3)	Complete response (%)	OI [a] Follow-up (%)	Median survival	Reference
HDAraC + HDMTX + others [b]	9	173	33	78	6 mo	Gill et al. 1987 [8]
COMET-A [d]	38	164	58	42	5 mo	Kaplan et al. 1989 [4]
Low-dose M-BACOD [e] + i.t. Ara-C	35	150	46	20 (PCP)	6.5 mo tot. CR=15 mo	Levine et al. 1991 [6]
12-wk regimen [f]	30	60	33	24	8 mo CR=15 mo [c]	Sawka et al. 1992 [21]
Infusional CDE [g]	16	87	75	36	17 mo	Sparano et al. 1993 [23]
"Novel" oral combination [h]	18	73	39	11	7 mo	Remick et al. 1993 [38]

[a] OI = Opportunistic infections; [b] Others = vincristine, L-asparaginase, prednisone, cyclophosphamide, adriamycin, etoposide; [c] CR = complete remission; [d] COMET-A = HD-cyclophosphamide, vincristine, HD-methotrexate, etoposide, cytarabine; [e] M-BACOD = bleomycin, adriamycin, cyclophosphamide, vincristine, dexametasone, HD-methotrexate; [f] 12-wk regimen = adriamycin, etoposide, cyclophosphamide, prednisone, methotrexate, bleomycin, vincristine, cytarabine; [g] CDE = cyclophosphamide, adriamycin, etoposide; [h] Novel oral combination = lomustine, etoposide, cyclophosphamide, procarbazine

Table 4. Prospective clinical trials in "low risk" patients with HIV-related NHL

Regimen	Eval. pts.	Prognostic factors	CR [d] (%)	OI [a] Follow-up	Median survival	Reference
MACOP-B [b]	11	No prior AIDS KPS [c] 100	64	?	7 mo total CR = 20 mo	Bermudez et al. 1989 [19]
M.D. Anderson regimen	12	SNC [e]	83	33 as cause of death	36% 5 yrs OS [f]	Lopez et al. 1990 [25]
MSKCC [g]	9	SNC [e]	56	?	6 mo	Straus et al. 1991 [26]
MACOP-B [b]	12	no prior AIDS high CD4 count no BM [h] involvement	58	?	CR 16 mo	Taillan et al. 1993 [24]
LNH-84 [i]	141	no OI [a] ZPS [l] ≤2	63	38 as cause of death	9 mo	Gisselbrecht et al. 1993 [28]
CHOP [m] IFN-α + AZT [n]	28	no OI [a] ZPS [l] ≤2 CD4 >50 cells/mm^3	64	?	21 mo	Huhn et al. 1993 [30]

[a] OI= Opportunistic infections; [b] MACOP-B = methotrexate, adriamycin, cyclophosphamide, vincristine, prednisone, bleomycin; [c] KPS = Karnofsky performance status; [d] CR = complete remission; [e] SNC = small non-cleaved cell; [f] OS = overall survival; [g] MSKCC= Memorial Sloan Kettering Cancer Center; [h] BM = Bone marrow; [i] LNH-84 = adriamycin, cyclophosphamide, vindesine, bleomycin, prednisone; [l] ZPS = Zubrod performance status; [m] CHOP = cyclophosphamide, vincristine, adriamycin, prednisone; [n] AZT = Zidovudine, IFN-α (Interferon-alpha)

Table 5. Prospective clinical trials in "high risk" patients with HIV-related NHL

Regimen	Eval. pts.	Prognostic factors	CR [b] (%)	OI [a] Follow-up (%)	Median survival	Reference
Low-dose CHOP [c]-like regimen + AZT [d]	29	intercurrent OI [a] ZPS [e] ≥ 3	14	44	3.5 mo	Tirelli et al. 1992 [29]
VCR-BLM [f]/wk	9	OI [a] ZPS [e] > 2 CD4 < 50 cells/mm^3	0	?	3 mo	Huhn et al. 1993 [30]

[a] OI = Opportunistic infections; [b] CR = complete remission; [c] CHOP = cyclophosphamide, adriamycin, vincristine, prednisone; [d] AZT= Zidovudine; [e] ZPS = Zubrod Performance Status; [f] VCR-BLM = vincristine-bleomycin

MACOP-B, a chemotherapy regimen that intensively delivers effective agents without prolonging chemotherapy-induced immunosuppression. However, in this study the prevalence of opportunistic infections during follow-up, a surrogate marker of immunosuppression, was not reported [24].

Encouraging results have been reported in HIV-SNC lymphoma, which generally occurred in patients with preserved immune function [13,14]. Lopez et al., using a regimen originally devised for non-HIV Burkitt's lymphoma, achieved a complete response rate of 83% with a 36% 5-year overall survival; most deaths (33%) were secondary to opportunistic infections [25]. Straus et al., administering a modified regimen initially designed to treat leukaemia, achieved a complete response in 5 of 9 patients (56%), but the median survival was comparable to that of retrospective series [26].

Within the French-Italian Cooperative Study Group a prospective study was performed in two different groups of HIV-related NHL. Patients with a previous history of opportunistic infections and a poor PS were treated with low-dose chemotherapy. Patients without these factors were eligible for an intensive and brief treatment with a slightly modified LNH-84 regimen [27]. In the "low-risk" category, complete responses were obtained in 63% of the 141 patients, a percentage not significantly different from that obtained in HIV-negative NHL (75%). Fourteen percent of the patients died during treatment, half due to treatment toxicity and half to disease progression. With a median follow-up of 28 months, the median survival and disease-free survival were 9 and 16 months, respectively. Deaths were caused by lymphoma (51%) and AIDS; 23 patients died of opportunistic infections in persisting complete remission. In multivariate analysis 4 factors were strongly associated with shorter survival: CD4 count <100 cells/mm^3, Zubrod PS <1, immunoblastic lymphoma, prior AIDS. For patients with a CD4 count >100 cells/mm^3 and Zubrod PS <1 the probability of survival at 2 years was 50% [28].

On the other hand, in patients at high risk low-dose chemotherapy with a CHOP-like regimen in association with AZT yielded a low complete remission rate (14%), without prevention of opportunistic infections (44%) and with a disappointing overall survival (3.5 months) [29].

Recently Huhn et al. reported on the results of a pilot study using induction therapy with CHOP for 4 to 6 cycles and maintenance therapy with IFN-α and AZT for 12 months in "normal-risk" patients (i.e., no opportunistic infections, Zubrod PS <3, CD4 count >50 cells/mm^3). A complete remission rate of 64% was achieved, with a median survival of 21 months. In the same trial, 9 patients in the "high-risk" group (with 2 or 3 poor prognostic factors) were treated with weekly vincristine and prednisone resulting in no remissions and an overall survival of only 3 months [30].

In the absence of randomized trials, controversy continues concerning the most appropriate regimens and the benefits of "more aggressive" vs "less aggressive" therapy. The recently activated EORTC AIDS and Tumor Study Group has undertaken a multicentre European study on NHL to compare chemotherapy regimens at different intensities in patients at low, intermediate and high risk. High risk has been defined as the presence of two or more of the following prognostic factors: CD4 less than 100 cells/mm^3, Zubrod PS ≥2 and diagnosis of AIDS. The results of this trial are awaited with interest (personal communication).

The occurrence of HIV-related lymphoma as a consequence of HIV warrants the initiation or continuation of antiretroviral therapy. However, since zidovudine is associated with myelodepression, it may be very difficult to administer this drug with combination chemotherapy, without haematopoietic growth factors. According to the preliminary results from a recent trial, Levine et al. employed the previously reported low M-BACOD regimen with concomitant dideoxycytidine (DDC) in a group of 21 patients, observing complete remissions in 14 (67%) with complicating opportunistic infections in only 2 patients (10%). Toxicity was unexpectedly mild, with 2/20 patients (10%) experiencing a granulocyte nadir between 500-750/mm^3, and 3 (15%) a nadir of less than 500 cells/mm^3. Grade 4 thrombopenia occurred in 1 (5%) and grade 1 or 2 paraesthesias in only 2 (10%) patients [31].

Combination treatment with chemotherapy and dideoxynosine (DDI) is being tested by the GICAT (Gruppo Italiano Cooperativo AIDS e Tumori) and the preliminary results are encouraging (personal communication).

Haematopoietic Growth Factors

Three phase I-II clinical trials have investigated the use of GM-CSF to decrease the myelosuppressive effects of cancer chemotherapy regimens in the treatment of HIV-related NHL. Kaplan et al. used GM-CSF with the CHOP regimen and found that delayed institution of GM-CSF (from day 4 to 13) was associated with a statistically higher mean nadir of the absolute neutrophil count, fewer chemotherapy cycles complicated by neutropenia and fewer days of hospitalization for fever and neutropenia when compared to patients who received the same dosage of CHOP chemotherapy without GM-CSF support. Complete responses were observed in 67% of control patients and 70% of GM-CSF treated patients, with median survival times of 9 and 11 months, respectively. However, the response and survival data must be interpreted with caution due to the small number of patients in the two groups. Although the median levels of serum HIV-p24 antigenaemia decreased one week after the first administration of chemotherapy in both groups, subjects treated with GM-CSF experienced an increase in p24 antigenaemia in the third week which was not seen in patients who received CHOP alone, suggesting stimulation of HIV replication. The clinical significance of this finding could not be determined [32].

A previous study showed 60% grade 3-4 haematologic toxicity in patients treated with a low-dose M-BACOD regimen. Following completion of this study, a phase I trial was performed that included GM-CSF with the modified M-BACOD regimen. Dose escalation of this regimen was found to be safe and possible, as reported by Walsh et al. [33]. In this study, when full-dose M-BACOD plus GM-CSF was given, only 18% of cycles were delayed for neutropenia on the day of scheduled treatment. The preliminary results of a trial at the NCI administering a modification of the proMACE/cytaBOM regimen (cyclophosphamide, etoposide, adriamycin, vincristine and methotrexate) with simultaneous zidovudine and GM-CSF in association with intrathecal methotrexate and cytarabine and inhaled pentamidine aerosol have been reported in abstract form. Eleven patients with untreated intermediate or high-grade systemic NHL with Karnofsky PS ≥30 and no active opportunistic infections were enrolled. All patients were evaluable for toxicity: 8 (73%) had grade 3-4 haematologic toxicity. Of the 8 patients who received more than 2 cycles of chemotherapy, 6 required dose reductions of at least 25% or dose delay of at least one week because of haematologic toxicity.

Constitutional symptoms related to GM-CSF were common. Complete remission was achieved in 43% of patients. Interestingly, no patients developed PCP during chemotherapy. Survival data were not reported [34].

The first prospective trial with a combination of chemotherapy and granulocyte-colony stimulating factor (G-CSF) has been recently reported by Tirelli et al. In this cost-effectiveness study 18 patients treated with intensive chemotherapy regimens (LNH-84 or CHVmP-VCR-BLM), G-CSF and AZT were compared with 19 patients treated with the same CT regimens without G-CSF and AZT. G-CSF significantly reduced the nadir WBC in patients with lymphocytes CD4 ≥200/mm^3, the mean delay between the CT cycles and the mean number of toxicity-related days of hospitalization. The cost of CT plus G-CSF and AZT vs chemotherapy alone did not increase, actually it decreased, but the data were not significant. Side-effects of G-CSF were uncommon and mild. In addition, a decreased incidence of mucositis was observed, while there was no positive impact on the overall response rate (78% in the G-CSF group vs 88% in the control group) [35].

Primary (P) Central Nervous System (CNS) Lymphoma

There have been no prospective studies on therapy for P-CNS AIDS-NHL. Most retrospective studies and case reports published to date described the use of radiation therapy as primary treatment for CNS AIDS-NHL [11,12]. Formenti et al. reported that whole brain irradiation, in doses ranging from 2200 to 5000 cGy and combined with partial tumour resection and systemic chemotherapy in some cases, resulted in complete remission in 50% of cases. The median survival time for the group was 5.5 months, and half of the patients died of opportunistic infections [36]. Baumgartner et al. reported the results of treatment in 29 patients with P-CNS AIDS-NHL. The therapy consisted of irradiation with 2130 to 5400 cGy; a small number of patients also underwent partial tumour resections and/or received systemic chemotherapy. The median survival time for this group was 4 months. A group of 26 other patients who received no treatment had a median survival time of 1 month. In 8 patients who completed radiation and were evaluated at autopsy, residual lymphoma was present in two (25%) and 87% died of opportunistic infections [37].

Goldstein et al. reported on 17 patients with AIDS-related primary CNS lymphoma treated with whole brain irradiation, using a variety of doses and treatment regimens. The mean survival was only 72 days. Survival was longer in patients with higher pretreatment Karnofsky scores. The correlation between dose and survival was not significant at completion of therapy, most patients showed improvement in Karnofsky score and had partial improvement in neurological symptoms. Post-treatment computed tomography showed tumour regression. Opportunistic infections rather than cerebral herniation or uncontrolled lymphoma were the most common cause of death also in this series [16].

In conclusion, the development of more effective therapy for primary CNS AIDS-NHL may require improvements in the treatment of HIV-associated opportunistic infections.

REFERENCES

1 Ziegler JL, Beckstead JA, Volberding PA et al: Non-Hodgkin lymphoma in 90 homosexual men. Relation to generalized lymphadenopathy and the acquired immunodeficiency syndrome. N Engl J Med 1984 (311):565-570

2 Knowles DM, Chamulak GA, Subar M et al: Lymphoid neoplasia associated with the acquired immunodeficiency syndrome (AIDS). The New York University Medical Center experience with 105 patients (1981-1987). Ann Intern Med 1988 (108): 744-753

3 Lowenthal DA, Straus DJ, Campbell SW et al: AIDS-related lymphoid neoplasia. The Memorial Hospital experience. Cancer 1988 (61):2325-2337

4 Kaplan LD, Abrams DI, Feigal E et al: AIDS-associated non-Hodgkin's lymphoma in San Francisco. JAMA 1989 (261):719-724

5 Roithmann S, Toledano M, Tourani JM et al: HIV-associated non-Hodgkin's lymphomas: clinical characteristics and outcome. The experience of the French Registry of HIV-associated tumors. Ann Oncol 1991 (2):289-295

6 Levine AM, Sullivan-Halley J, Pike MC et al: Human immunodeficiency virus-related lymphoma - prognostic factors predictive of survival. Cancer 1991 (68):2466-2472

7 Pedersen C, Gerstoft J, Lundgren JD et al: HIV-associated lymphoma - histopathology and association with Epstein-Barr virus genome related to clinical, immunological and prognostic features. Eur J Cancer 1991 (27):1416-1423

8 Gill P, Levine A, Krailo M et al: AIDS-related malignant lymphoma: results of prospective treatment trials. J Clin Oncol 1987 (5): 1322-1328

9 Monfardini S, Tirelli U, Vaccher E et al: Malignant lymphomas in patients with or at risk for AIDS. JNCI 1988 (80):855-860

10 Levine AM, Wernz JC, Kaplan L et al: Low-dose chemotherapy with central nervous system prophylaxis and zidovudine maintenance in AIDS-related lymphoma. A prospective, multi-institutional trial. JAMA 1991 (266):84-88

11 Levine A: Epidemiology, clinical characteristics and management of AIDS-related lymphoma. Hemat/Onc Clin of North Amer 1991 (2):331

12 Pluda J, Broder S, Yarchoan R: Therapy of AIDS and AIDS-associated neoplasms. In: Pinedo HM, Longo DL and Chabner BA (eds) Cancer Chemotherapy and Biological Response Modifiers Annual 13. Elsevier Science Publishers BV, Amsterdam 1992 pp 395-439

13 Northfelt D and Kaplan LD: Clinical aspects of AIDS-related non-Hodgkin's lymphoma. Curr Opin Oncol 1991 (3):872-880

14 Boyle M, Swanson CE, Turner JJ et al: Definition of two distinct types of AIDS-associated non-Hodgkin lymphoma. Br J Haem 1990 (76):506-512

15 Biggar RJ, Horm J, Goedert JJ, Melbye M: Cancer in a group at risk of acquired immunodeficiency syndrome (AIDS) through 1984. Am J Epidemiol 1987 (126):578-586

16 Goldstein J, Dickson DW, Moser FG et al: Primary central nervous system lymphoma in acquired immune deficiency syndrome. Cancer 1991 (67): 2756-2765

17 Ziegler JL: "Biologic" differences in acquired immune deficiency syndrome-associated non-Hodgkin's lymphomas? J Clin Oncol 1991 (8):1329-1331

18 Kalter SP, Riggs SA, Cabanillas F et al: Aggressive non-Hodgkin's lymphomas in immunocompromised homosexual males. Blood 1985 (3):655-659

19 Bermudez MA, Grant KM, Rodvien R, Mendes F: Non-Hodgkin's lymphoma in a population with or at risk for acquired immunodeficiency syndrome: Indication for intensive chemotherapy. Am J Med 1989 (86):71-76

20 Monfardini S, Vaccher E, Foà R, Tirelli U: AIDS-associated non-Hodgkin's lymphoma in Italy: intravenous drug users versus homosexual men. Ann Oncol 1990 (1):203-211

21 Sawka CA, Shepherd FA, Brandwein J, Burkers RL, Sutton D, Warner E: Treatment of AIDS-related non-Hodgkin's lymphoma with a twelve week chemotherapy program. Leukemia and Lymphoma 1992 (8):213-220

22 Matsushima Y, Kanzawa F, Hoshi A: Time-schedule dependency of the inhibiting activity of various anticancer drugs in the clonogenic assay. Cancer Chemother Pharmacol 1985 (14):104-107

23 Sparano JA, Wiernik PH, Strack M, Leaf A, Becker N, Valentine ES: Infusional cyclophosphamide, doxorubicin, and etoposide in human immunodeficiency virus and human T-cell leukemia virus type I-related non-Hodgkin's lymphoma: a highly active regimen. Blood 1993 (10):2810-2815

24 Taillan B, Garnier G, Ferrari E et al: MACOP-B chemotherapy for the treatment of high-grade lymphomas in patients with HIV-1 infection. Acta Haematol 1993 (89):10-12

25 Lopez TM, Hagemeister FB, McLaughlin P et al: Small noncleaved cell lymphoma in adults: superior results for stages I-III disease. J Clin Oncol 1990 (4):615-622

26 Straus DJ, Wong GY, Liu J et al: Small non-cleaved-cell lymphoma (undifferentiated lymphoma, Burkitt's type) in American adults: results with treatment designed for acute lymphoblastic leukemia. Am J Med 1991 (90):328

27 Coiffier B, Gisselbrecht C, Herbrecht R et al: LNH-84: a multicenter study of intensive chemotherapy in 737 patients with aggressive malignant lymphoma. J Clin Oncol 1989 (7):1018-1026

28 Gisselbrecht C, Oksenhendler E, Tirelli U et al: Human immunodeficiency virus-related lymphoma treatment with intensive combination chemotherapy. Am J Med 1993 (95):188-196

29 Tirelli U, Errante D, Oksenhendler E et al: Prospective study with combined low-dose chemotherapy and zidovudine in 37 patients with poor-prognosis AIDS-related non-Hodgkin's lymphoma. Ann Oncol 1992 (3):843-847

30 Huhn D, Weiss R, Nerl C et al: HIV-related non-Hodgkin's lymphoma: CHOP-induction and AZT/IFα-maintenance therapy. Proc ASCO 1993 (12):52 (abstract # 12)

31 Levine AM, Katz-Willson E, Espina B et al: Low dose m-BACOD with concomitant dideoxyctidine (ddC) in AIDS related lymphoma. Blood 1992 (80/1 suppl 1): 328a (abstract # 1301)

32 Kaplan LD, Kahn JO, Crowe S et al: Clinical and virologic effects of recombinant human granulocyte-macrophage colony-stimulating factor in patients receiving chemotherapy for human immunodeficiency virus-associated non-Hodgkin's lymphoma: results of a randomized trial. J Clin Oncol 1991 (6):929-940

33 Walsh C, Wernz JC, Levine A et al: Phase I trial of m-BACOD and granulocyte macrophage colony stimulating factor in HIV-associated non-Hodgkin's lymphoma. JAIDS 1993 (6):265-271

34 Hahn SM, Pluda J, Shay L et al: Treatment of AIDS-related non-Hodgkin's lymphoma (NHL) with chemotherapy, AZT, and granulocyte-macrophage colony-stimulating factor (GM-CSF). VII International Conference on AIDS, Florence 16-21 June, 1991, p 274 (abstract WB 2368)

35 Tirelli U, Errante D, Vaccher E et al: Treatment of HIV-related non-Hodgkin's lymphoma (NHL) with chemotherapy (CT) and G-CSF: reduction of hospitalization and toxicity with concomitant overall reduction in the cost. Proc ASCO 1993 (12):53 (abstract # 13)

36 Formenti SC, Gill PS, Lean E et al: Primary central nervous system lymphoma in AIDS: results of radiation therapy. Cancer 1989 (63):1101-1107

37 Baumgartner JE, Rachlin JR, Beckstead JH et al: Primary central nervous system lymphomas: natural history and response to radiation therapy in 55 patients with acquired immunodeficiency syndrome. J Neurosurg 1990 (73):206-211

38 Remick SC, McSharry JJ, Wolf BC et al: Novel oral combination chemotherapy in the treatment of intermediate-grade and high-grade AIDS-related non-Hodgkin's lymphoma. J Clin Oncol 1993 (9):1691-1702

MIX
Papier aus verantwortungsvollen Quellen
Paper from responsible sources
FSC® C105338

If you have any concerns about our products,
you can contact us on
ProductSafety@springernature.com

In case Publisher is established outside the EU,
the EU authorized representative is:
Springer Nature Customer Service Center GmbH
Europaplatz 3, 69115 Heidelberg, Germany

Printed by Libri Plureos GmbH
in Hamburg, Germany